Practical Considerations for Successful Crown and Bridge Therapy

- BIOLOGIC CONSIDERATIONS
- PSYCHOLOGIC CONSIDERATIONS
- PREVENTIVE FACTORS

HAROLD R. HORN, D.D.S., F.A.C.D.

Formerly Assistant Clinical Professor, Department of Denture Prosthesis, and Research Fellow, Graduate and Postgraduate Prosthodontics, New York University College of Dentistry; Faculty, First District Dental Society Continuing Education Program, New York; Member, American Prosthodontic Society and Dental Materials Group of the International Association for Dental Research

W. B. SAUNDERS COMPANY • Philadelphia • London • Toronto

W. B. Saunders Company: West Washington Square
Philadelphia, PA 19105

1 St. Anne's Road
Eastbourne, East Sussex BN21 3UN, England

1 Goldthorne Avenue
Toronto, Ontario M8Z 5T9, Canada

Library of Congress Cataloging in Publication Data

Horn, Harold R

Practical considerations for successful crown and bridge therapy.

Includes index.

1. Crowns (Dentistry) 2. Bridges (Dentistry) I. Title.

RK666.H77 617.6'92 76-8577

ISBN 0-7216-4783-9

Practical Considerations for Successful Crown and Bridge Therapy ISBN 0-7216-4783-9

Last digit is the print number: 9 8 7 6 5 4 3 2

DEDICATION

This book is dedicated to my son, Richard.
May the "bugs" that got me get him. . .

FOREWORD

Early in his book Dr. Horn appropriately notes that "bridges don't belong in the mouth." They are inert matter placed into a viable, biological environment. Their tolerance by the oral tissue, and thereby the longevity of the restoration, is made possible only by the capability of the dentist to meld an intelligent application of scientific fundamentals into technical skills. Herein lie the challenges, intrigue and rewards of restorative dentistry. It is in that context that this book was born.

Invariably, any text is a reflection of the character of the author, and mirrors his conceptual thinking; this one is no exception. It is not intended to be a comprehensive treatise on the technical steps involved in abutment preparations and the fabrication of crowns and bridges. The reader who is looking for detailed information of that type will need to seek out the numerous books written with that objective in mind.

Rather, the principal thrust is upon prevention, prevention in a dual sense. First, that numerous problems associated with crown and bridge prostheses can be prevented before they arise; therefore, little emphasis is placed upon what to do after failures caused by ignorance or neglect do occur. Second, good restorative dentistry is indeed preventive dentistry. The helpful hints with which the book is laced stress the parameters involved in the selection and use of materials and technology *before* the restoration is fabricated and inserted.

It is a book with which the dentist should feel comfortable. He is not talked down to, nor is he overwhelmed by scientific jargon. The principles and theories are presented in a palatable, integrated manner. Obviously, it is written for the dentist by a dentist who has a deep concern for, and understanding of, the frustrations of the practitioner.

There will be some who may not agree with all that is said, or with the emphasis placed upon certain topics, such as the selection of cements and cementation. However, Dr. Horn has drawn upon his experience as an outstanding clinician and teacher, and has gone to great effort to successfully get his ideas into clearly understandable words; many of the areas stressed are ones too frequently neglected in other texts on crown and bridge therapy.

To the reader who is interested in a commonsense discourse on the harmonious interaction of certain biological, physical and esthetic considerations that pertain to the construction, placement and maintenance of crowns and bridges, this book should prove invaluable.

RALPH W. PHILLIPS, M.S., D.SC.
Associate Dean for Research
and Research Professor of
Dental Materials
Indiana University School of Dentistry

PREFACE

Twenty years ago a small gold inlay was cemented into my lower left second molar. It was painful. For one year it was sensitive to thermal changes, and during that time I dared not partake of ice cream or any cold beverage. One day, while my own tooth was throbbing with pain, I cemented a few gold crowns into the mouth of a young adult patient. Pain and tears ensued. Our suffering was parallel. The pain initiated by cementation with an irritating acid cement was indelibly etched in my mind.

As time went by I recognized that there was little or no pain involved with cementations to older and less vital teeth, or to teeth protected with cavity varnish. Also, I recognized cement as the enemy of the dentist in his attempts to place crowns and bridges into the mouth accurately. Although cement was absolutely necessary, it was a necessary evil! Cementation not only caused pain but also raised bites and spoiled margins.

Nevertheless, the die was cast, and my interest was henceforth directed to the collection and organization of information related to the cementation procedure and to the challenge of coping with this "weak link" in the chain of fixed restorative procedures.

I searched for and experimented with various additives for both the universal zinc phosphate cement and zinc oxide and eugenol cement. I could hardly define my direction, but on an empirical basis I was ready to try anything for modification or improvement of cementation. Hand cream, talcum powder, antiseptics, lanolin, and "everything but the kitchen sink" were thrown into cement mixtures in my search for something or other. Ultimately, with the help of concurrent scientific reading, my path of investigation led to the benzoic acid derivatives. It was known that these substances influenced the physical and chemical characteristics of zinc oxide and eugenol cements. Quite by accident, I detected an unusual phenomenon when certain parahydroxybenzoates were added to a slurry of zinc oxide and eugenol. I was anxious to translate this finding into practical utilization, and to present the results to the dental profession. But this is easier said than done. The average dentist in his daily practice is always searching for more effective therapy and technique. Actually, whether he knows it or not, he is involved in a form of clinical research. Occasionally, as a result of an unusual occurrence, an accident, or an interesting observation, the dentist is stimulated into a research endeavor. His investigation may have the potential for meaningful conclusions. But at this point, how shall he proceed? The average dentist is not well informed about the details of research protocol. He may not know how or where to present new ideas, innovations, and clinical discoveries. In fact, dental educators have been long remiss in providing instruction in research methodology, scientific writing and oral presentation.

It was my good fortune at that time to meet Mr. John O. Semmelman of Dentsply International. He introduced me to the Dental Materials Group of the International Association for Dental Research and suggested that I present my research with zinc oxide and eugenol additives at their next meeting. I submitted an abstract that was accepted for presentation. But I doubt whether I would have been able to prepare data and format at that time without the understanding and help that I received from Dr. Harry Blechman, former Dean of New York University College of Dentistry. He, literally, took me by the hand and guided me into the creation of a scientific presentation. I am thankful to him not only for what he did to help me but also for the way he did it. His patience and humility as a teacher overcame other pessimistic influences that might have restrained me. This was the beginning. The seed was planted that would ultimately evolve into the creation of this text.

Subsequently I encountered a number of individuals to whom I owe a debt of gratitude for contributing to my development and knowledge in the field of restorative dental materials and fixed prosthodontics. Dr. I. Kenneth Adisman, my mentor and educator, has led me into many worthwhile endeavors. The late Dr. Eugeñe Molnar of Chicago has shared information with me that couldn't be obtained anywhere else.

I am especially thankful to Dr. Ralph W. Phillips, from whom I learned much about "the responsibility of being the best" and even more about the science of dental materials. In 1963 he introduced me into a conspiracy with Gerhard Brauer aimed at improving the physical properties of zinc oxide and eugenol cement. The ortho-ethoxybenzoic acid (EBA) cements were a direct result of the research activities of Gerhard Brauer and co-workers at the National Bureau of Standards. I will always be grateful to him for allowing me the privilege of evaluating the EBA cement in the final cementation of crowns and bridges.

When teaching postgraduate and continuing education courses, I have often presented material about EBA cements taken from the ever-increasing volume of research reports on this cement published in the current dental literature (1964). This aroused a lot of interest among dentists interested in fixed prosthodontics—especially because there was also at that time an increasing emphasis being placed on biologic considerations in restorative dentistry. Sad to say, it was embarrassing to me when I couldn't answer the question that had no answer: "Where may EBA cement be obtained?" For a very good reason, manufacturers were not interested. It was too expensive. The ortho-ethoxybenzoic acid cost about 80 dollars a pound. Also, apprehension, skepticism, and fear of change played their usual roles in the prevention of progress. Ultimately, and fortunately for the dental profession, one manufacturer had the courage to step in where others feared to tread, and after conferences with the National Bureau of Standards and the United States Department of Commerce, Mr. Harold A. Opotow began to manufacture the first EBA cement in 1965. This cement was presented to the dental profession as the exact formulation that had been developed at the National Bureau of Standards and tested and documented in the dental literature.

I have come to know Mr. Harold Opotow not only as a man with great courage and pioneering ability but also as a truly unique dental scientist. Conferring with him and bouncing ideas off his "know-how" intellect has greatly increased my understanding of various dental products, manufacturing procedures, and formulation problems.

Having contributed, through clinical research and teaching, to the development of a biologically compatible final cement for crowns and bridges, I then proceeded to work on a new type of material. A non-setting temporary cement that would seal and sedate prepared abutment teeth over a trial period was urgently needed for the modern and more sophisticated practice of fixed prosthodontics. Dentists were then recognizing that biological evaluation of a fixed restoration is accomplished by temporary cementation. A formulation containing zinc oxide and eugenol was developed that set to a rubbery consistency and allowed easy, non-traumatic removal of fixed bridges after a period of evaluation. The details related to its utilization are presented in Chapter 11.

Subsequently, I presented lectures and seminars dealing with the installation of crowns and bridges, cementing materials, and associated phenomena. When this teaching expanded to a two-day course in the Continuing Education Program of New York's First District Dental Society, I realized that the subject matter being presented was actually the heart and core of effective crown and bridge therapy. Biologic considerations, preventive factors, and the psychologic considerations of esthetics represented a large portion of crown and bridge prosthodontics that was unavailable in book form until the creation of this text.

* * * * * *

This book will do for you exactly what its title promises: it will help you be successful in crown and bridge endeavors.

As you will see, it is different from other books in this field. Books on fixed restorations usually concentrate on treatment planning, preparation, impression and casting technique, and occlusion. You will find none of these here. Instead, this book will give you scientifically based information to improve your grasp of the factors leading to healthier, more comfortable, and better-looking crowns and bridges.

HAROLD R. HORN

CONTENTS

one

Introduction

If we are to achieve results never before accomplished, we must expect to employ methods never before attempted.

Sir Francis Bacon

What Is Crown and Bridge Therapy?

Methods of preparing abutment teeth and the procedures involved in fabricating crowns and fixed partial dentures are included in the curricula of all dental schools teaching fixed prosthodontics. The dentist is educated on various levels and by various means to cope with technical procedures such as impression making, waxing, casting, and soldering. He is also instructed explicitly in the utilization of tooth-reduction apparatus to sculpture abutment teeth to certain predetermined outline forms. Texts and journals supply an abundance of information on oral diagnosis, fixed partial denture design, periodontal considerations, and occlusion. This is probably the first crown and bridge book that does not tell how to prepare an abutment tooth and cope with the mechanics and philosophies of occlusion.

Technology is not treatment. Several recent books tell the dentist how to make better crowns and bridges. This is not one of them! Instead, this book will be a guide to more effective crown and bridge *therapy*. Therapy is treatment. Its ultimate effectiveness occurs after the fixed prostheses have been fabricated and installed in the mouth. Is the patient's oral condition benefited or improved in any way by impressions, casting, and other technical considerations? Hardly. Actually, the full therapy derived from crown and bridge procedures begins only when a fixed prosthesis is installed in the patient's mouth and the benefits inherent to its conception are inaugurated. The mechanical end-results must be fitted to and coordinated with living tissues; therefore, fixed restorations are truly therapeutic agents which operate under the anatomic, physiologic and psychologic limitations of the individual patient. There are various considerations before and after final cementation that enhance the *treatment benefits* that accrue to the patient as a result of combining technical procedures with biologic, psychologic, and preventive factors. Successful crown and bridge therapy, therefore, denotes something other than the mere replacement of missing teeth by artificial substitutes. It is the treatment provided by the dentist that utilizes fixed restorations to repair, restore and modify components of a dentition to enhance function, esthetics, and the preservation of hard and soft tissues. Successful crown and bridge therapy is no longer judged by mechanical perfection and longevity (based on the ability of the oral structures to withstand abuse), but by the achievement of the preventive objective, esthetics, and biologic considerations.

What is Wrong with Crowns and Bridges Today?

As mentioned before, every dentist has been instructed in the mechanics of crown and bridge technology. Lectures, periodicals, and textbooks keep him informed of new and old crown and bridge procedures. Yet, the proof of the pudding—the end result—the patient treated with crowns and bridges, attests to the many failures of this branch of dentistry. Crowns and bridges should look like real, natural teeth, but they seldom do. Artificiality seems built in. They scream falseness. Abutment preparations threaten the vitality of pulps and too often contribute to their demise. Restorations may fit poorly or loosen prematurely. Soft tissues reflect abuse by pontics and poor margins. A proliferation of facts and fallacies related to new materials and procedures for impression making and veneering may confuse the dentist. Temporary cementation presents embarrassing problems. Final cementation may raise bites, cause pain, and ruin margins. Neglected factors for prevention lead to poor sanitation, periodontal conditions and caries.

This book is compiled for those dentists who have experienced enough problems, failures, and frustrations to realize that successful crowns and bridges depend not only on the technology of abutment preparation, occlusion, and fabrication but also on biologic, psychologic, and preventive considerations. These influence the restorative therapy to yield healthy abutment teeth, compatible gingival tissues, and esthetic restorations.

This book will be concerned with the biologic, psychologic, and preventive considerations necessary to improve or modify the aforementioned inadequacies, and to accomplish successful crown and bridge therapy.

BIOLOGIC, PSYCHOLOGIC AND PREVENTIVE CONSIDERATIONS

Biologic Considerations

Biologic considerations have been emphasized repeatedly in recent years. As a result, the present day concept of fixed restorative dentistry differs from that of the past. Today dentists are more keenly aware of the need to protect the vital pulp from chemical irritation, microleakage, and the toxic effects of dental restorative materials that may contribute to its demise. There is increasing concern for the control of pain and the maintenance of pulpal health after abutment preparations have been accomplished. Temporary cements are selected for their sedative ability and pulpal compatibility. Final cements should meet biologic requirements. Other considerations exist. How do the soft tissues respond to the placement of crown margins and to contact with pontics? Are impression procedures harmful to the pulp? What is a biologic installation? What are the roles of cavity varnish, calcium hydroxide liners, and polycarboxylate cement in fixed restorative dentistry? Certain biophysical factors contribute to the successful retention of fixed restorations. Why is it important to recognize them?

Specifically, biologic considerations in crown and bridge therapy deal with various aspects of restorative dental materials and procedures and the responses they elicit from pulpal and gingival tissues: the management, protection, repair, and recontouring of prepared abutment teeth; the control of pain; the biophysical factors governing retention; the bio-assessment of fixed bridges prior to final installation (temporary cementation); antibacterial values; and the role of cavity liners and medicaments.

Psychologic Considerations

Psychologic considerations are mostly those related to the esthetics of restorative dentistry. The cosmetic factors that enhance the natural appearance of a restored dentition should be clearly understood by the dental practitioner, not in vague overall classifications, or theory or concept, but in specific details as they pertain to each individual tooth in its surroundings. Every possible consideration should be given to make fixed restorations look more natural. This is a great challenge to the dentist. How can he compete with Mother Nature? Most crowns and bridges have a certain amount of built-in artificiality. Even when color is blended to perfection, and shape, form and position are pleasing, lack of translucency and different degrees of light transmission and throwback cause a false look.

The psychologic makeup of every patient requires that fixed repairs not only look as good "as they were before" but also give him or her comfort and security about durability. The patient wants them to be long lasting; in fact, longer lasting than the originals they replace. To accomplish this, preventive measures, including sanitation and nutrition, should be considered but unfortunately are often overlooked.

Therefore, although the psychologic considerations in crown and bridge therapy deal mainly with esthetics, they also deal with the initiation and propagation of comfort, the security of durability, and the appreciation of preventive measures toward this goal. Also of importance is the role of nutrition as both a psychologic and a preventive factor in crown and bridge therapy that influences not only durability but function as well. There are also some psychologic considerations in impression making (see Summary, Chapter 3) and in the terminology describing "permanent" cementation (see Chapter 12).

Preventive Considerations

In recent years it has become increasingly evident to the dental profession that to fulfill its obligation of oral health to the public, it must modify its concern with the repair of disease or damaged tissues and concentrate its efforts on the prevention of disease.

The basic treatment for all dental patients should be prevention, and what is not preventable must be repaired. Although crown and bridge therapy is a dental service dealing with the failure of prevention, this book tells what can be done at the chairside in certain crown and bridge procedures to prevent oral disease.

Control, prevention and elimination of dental disease are the ideals of the dental profession. Consideration for prevention should heavily influence all plans for therapy and technique in every aspect of dentistry. Patients receiving crown and bridge therapy should be motivated to maintain and perpetuate the benefits of this treatment.

The dentist should endeavor to incorporate as many preventive factors as possible into restorative treatment.

Preventive considerations in crown and bridge therapy are as follows:

1. Oral hygiene. The removal of plaque should be a continuous and never-ending endeavor.
2. Sanitation. The interproximal spaces and the areas under pontics should be designed for easy cleansing.
3. Nutrition. Control of food habits is required to maintain the health of the bone and tissues that frame the fixed prosthesis.
4. Biologic evaluation of bridges prior to final cementation. This tentative placement to assay tissue reactions, fit, and contact points is called temporary cementation.
5. Antibacterial and anticariogenic factors. Since all restorations have a potential for leakage, a cement with antibacterial properties may function as a secondary line of defense against bacterial invasion. Silicophosphate cements possess anticariogenic properties by virtue of the fluoride they contain.
6. Microleakage. An improvement of the marginal seal will help prevent caries.
7. Periodontal conditions—the contours and placement of crown margins and other soft tissue considerations.
8. Oral habits—fingernail biting, lip biting, pipe smoking, tongue-thrusting, abnormal swallowing.

The preventive concept in dentistry includes the prevention of the extension of oral breakdown through effective crown and bridge therapy. The extent to which this health goal is realized is the measure of fixed prosthodontics' contribution to preventive dentistry.

Crowns and Bridges Do Not Belong in the Human Mouth

Actually, crowns and bridges do not belong in the human mouth! They are foreign bodies. They are inert, dead matter installed in a warm, moist, living system. They are not rejected because they are mechanically bonded into position with the aid of a luting agent. They are tolerated, therefore, and the mouth becomes their *storage place* when certain biophysical requirements are met. However, rejection may manifest itself in the form of periodontal disorder, occlusal imbalance, pulpal demise, premature loosening, and psychologic failure (poor esthetics).

The installation method, cementation, provides the linkage between the mechanical fabricate and the oral environment. This linkage poses many problems. The cementation procedure has been called the Achilles heel of fixed prosthodontics. It is a critical maneuver that has the potential to sabotage the most perfect fixed prosthesis. It may cause pain, occlusal disharmony, and marginal discrepancies. Occasionally, crowns and bridges loosen prematurely despite the use of so-called "permanent" cement. Conversely, restorations cemented with temporary cement are often difficult to remove prior to final cementation.

Unfortunately, the installation of crowns and bridges has heretofore been a mechanical problem exclusively, segregated from the influence of biologic requirements. A new approach is necessary; a biologic approach *based on research evidence rather than on custom, habit, empiricism and folklore.*

Research Evidence that Has Changed Our Ways

In the past few decades many findings of importance to crown and bridge installation have evolved from research endeavors. Each finding has contributed knowledge beneficial to the dentist. However, they all magnify the challenge of accomplishing successful crown and bridge therapy. The following are some of the results of research that have changed our ways:

1. Castings do not seat completely during cementation.[1] A cement line always exists despite all efforts to reduce it to a minimum. It remains continuously exposed to the oral fluids. The dentist must face the challenge of keeping the resultant film of cement as small as possible so that previously established margins and occlusal relationships will not be disturbed.

2. No dental material is capable of *true* adhesion to prepared tooth structure. This includes polycarboxylate cement.

3. Thermal changes in the oral environment cause leakage and percolation between tooth structure and restorative materials.[2] This

allows the ingress of microorganisms. *Note:* The ice cream and hot coffee habit seems to be too deeply ingrained in people to change. It may take centuries to modify the human habit of eating hot and cold foods at the same time. Many dental organization dinners terminate with ice cream and coffee. It appears that dentists should practice what they preach.

4. Zinc phosphate cements irritate the pulp, are soluble in oral fluids, and do not provide a lasting seal.[3, 4] Also, the acidity of this cement prevails longer than previously believed.

5. Cavity liners are only partially effective in protecting against marginal leakage and the irritation from acid cements.[5]

6. Chemical agents employed for cavity sterilization may be injurious to the pulp.[6]

7. Dental caries is of bacterial origin. Therefore, antibacterial cements, bases, and liners may be helpful in limiting the proliferation of organisms on dentin if they do not themselves irritate or damage the dentin.

The Best Way to Spoil a Fixed Restoration

Crowns and bridges are often adjusted in the mouth to meticulous fit and comfort. Margins are where they should be; pontics harmonize passively with the tissue of edentulous areas; contacts are perfect; occlusion is adjusted—the bite is right! Temporary cementation is over. The period of trial and assessment has led to beneficial modifications. Now, the chips are down! The time has come for final installation. And with it should come the recognition and realization that *the best way to "spoil" a fixed restoration is to cement it!* Although stated with tongue in cheek, the realization is more sad than funny. Cementation may raise the occlusal level and spoil the bite. How annoying at this time to have to regrind the previously perfected bite. Margins are no longer where they were before. Occlusal and marginal preciseness go hand in hand. If margins are moved, so is the occlusion. Contact areas and pontics may no longer be in the same position. Added to these negative potentials is the change in many instances from comfort to pain that may occur because of chemical irritation from the cement or because of the hydraulic pressure engendered during seating of the restoration.

After solving all of the problems of technique and fabrication in crown and bridge prosthodontics, the dentist is further challenged to cement these restorations in painlessly, and to keep the resultant film of cement to a minimum so that previously established margins and occlusal relationships will not be disturbed.

How to Evaluate a New Dental Restorative Material

A large amount of crown and bridge therapy is expressed in the application and manipulation of various restorative dental materials. In fact, dental materials may be considered the "building blocks" of restorative dentistry. However, in past decades the study of dental materials has been a rather dull subject—a drudgery of information needing commitment to memory. Oral surgery and operative techniques appeared far more glamorous to the dental student and the young dentist. In fact, some dental schools did not deem it necessary to have a teaching department of dental materials, but required each separate branch of dental education to instruct in the use of related materials.

This picture has now changed, perhaps because of the exciting new developments that have trickled down to dentistry from space-age technology, or perhaps because of a new breed of researchers and writers who stressed and illuminated the practical, bread-and-butter aspects of the new materials. How lucky is the dentist of today! His predecessor never heard of composite fillings, cyanoacrylates, EBA cement, acid etching, pit and fissure sealants, aluminous porcelain, polycarboxylates, and spherical alloy.

New materials are always especially interesting to dentists. They promise the accomplishment of a new procedure or the more effective utilization of an old one. However, new dental materials are often unsatisfactory and do not live up to expectations. Somehow they never seem to be what they are "cracked up" to be. Much too often they lead to disappointment. This may be so for a number of reasons, but in many instances it is due to lack of knowledge related to the handling and manipulation of the material. Dentists are inclined to plunge into the use of a new product without digesting the pertinent information regarding effective use. Occasionally, after a number of failures the dentist will be guided by the old saying, "When all else fails, go back and read the directions."

Many new dental materials and procedures are presented at conventions and in the dental journals. Alluring new packaging, new sales gimmicks, and new slogans are used to attract attention. The dentist is beguiled by claims and counterclaims that blare from journal advertisements. He is occasionally exposed to misinformation and slanted views regarding new materials and techniques. He must face the monumental task of evaluating both manufacturers' claims and research reports of new developments. It is difficult for the average dentist to make meaningful decisions with regard to numerical values, statistics, and physical and chemical properties.

Perhaps the following classification of materials and the "triad of evaluation" will be helpful in the understanding and selection of new dental products.

CLASSIFICATION OF RESTORATIVE DENTAL MATERIALS

1. Materials stored permanently in the mouth—for example, gold, porcelain, resin, cement, liners, bases, and amalgam.

2. Materials that enter the mouth for a short period of time—for example, impression material, wax, silicone grease, and temporary cement.

3. Materials that never enter the mouth—for example, casting investment, artificial stone, flux, tripoli, and rouge.

THE TRIAD OF EVALUATION

Any new dental material presented to a dentist for his consideration should be subjected to a series of critical questions to determine its merit and the feasibility for its utilization. Regardless of the type of product—filling material, cement or denture base material—questions should be posed according to a "Triad of Evaluation" (Fig. 1–1). This starts with physical testing, proceeds to biologic testing, and concludes with clinical testing.

Physical Testing and Evaluation

In the development of a new dental material, physical testing is one of the first considerations. After all, if a material does not function well mechanically, why go any farther? Why bother to test it biologically and clinically? So physical testing is of initial concern. In applying the *triad of evaluation* the dentist should ask these questions when confronted with a new material:

1. Where, and by whom, was it developed?
2. Who did the physical testing?
3. Where are the results documented in dental literature?

The dentist's best friend in the physical evaluation of dental materials is the American Dental Association's *Guide to Dental Materials and Devices* and the specifications for dental materials therein. The specifications are designed to evaluate materials on the basis of physical and mechanical properties determined in the laboratory.

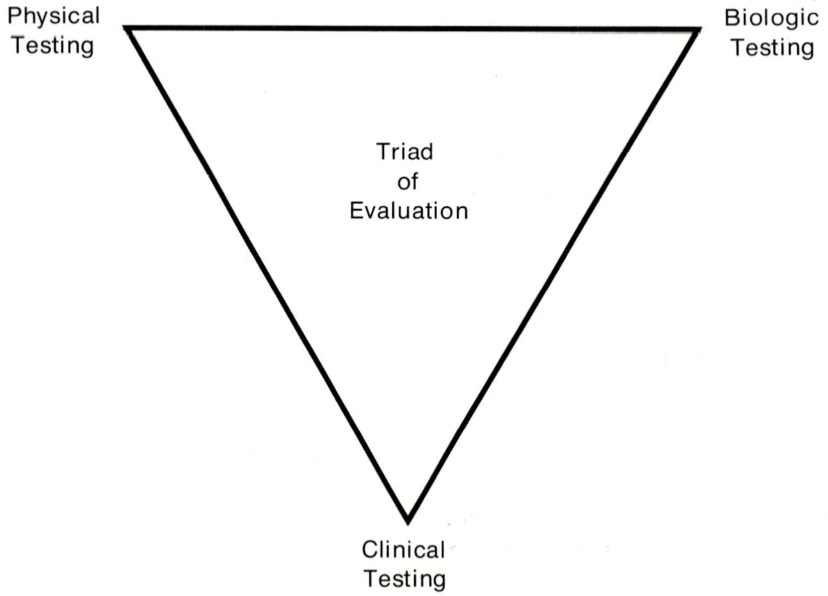

Figure 1–1 New restorative dental materials are evaluated by reference to physical, biologic and clinical testing.

The tests simulate actual service conditions as closely as possible. However, the true value of the laboratory test is measured by the degree of correlation between data obtained from laboratory tests and the behavior of the materials in service. If a product is tested and found to comply with the specification, its name is placed on the *List of Certified Dental Materials*, which is published periodically in *The Journal of the American Dental Association*. This should be the dentist's "buyer's guide" for the materials used in dental practice. However, the products appearing on this list will produce satisfactory restorations only if used correctly. The manufacturer's directions should be strictly adhered to in using a specific product. For successful results, the handling or manipulation of a material is as important as the material itself. Dentists who accept the ambiguous wording in the advertising of some dental products are overlooking one of the most important and costly programs of the American Dental Association—the Dental Materials Certification Program.

Biologic Testing and Evaluation

The crowning tenet of Anglo-Saxon law—that a person is innocent until proved guilty—cannot and does not apply to dental materials and devices. There is a special concept of justice and evaluation for these materials. It starts with the assumption that every product is dangerous until proved safe.

Just about anything put in or on the human body for medical or dental purposes is capable of doing some harm under some circumstance. As a result, the real issue is not absolute guilt or innocence but a choice of balancing potential harm against potential benefits.

Biologic evaluation of a new dental material has become absolutely imperative to the protection of and the maintenance of the health of patients. It is possible for a dental material to be perfect from a mechanical standpoint and yet be too toxic or irritating to be applied in the human mouth. The development, study, and physical testing of new materials is not enough. The dentist must be alerted to ask the following questions:

"Where was this new dental material tested biologically?"

"Who did the biologic evaluation?"

"Where is it documented in the literature so that I may read about it?"

Just a few decades ago, restorative dental materials simply had to satisfy certain physical and chemical requirements before they were certified for use in patients. Today, they must also satisfy certain biologic requirements. In other words, restorative materials should not be injurious to living tissues by virtue of their chemical action or other irritational effects. Unfortunately, many restorative materials have been shown to be injurious. For example, acid cements, acrylic monomer, and composite resin fillings. Their use is only justified when appropriate liners and bases are utilized in a protective way.

The biologic evaluation of materials used in dentistry includes:

1. Screening for toxic or other untoward effects of the materials.
2. Clinical evaluation of materials that have been screened.

The testing and requirements for the biologic evaluation of a dental material are based on the intended use of the material and include tests for acute systemic toxicity and mucous membrane irritation, short-duration tests for inflammatory reactions and irritation of the pulp, and long-duration tests for tumor production and chronic inflammatory reactions.[9]

In the recommended standard practices for biological evaluation of dental materials published by the Council on Dental Materials and Devices of the American Dental Association the toxicity of a material is defined as "the measure of functional or structural injury to living tissue that will probably occur by exposure of the tissues to a given concentration of the material."[9]

More foreign materials are introduced into the human organism in dentistry than in any other branch of the healing arts. Many different symptoms are recognized as side effects caused by amalgams, synthetic substances, and rubber. Some of these side effects occur only when the causative material is subject to solution. Even traces of some substances may cause strong allergic reactions. For example, in some alloys a very small amount of copper may dissolve out and produce reactions such as eczema, impaired vision, abdominal pain, depression, and tremor. Occasionally, a patient may react with similar disturbances to a minute amount of mercury contained in an amalgam. Various substances from the materials used in fixed and removable prostheses may produce oral manifestations. The untoward reaction may appear only after the passage of time, and the only remedy is the removal of the offending prosthesis.

Clinical Testing and Evaluation

Clinical research, the direct use of the human mouth for evaluation, presents many problems. Because of the many inherent variables, it is the most difficult type of dental research.

After physical and biological evaluation, a new dental material should be judged for its ability to perform in a practical situation. Its ease of manipulation, its handling characteristics, and all other features that become apparent in the course of utilization should be observed and documented.

Here the questions are "Who used the new material in clinical research?" and "Where are the results documented so that I may read about them?"

An example of the application of the triad of evaluation: New material—EBA cement

1. Physical evaluation
Civjan, S., and Brauer, G. M.: Physical properties of cements, based on zinc oxide, hydrogenated rosin, o-ethoxybenzoic acid, and eugenol. J. Dent. Res. *43*:281, 1964.

2. *Biological evaluation*
Phillips, R. W., and Love, D. R.: The effect of certain additive agents on the physical properties of zinc oxide-eugenol mixtures. J. Dent. Res. *40*:294, 1961.

3. *Clinical evaluation*
Horn, H. R.: The cementation of crowns and fixed partial dentures. Dent. Clin. North Am. March 1965, p. 65.

THE ERRATIC BEHAVIOR OF RESTORATIVE MATERIALS

The results of the physical testing of dental materials may be different in one part of the country than in another. Published dental research reports on identical dental material often show large differences in some physical properties, depending on the geographical area in which the research was done. Without a doubt there are discrepancies in batches and manufacturing procedures and raw materials, but other considerations should not go unrecognized. For example, are dental materials modified by storage through long-range transportation that passes through changing zones of rising humidity and falling barometric pressure, or changes in the earth's electromagnetic field, or areas where there is release of radiation from nuclear power plants? The ability of radiation to penetrate materials and change their physical and chemical properties is used to modify and improve certain characteristics of plastics, wood, and rubber. Many dental materials are sensitive to radiation. Radiation that cannot be seen, felt, or heard may change chemical and physical properties of restorative dental materials. Research has determined the effect of radiation exposure on certain resin adhesive systems. In these, radiation caused crosslinking, resulting in increased tensile strength and modulus of elasticity, decreasing elongation and increasing embrittlement.[7]

Radiation leakage from an ultraviolet light designed to harden resins applied to a tooth caused the Food and Drug Administration to temporarily halt distribution of the device. The activator light not only caused the resins to polymerize but also caused injury to some patients from the stray radiation. To correct the situation it was necessary to modify old and new activator light units with appropriate shielding against radiation leakage. Color television, microwave ovens, fluoroscopes, radioisotopes, luminous watch dials, and laser devices are just a few of the increasing sources of radiation that may be harmful not only to humans but also to the materials used in restorative dentistry.

The x-ray machine is the greatest radiation hazard.

The source closest to home, however, the x-ray machine in the dental office, is probably the biggest culprit! In many dental offices the scatter of x-ray radiation freely contacts resin filling materials, impression pastes, and cements that are on shelves or in cabinets in the same room. Does this affect the polymerization involved in the utilization of many of these materials? Does it play a part in the occasional *erratic behavior of certain dental materials?*

A color television set has the potential for giving off harmful x-rays. Actually, a color television set (and the black-and-white to a lesser degree) is a low voltage x-ray machine and emits radiation. Television provides entertainment and distraction for the dental patient in the waiting room and occasionally in position in front of the dental chair in the smaller treatment room. Here at close quarters any radiation emitted may influence various dental materials (as well as the dentist and patient). Excessive emissions from the back of a television set on the other side of a thin wall may penetrate the wall and contact and modify any restorative materials in storage nearby. As a safety precaution, both people and dental materials should always be at least eight feet away from the television set.

To preserve the true identity and characteristics of restorative dental materials, medicaments and chemical solutions used in the dental treatment room, *they should be placed so that they are protected from radiation.*

Thermal changes also influence various dental materials, especially high temperatures. Some new adjunctive materials require refrigeration, and it is not unlikely that in years to come all dental offices will have a small refrigerator to protect and maintain materials at an optimum level of performance.

Another consideration is the reaction between certain dental materials. For example, bottles of *acrylic resin monomer and polymer should not be stored in the same cabinet or on the same shelf with the eugenol component of a zinc oxide and eugenol cement.* If they are, there may be a very definite slowdown in the rate of polymerization of the resin material. Fumes, or even slight traces of the volatile eugenol confined in the same enclosure with acrylic resin, may not only inhibit polymerization but also change other physical properties and predispose the resin to discoloration (see Chapter Six).

Keep all eugenol-containing impression materials and cements in a storage area apart from other dental products.

Physical properties of dental materials tend to change from batch to batch of a given manufacturer and from brand name to brand name. Although materials tested may yield different data in different laboratories, manufacturers are seldom to blame for such changes in their products. Variations in the basic ingredients furnished by the supplier are usually responsible for the erratic behavior of some materials. Also, with the conglomerate acquisitions of dental companies and the subsequent changes in manufacturing methods, policies, and personnel, a "name brand" dental material may differ from the original product.

DATING DENTAL RESTORATIVE MATERIALS

Since the shelf life of many dental restorative materials presents a problem, the date of manufacture should be noted on the product. Actually, other dates may be important as well, such as the date of packaging, the date of shipping, and perhaps an estimated date of expiration. The user of a dental material has no way of knowing how old it is, or how long the material was on the shelf in the dental supply depot before he purchased it. It is also possible for a material to remain stored on the shelf in the dentist's office for an exceptionally long period of time. It is easy for the dentist to forget how long ago a particular product was purchased. If all materials were dated, the dentist would be able to determine the time interval between manufacture and utilization, and this would guide him in adjusting his technique in handling the material. For example, composite resins and some silicone impression materials exhibit a much slower setting time toward the end of their shelf life. Other properties may also be modified. If the extent of shelf life can be recognized by a date on the container, the dentist can adjust accordingly.

Many foods and drugs have expiration dates. Some day in the near future the dental materials for oral health will also be dated. *Until then, it is advisable for the dentist to mark the date of receipt on every package of dental material that arrives in the office.* At least he will always know how long a product has been *on his shelf.*

A FEW WORDS TO REMEMBER ABOUT TERMINOLOGY

Civilization as it is known today is based on understanding and adequate communication. Over the years there have been proposals for a universal language to alleviate the confusions and misunderstandings of multilingual philosophies. Although a universal language may not be feasible in this day and age, there is no doubt that the idea has merit. In the art and science of fixed prosthodontics many words and terms have special connotations. Therefore, a standardized nomenclature is important. For example, a uniform terminology permits authors to discuss their concepts and techniques and be sure that they are understood, regardless of the geographic location or the specialty of the reader. Also, the results of research may be interpreted and presented more effectively with an exacting nomenclature. The teaching of crown and bridge prosthodontics is improved when the barriers of poor communication are broken. The Academy of Denture Prosthetics recognized the problem and published the first *Glossary of Prosthodontic Terms* in 1956. Revised editions of this publication have helped many dentists use the proper scientific terminology and increased their awareness of the various connotations of terms.

Many similar terms have subtle differences that require precise defining. For example, what is the difference between a resin and a rosin? Although every rosin is a resin, not every resin is a rosin. Rosin is a resinous material obtained by chemical means from a pine tree. However, the words resin, polymer, and plastic all mean the same thing. Also, to glue, adhere, bond, lute, or cement designates a similar action. Similarly, the words cap, crown, and jacket all imply the complete coverage of a prepared tooth.

Three-quarter crowns, inlays, or onlays may be utilized in crown and bridge therapy depending on various factors, such as esthetics, alignment, thinness of tooth structure, span involved and susceptibility to caries. Although the three-quarter crown is a very adequate restoration, it may darken a thin anterior tooth and block out some of its translucency, thereby compromising the esthetic effect. For uniformity of discussion and for a better grasp of concepts and philosophies involved in the crown and bridge therapy presented herein, *reference in this book will be limited to the complete crown.* The complete crown is defined as "a restoration that reproduces the entire surface anatomy of the clinical crown and fits over a prepared tooth stump."[8]

The prime function of words is communication. It is important to select the right word to convey the exact intended meaning that will be understood by the most people. This may be accomplished more successfully with simple words that are easily understood. Simple words are the ideal tools for communication.

THE IMPORTANCE OF DENTAL CEMENTS

Although dental materials may be the "building blocks" of fixed restorative dentistry, dental cements provide the matrix that "puts it all together." At numerous occasions throughout crown and bridge therapy the dentist reaches for one cement or another: to line, base, and patch; to sedate pain; to hold protective coverage, pins, and posts; to evaluate biologically; and finally to install. The most carefully accomplished and adjusted occlusal rehabilitation based upon the most intricate gnathological concepts may be reduced to failure by the introduction of a dental cement that is too thick or is poorly handled.

Much of the success of crown and bridge therapy depends on the selection and effective utilization of an appropriate cementing material.

It is important to take a fresh look at the functions of a crown and bridge cement and to redefine the benefits to be obtained from this material (Chapter 9). The dentist must recognize the need for the selection of a cement based on the biophysical factors involved (Chapter 7). He must know the basic characteristics of the various crown and bridge cements and the details pertinent to their effective utilization (Chapter 8). He must also be aware of associated phenomena such as microleakage, hydraulics, capillary action, viscosity, surface tension, adhesion, wettability, filtration, and venting (Chapter 9).

THE END OF THE INTRODUCTION

This book will be concerned with the birth of fixed restorative therapy, with biologic, psychologic, and preventive considerations, with restorative dental materials, and with the ultimate juxtapositioning of a mechanical fabricate into a dynamic biologic environment.

Also, please note that many of the commercial products and dental materials that are mentioned in this book are identified as to origin and utilization in the appendix that follows the text. This will include the name and address of the manufacturer, the nature of the material, why it is used, and comments based on the author's opinion and experience in handling the material, and also on research evidence from dental literature.

REFERENCES

1. Jorgensen, K. D.: Factors affecting the film thickness of zinc phosphate cements. Acta Odont. Scand. *18*:479, 1960.
2. Nelson, R. J., Wolcott, R. B., and Paffenbarger, G. C.: Fluid exchange at the margins of dental restorations. J. Am. Dent. Assoc. *44*:288, March, 1952.
3. Brännström, M., and Nyborg, H.: Dentinal and pulpal response. Odont. Revy *11*:37, 1960.
4. Norman, R. D., Schwartz, M. L., and Phillips, R. W.: Studies on solubililty of certain dental materials. J. Dent. Res. *36*:977, December, 1957.
5. Langeland, K.: Biologic considerations in operative dentistry. Dent. Clin. North Am. March, 1967, p. 125.
6. Seltzer, S., and Bender, I. B.: Modification of operative procedures to avoid postoperative pulp inflammation. J. Am. Dent. Assoc. *66*:503, April, 1963.
7. Tilmans, A., and Krokosky, E. M.: Radiation effects on epoxies. J. of Materials *6*:465, 482, June, 1971.
8. Boucher, C. O.: Current Clinical Dental Terminology, St. Louis, The C. V. Mosby Co., 1963.
9. Council on Dental Materials and Devices: Recommended standard practices for biological evaluation of dental materials. J. Am. Dent. Assoc. *84*:382, February, 1972.

two

The Prepared Abutment Tooth

It may appear that we are belaboring the idea of promoting the biologic approach to all problems in dentistry, but that is, and will continue to be, the true justification for the continued existence of the profession.

Arthur Elfenbaum

Be kind to vital abutment teeth. They have suffered enough! The ultimate success of crown and bridge therapy depends upon the health of the teeth that support fixed prostheses. Few teeth take as much abuse, and abutment teeth deserve all the consideration they can get. They come in all sizes and shapes, and range from the perfectly healthy tooth in occlusal harmony to the tooth that is traumatized, containing one or more fillings or carious areas.

The preparation of an abutment tooth for a fixed restoration should involve the benevolent sculpturing of the tooth to a predetermined form by the dentist. However, this is more often as not expressed as a violent attack on the integrity of the tooth with fast and furious tooth reduction apparatus that just about annihilates the tooth and amputates to within a whisker of the pulp. Further annoyances that have the potential for contributing to the demise of the abutment tooth are as follows:

1. Application of irritating medicaments and chemicals.
2. Poorly fitted protective coverage.
3. Poorly cemented protective coverage.
4. Application of hot impression materials and pressure.
5. Indiscriminate blasting of air on the tooth.
6. Trauma from high or poorly adjusted occlusion.
7. Trauma from the forces applied to remove temporarily cemented restorations.
8. Irritation from acid cementing materials.
9. Hydraulic pressures inaugurated in cementation.

Abutment teeth are also abused by the following:

1. The burden of partial dentures.
2. Orthodontic procedures.
3. Bruxism.
4. Thermal changes.
5. Accidental fracture.

It is a tribute to the inherent toughness and tenacity of certain living human processes that many teeth that have been poorly treated and subjected to every lack of consideration still survive. However, many don't survive, and don't prevail in the mouth as the much desired healthy, vital abutment tooth. Much too often, failure manifests itself to the patient initially as a toothache or endodontic procedure and later, and more embarrassing to the dentist, as the slow, insidious biologic undermining of an extensive fixed restorative measure.

Much of the success of fixed restorative dentistry today depends on the marvelous defensive and reparative powers of the dental pulp. A pulpal reaction is unavoidable in the most careful abutment preparation even though the pulp is resistant to external effects and is tolerant of a large amount of trauma. The dental pulp reacts to every injury. The issue is whether the reaction is reversible or not. Will it recover? Or will it break down and become necrotic and ultimately develop an abscess? There is no way to predict which way a pulp will go. Some with irreversible lesions may survive for years if they don't become infected. Therefore, the dentist should give the pulp (and the patient attached to it) every possible consideration related to the healing potential of the pulp. *He should try to reduce the odds of inducing irreversible pulp damage.*

How? By avoiding drugs and medicaments that may cause more harm than benefit. By repairing and recontouring the abutment tooth with non-irritating and adhesive restorative materials. By providing well-fitting protective coverage cemented with a zinc oxide and eugenol cement. And by recognizing the factors that contribute to pain or comfort. Proper healing due to the inherent reparative capacity of the pulp is more likely to take place if the "tincture of tenderness" is applied. However, there is no explanation for the mysterious death of a pulp that occurs despite the best treatment.

Crown and bridge therapy is more successful if prepared abutment teeth are maintained in a healthy, vital condition. *A vital abutment tooth is stronger, more elastic, and less likely to fracture under the stress of function than a non-vital abutment tooth.* Although endodontically-treated teeth with posts, pins, or cores make very adequate abutments, they must be considered second-best to vital teeth.

Every effort should be extended to provide for the maximum health and longevity of prepared tooth structure. Guidance in obtaining this objective during the mechanical preparation of the tooth may be found in various technical crown and bridge textbooks. However, the biologic considerations that influence the health of the prepared vital abutment tooth are examined herein in the following categories:

1. Beware of drugs and medicaments
2. Repair of abutment tooth contour
3. Protection of the abutment preparation
4. Factors that influence pain and comfort

BEWARE OF DRUGS AND MEDICAMENTS

There are cycles of thought and theory on many aspects of dentistry. One subject that has been on the "merry-go-round" for many years is the relationship of pulpal health and applied medicaments. For many years various chemical agents were applied to cut tooth structure for "cavity sterilization." Subsequently research reports pointed out that the various agents applied were harmful and not beneficial. It became necessary to weigh the necessity of destroying bacteria on the tooth on the one hand against provoking inflammation of the pulp on the other. The unmedicated pulp won out. Drugs contributed more damage than benefits.

Nevertheless, dentists like to doctor teeth. It is surprising that, despite research to the contrary, many clinicians feel compelled to apply various medicaments to prepared tooth structure. A few decades ago, this was termed the "cavity toilet." Silver nitrate, alcohol, phenol, hydrogen peroxide and various other agents were routinely swabbed on prepared teeth either singly or in combination to destroy microorganisms and to seal dentinal tubules. Modern research has flushed these procedures down the drain. It has determined that *any medicament capable of killing germs may also be capable of harming the pulp.* Sterilization of tooth structure with drugs prior to repair does more harm than good. Also, some of these agents such as silver nitrate *are more apt to open the dentinal tubules* than to seal them. Silver nitrate has been shown to be irritating to the pulp in numerous studies.[1,2,3] Phenol is a poor sterilizing agent and is also cytotoxic. It is an undesirable and detrimental agent for application to dentin.[4] Alcohol injures odontoblasts. It denatures the protein of the protoplasmic processes. Hydrogen peroxide solutions are potentially damaging.[5,6]

It all boils down to lukewarm water. The best "cavity toilet" material to apply to any prepared tooth structure is lukewarm water. There is no research evidence to substantiate that any drug or medicament available today is of greater benefit to tooth structure than lukewarm water.

More recently, the cycle of thinking along these lines has been rotated through the efforts of Brännström and Nyborg.[7] A new interest has been awakened in the need for cavity medication. They have suggested that the diffusion of bacteria trapped under a restoration or entering through microleakage may be *the real cause of pulpal inflammation* rather than the chemical irritation of the restorative material. Brännström and Nyborg have contributed a substantial amount of documented research[7-12] showing that enormous amounts of viable bacteria were existing between prepared tooth structure and restorative materials. They theorize that the microorganisms were there to begin with, or were carried in on the filling material, or they entered after the restoration was placed through microleakage. To contend with this problem, they experimented with a new microbicidal solution called Tubulicid* and found that this material had the ability to successfully remove the bacteria without detriment to the dentin and pulp. It is a fluoride-containing, surface-active solution. The question that arises is, "Why is Tubulicid able to kill germs without harming the tooth unlike other antibacterial agents?" And the answer may be—that selectively, only at an optimum level of germicidal concentration, not too strong, and yet just strong enough, an antimicrobial agent may function with benefits and no harm. In other words the germicides used in the past may have been too strong. Milder antibacterial materials may act against microorganisms without harming the pulp. It should be noted that one of the best mild antiseptic materials is a mixture of zinc oxide and eugenol. Nevertheless, regardless of this conjecture and the published research showing the merits of Tubulicid[7, 11] the product is not available in this country. One of its components, dodecyldiamino-ethyl glycine, may not be approved by the Food and Drug Aministration for import. Nevertheless even if it were available, it would not seem to be a clinical necessity for modern crown and bridge therapy, especially if a zinc oxide and eugenol final cement is utilized, since bacteria may not survive and increase in number to even a small extent with this material.[43]

Another material, a cavity liner called Tubulitec,** has been repeatedly suggested for the prevention of bacterial growth and for protection under several restorative materials.[7–9, 13–17] This liner contains polystyrene in chloroform, calcium hydroxide, zinc oxide, a flourine salt, and an antiseptic, thymol iodine. Although various reports by the same investigators have shown that Tubulitec prevents bacterial invasion, some doubt has been cast on the antibacterial efficacy of thymol iodine and on whether or not it and the fluorine salt can emanate from a hardened dry resin film sufficiently for the benefit of the adjacent tooth structure (see Chapter 10). Nevertheless, regardless of other considerations, Tubulitec does provide as effective pulp protection as any other chloroform-contained cavity liner. It is desirable to use more than one layer of the liner, especially under composite resin filling materials.

Will tooth structure once sterilized by a medicament remain sterilized? Or will microleakage allow the entrance of new bacteria? Or are new bacteria introduced on the restorative material itself? An effective and long-lasting antimicrobial effect may only be obtained if a varnish, liner, or restorative material with free antibacterial activity is placed and allowed to remain in contact with the prepared tooth structure. Then, all old bacteria, and any new ones that enter by seepage, will find the locale an unsuitable area for proliferation. Ultimately, formulations of zinc oxide and eugenol with an appropriate

---

*Dental Therapeutics AB, Nacka 1, Sweden; Premier Dental Products, Norristown, Pa. 19401.

**Buffalo Dental Manufacturing Company, Brooklyn, NY 11207.

additive may be tailored to more completely fulfill this requirement.

Once again a cycle of thought and theory has been completed but the "merry-go-round" goes on. It is important for dentists to be cognizant of the research developments pertaining to pulpal protection, but today in dentistry lukewarm water should still be considered the best "abutment toilet" for successful crown and bridge therapy.

CORTICOSTEROIDS AND ANTIBIOTICS

In more recent years it seemed cogent to utilize antibiotics and corticosteroids for their benefits to prepared tooth structure. Rationales for administration of these materials, either singly or in combination, have been touted to the dental profession. Textbooks dealing with restorative dentistry tell the dentist to apply various corticosteroid ointments routinely in the temporary cementation of fixed restorations.[18, 19] This should not be done. Dental journal reports and advertisements propose the use of antibiotics in crown and bridge cements as well as in root-canal filling materials. This should not be done. Unfortunately, little or nothing is mentioned about the precautions and the contraindications to the use of these drugs. Corticosteroids are known to hide symptoms useful in diagnosis. They encourage bacteremia,[20] and are not known to have the ability to heal any condition.[21] Corticosteroids may reduce pain, but will also interfere with dentin bridging if an exposure is present. Steroids and antibiotics should not be recommended to dentists, or in turn to patients, without emphatic designation of the precautions and contraindications concomitant to their use.

The routine use of steroids for application to tooth structure is not justified.

Crowns and bridges, as well as all other types of restorations, exist with the potential for microleakage. A substance *may leach out* from under or between a restoration and a prepared tooth just as readily as one *may leak in.* Antibiotics and corticosteroids are no exceptions. However, if one of these materials leaches into the oral cavity, *the patient's well-being is threatened.* Sinkford and Harris[22] noted: "So potent an agent as hydrocortisone used topically in the oral cavity with such a varied bacterial flora could be potentially dangerous to the incipient rheumatic, to the individual with resistance lowered by viral infection, or to others with particularly vulnerable organs such as lungs and kidneys."

Antibiotics also have been shown to be of limited value for abutment therapy. If used in large enough amounts in a dental cement, the irritational characteristics of the cement are increased and the potential for sensitization is always present. A systemic reaction to a polyantibiotic root-canal dressing has been reported.[23] It has also been demonstrated that an antibiotic may sensitize an individual via the root canals of teeth;[24] this causes serious complications.

The path of administration of an allergenic drug influences the probability of sensitization. *Topical application is the manner most likely to sensitize.* Parenteral injection is the next most likely, and oral administration is the least likely.[25]

A "wonder drug" is only wonderful if used in the right doses for the proper length of time against organisms known to be sensitive to it. Regardless of how miraculous the cures a drug can effect, it is still likely that some patient will suffer undesirable consequences. With any drug, the benefits must be weighed against the risks involved. A drug that may have a life-threatening effect should not be used to treat a relatively minor condition.

The topical use of antibiotics should be avoided in crown and bridge therapy.

Corticosteroid preparations have been suggested for the control of sensitive dentin and pulpal reactions. The use of these drugs in these situations must still be considered *experimental* or *empirical.*[26] If they are used nevertheless, the dentist must ascertain by a careful history that the patient is not receiving systemic corticosteroids from his physician. Accidental dual administration may exaggerate the adverse effects of the drugs. Also, topical applications should be avoided in patients suffering from diabetes, hypertension, peptic ulcer, tuberculosis or viral infections.

A five year report[27] on the pharmacologic treatment of painful pulpitis showed a corticoid-antibiotic mixture applied as a pulp-capping agent to have no more efficacy than a starch control.

SUMMARY

Over the years drugs and medicaments have been applied to cut tooth structure for the following reasons:

1. To kill microorganisms.
2. To seal and occlude the dentinal tubules to keep out microorganisms.
3. To prevent or eliminate inflammation (i.e. antibiotics, corticosteroids).

Are they successful? Langeland[28] says it this way, "there is no medicament available today which will selectively kill bacteria—protoplasmatic in their nature—without also causing damage to the odontoblast processes." He continues, "none of the suggested medicaments such as silver nitrate, fluoride, or cyanoacrylate derivatives, has been able to cause an occlusion of the dentinal tubules."

It has been shown convincingly that the histologic evidence of inflammation in the dental pulp is not altered by treatment with corticosteroids, or combinations of corticosteroids and antibiotics.[29] All things considered, the dramatic reduction in pulpal pain is the only positive benefit that may be derived from the use of a corticosteroid. This factor alone hardly justifies their general use in pulp therapy since the disappearance of the pain may just serve to conceal a severe inflammatory response.

REPAIR OF ABUTMENT TOOTH CONTOUR

Not every prepared abutment tooth resembles the textbook picture of a perfectly prepared tooth. Many have discrepancies such as voids and undercuts due to the removal of carious areas and old fillings or inlays (Fig. 2–1). Some "patching" must be accomplished to repair the walls of the preparation so that impression making and other procedures may be facilitated. In past years, undercut areas and other remaining concavities were brought back to contour by filling them with zinc phosphate cement. Since this cement was not adhesive to tooth structure, it fell off prematurely in many instances, much to the chagrin of the dentist and the patient. After a tooth has been reduced to the depth of crown preparation, any further encroachment into it for undercuts to mechanically retain the zinc phosphate cement would be hazardous. Also, since zinc phosphate cement is irritating when applied close to the pulp, it often contributes to pain and occasionally to the death of the tooth. Zinc oxide and eugenol, with its ability to soothe and sedate tooth structure, was utilized by some dentists to repair abutment teeth, but this material is not hard enough to give an appropriate surface; nor does it adhere any better to the prepared dentin. It also inhibits the polymerization of any subsequent application of acrylic resin protective coverage.

In recent years, calcium hydroxide formulations have been used to fill undercut areas on prepared abutment teeth. Materials such as Dycal* and Hydrex** are used to effectively "spackle" the walls of

*L.D. Caulk Company, Milford, DE 19963.
**Kerr Manufacturing Company, Romulus, MI 48174.

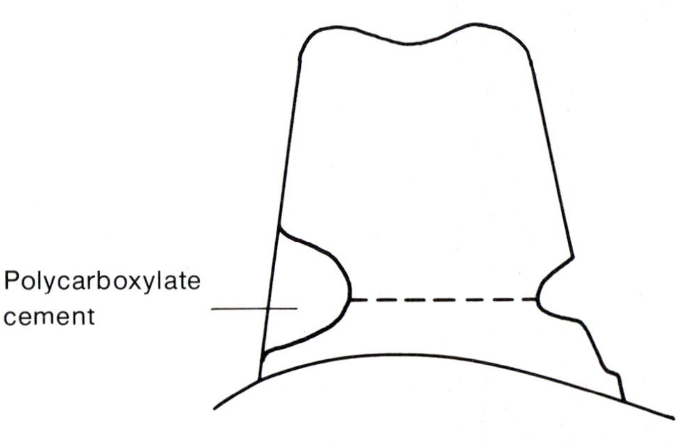

Figure 2–1 Prepared vital abutment tooth after removal of old fillings and caries. The lingual area has been filled with polycarboxylate cement and now presents a smooth surface. The buccal undercut area requires a similar repair. A non-vital tooth would have a potential for fracture along the broken line.

abutment preparations. They do not irritate tooth structure or inhibit the polymerization of acrylic resin crowns. In fact, they are especially suitable for application to deep areas that may be suspected of pulp exposure. However, although calcium hydroxide has been considered to be a very suitable material for effective abutment repair, it is less than perfect for this purpose. It does not supply a hard enough surface in many instances, and it has no adhesive ability.

Materials for Abutment Tooth Repair

Two modern dental materials have the physical and biologic properties required for effective abutment repair. They are polycarboxylate cement and composite resin filling material.

The composite resin material is stronger and should be selected for use where strength is required. It has found widespread utilization in the repair of non-vital abutment teeth, and is used effectively with pins and cores. However, in vital teeth, pulp protection is necessary. The polycarboxylate cement is the more adhesive of the two and has more biologic compatibility. They both require the dentist to have intimate knowledge of their handling characteristics and physical and biologic properties.

Polycarboxylate Cement

Of all available dental cementing materials, *polycarboxylate cement is the most adhesive to prepared tooth structure.* Although the original claims of true adhesion to dentin as well as enamel have not been substantiated *in vivo,* it does adhere to dentin far better than does zinc phosphate cement or any other available cement. It is, therefore, the most suitable cement with which to fill in cavities, undercuts or irregularities in the contour of an abutment preparation. Unlike zinc phosphate cement, it will not fall off during subsequent procedures such as impression making and the temporary cementation and removal of temporary coverage. Unlike an irritating acid cement such as zinc phosphate cement, polycarboxylate is kind to dentinal and pulpal tissues. Unlike zinc oxide and eugenol cement, it will not inhibit the polymerization of acrylic resin temporary coverage. Unlike calcium hydroxide formulations, it presents a hard surface on setting that may easily be formed flush with the remaining preparation.

One shortcoming of the polycarboxylate cement is its *early solubility.* Immediately after placement, and while going through the early stages of setting (polymerization), *it is very sensitive to contact with water.* The dentist must protect it from moisture or the material will dissolve away and present a weakened and irregular surface. Setting time will also be prolonged. Also, after placement to restore contour, any contact with lip, cheek, or tongue results in distortion and stringing out of the cement. This should be avoided. The cement may be placed and shaped with a plastic instrument dipped in alcohol.

In a very deep concavity on a prepared tooth that is sensitive, a very small amount of zinc oxide and eugenol cement such as Temrex Cement* may be applied and then covered with a mix of a polycarboxylate cement such as Durelon.** The zinc oxide and eugenol cement obtunds pain and will soothe and sedate a sensitive tooth. Polycarboxylate cement will not; but it is an adhesive and strong cover for the weaker but sedative material. In a deep cavity on a prepared abutment tooth that has a pulpal exposure or is suspected of having a microscopic exposure, a calcium hydroxide paste such as Kerr's MPC† or Pulpdent‡ may be applied and covered with polycarboxylate cement. Polycarboxylate cement is not recommended for direct pulp capping since it does not stimulate dentinogenesis and it is not bactericidal.[30]

Polycarboxylate cement is not adhesive unless it is applied in a thin-flowing glossy state. However, it is difficult to place a thin mix of this cement on an abutment tooth and maintain the desired contour. The cement flows with gravity and slumps. This is a real problem with upper teeth. Note the following suggestions:

1. Prepare for two small mixes of the polycarboxylate cement. Mix and apply the first to the depth of the concavity and fill half of it. After it loses its gloss and starts to harden, mix and apply the second mix to establish contour.
2. A plastic filling instrument dipped in Campho-Phenique§ or alcohol may be used to shape and contour the cement without stickiness and stringing out.

A shortcoming of carboxylate cement is its tendency to absorb moisture and swell slightly. As a result, if a large area of an abutment tooth is repaired to contour with this cement, the area may swell from contact with saliva during the procedures prior to final cementation. This may cause a casting made from an impression before the swelling occurred to fit very tightly or not at all. This problem may be solved by using a sandpaper disc very slightly on *the cement component* of the repaired abutment tooth prior to fitting the casting.

In summary, the polycarboxylate cement is the most ideal material to repair and recontour the prepared abutment tooth for the following reasons:

1. It stays in place without undercuts to hold it.
2. It is non-irritating to the pulp.
3. It sets to a smooth, hard surface.
4. It does not inhibit the polymerization of acrylic resin temporary coverage.

More information about polycarboxylate cement will be found in Chapter 8.

---

*Interstate Dental Company, Inc., New Hyde Park, NY 11040.
**Premier Dental Products Company, Norristown, PA 19401.
†Kerr Mfg. Company, Romulus, MI 48174.
‡Pulpdent Corporation of America, Brookline, MA 02147.
§Glenbrook Laboratories, New York, NY 10016.

Pulp Exposure During Abutment Preparation

To allow for the proper contour and size of the finished crown restoration, a large amount of tooth structure must be removed. In accomplishing this, the dentist is between the devil and the deep blue sea! If he doesn't remove enough tooth substance, the ultimate crown will be too fat and overcontoured; if he removes enough tooth substance, an exposure may result! This unfortunate occurrence usually hurts a sensitive dentist far more than it does the patient. What can be done if an exposure occurs as a result of tooth reduction? After all, x-ray guidance is not three-dimensional. The anatomy of the buccal or labial extent of a pulp chamber may not be readily determined. Much too often, concern for esthetics motivates excessive tooth reduction on these surfaces. Of course, root canal therapy can be started at once. In the majority of cases it would be the best procedure and is what usually happens. However, although pulp capping may be more feasible for an exposure inside a cavity, an exposure on the surface of a preparation that is aligned with other surfaces and possibly with other teeth is a difficult and very complex problem. Any material used to cap (cover) the exposure will create a bump on the tooth surface and therefore an undercut that will not allow for the draw and insertion of a crown. More than likely, it will also fall off. Pulp capping is contraindicated if the mechanical exposure is *large* and the deeper structures of the pulp have been contaminated. However, when a small "pin point" exposure or small "pink colored area" of suspected exposure is present, there may be some hope for recovery. The cells of the pulp are the judge and jury that will decide whether or not their repair capacity has been exceeded by injury. Therefore, in selected cases, according to the position and size of the exposure and other considerations, pulp capping may be accomplished. Of course, endodontics may be resorted to later if the pulp capping is not successful.

1. Isolate, control bleeding and apply a small amount of a calcium hydroxide paste to cover the exposure in the usual manner. Calcium hydroxide is the drug of choice for pulp capping. However, isobutyl cyanoacrylate monomer has an interesting potential for pulp capping. It produces immediate hemostasis when applied to an exposure.[31]

2. Cover the complete tooth surface (usually the labial or buccal), including the calcium hydroxide paste, with a thin-flowing glossy mixture of polycarboxylate cement. For the first time in dentistry, a cement is available that will firmly adhere to cut tooth structure. Polycarboxylate cement also sets to a strong, hard surface and has biologic compatibility with the tooth. In this instance, and for the purpose, zinc phosphate cement would not be adequate, because it does not adhere to the tooth without mechanical undercuts and, therefore, may fall off readily. Also, it is far too acidic and irritating at close range to the pulp. The pul-

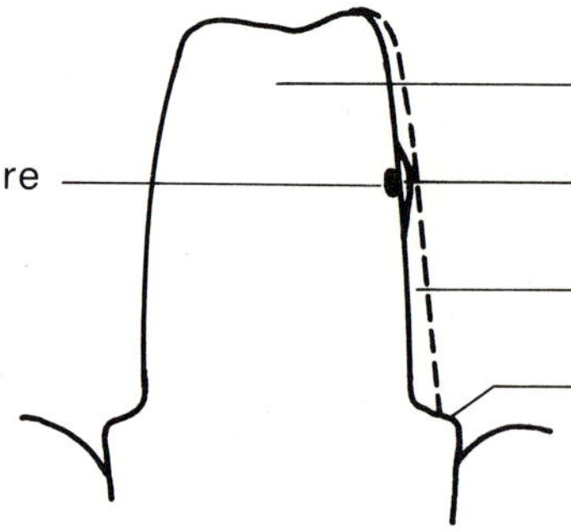

Figure 2–2 A tooth prepared with a substantial buccal shoulder and an exposure capped with calcium hydroxide. The entire buccal surface is covered with polycarboxylate cement to protect the pulp capping and to present a surface devoid of undercuts. The buccal full shoulder depth is decreased by the thickness of cement.

pal response to the application of a carboxylate cement is as benign as to zinc oxide and eugenol cement.

3. Recontour hardened cement and adjacent tooth surfaces to a new outline form (Fig. 2–2).

Dental pulp undergoes many changes throughout life. Pulpal reaction in an older patient is decidedly different from that in a young person. The pulp changes not only with age but also with a variety of other stimuli. Despite the effects of caries, attrition, abrasion, erosion and trauma, the dental pulp may remain normal. Even exposed pulps may heal and remain normal. Where there's vitality, there's always hope for recovery.

Composite Resins

Composite resins are not only effective as filling materials; they may also be used as fissure sealants, as "cover-up paint" for tooth erosion, in Class IV angle repairs, and in crown and bridge prosthodontics to *build up and shape the remains of a tooth for a crown* and as a *final cementing material* for crowns and bridges.

Composite resins usher in a new and magical era of effective tooth repair. For many years there was second-rate acrylic resin trying to replace third-rate silicate cement, now there is first-rate composite resin and the magic of acid etching. Composite resins have been tried and proved and improved over the past 10 years. If any dentist has not had the pleasure of matching composite resin with tooth structure or marveled at the efficacy of acid etching in bonding a resinous material to enamel, he is missing much.

These are new tools of the trade—but they are not perfect. They require understanding and practical clinical experience for successful utilization. An abundance of literature and many lectures have extolled the mechanical properties of composite resins. Multicolor full-page advertisements have pitted the physical properties of one composite material against those of others. Here, the dentist is bombarded with an abundance of information that he can do without, because a *comparison of physical properties is not meaningful to successful clinical applications.* Composites are composites. All true composites have a similar range of physical properties and, of course, these should be known to the dentist who plans to use them.

So, in a nutshell, composites are beefed-up plastic materials. They are fortified resins. Therefore, they are harder and stronger. They don't shrink as much on polymerization as acrylic resin does. Nor do they expand and contract as much with thermal change as acrylic does. Also, resistance to abrasion is more than twice as good as unfortified resin, and there are fewer color problems. Composites match tooth structure more effectively.

The consideration of characteristics and *features other than physical properties* is meaningful to practical use. For example, let's pose a few questions that physical property measurements can't answer.

1. Can freshly mixed composite resin be bonded to hardened composite resin?

   Hardened composite resin presents a surface with a large amount of glass-like material that cannot easily be bonded to fresh composite resin. The matrix of resin that is available for contact with a new mix of unpolymerized resin is minimal. Therefore, bonding new composite to old is not readily accomplished. Grinding the old surface to knock out some of the glass-like particles and present more resin material for attachment may be of some help, but successful bonding is questionable. However, many of the newer versions of the composites have a pure resin bonding component that allows for very effective attachment of new to old composite.

2. Will a zinc oxide and eugenol base prevent a composite resin from hardening?

   Many of the composite resins will set hard and effectively over zinc oxide and eugenol. Some will not. There is some confusion and misunderstanding regarding this problem. The directions for composites such as Adaptic,* Love** and HL-72† indicate compatibility with zinc oxide and eugenol. Powder and liquid type composites such as Blendant‡ should not be placed over eugenol-containing bases. It has been reported that despite a hard set, some of the physical properties of a composite resin are slightly modified when placed over zinc oxide and eugenol. However, the slight loss of physical values is far overshadowed by the biologic benefits to be derived from therapy with zinc oxide and eugenol. Also, it may be well to note that an EBA cement that has approxi-

*Johnson & Johnson Dental Products Company, East Windsor, NJ 08520.
**Stratford-Cookson, College Park, GA 30337.
†Lee Pharmaceuticals, South El Monte, CA 91733.
‡Kerr Manufacturing Company, Romulus, MI 48174.

mately two-thirds less eugenol in the liquid component may be less likely to influence the physical properties of a composite resin material. The zinc oxide and eugenol cement should be thoroughly hardened before the composite resin is placed.

3. Does acid-etch bonding of a resin work as well on deciduous teeth as it does on permanent teeth? How about non-vital teeth?

   No. Less mechanical retention results when resins are bonded to deciduous teeth as compared to permanent teeth. Etching does not produce the deep dissolution of the prism cores necessary for proper adhesion.
   The acid etching is effective in preparing the surface of a non-vital tooth for bonding with resin.

4. Can toothpaste be harmful to composite resin restorations? And, if so, which ones?

   Yes. Toothpastes that contain chloroform. *Accepted Dental Therapeutics* lists three popular brands of toothpaste that *contain up to 3 per cent chloroform.* They are Ultra Brite, Close Up and Macleans. The repeated application of chloroform is deleterious to a resin surface. The resin matrix of a composite resin filling material may be harmed by contact with chloroform. Discoloration and accelerated wear are manifestations of the chemical attack.

5. Should zinc phosphate cement liquid be used for acid etching?

   No. Not without some controlled dilution. The phosphoric acid liquid component of a zinc phosphate cement is too concentrated (approximately 65 per cent) for effective utilization as an acid etchant. Also, it is too fluid and colorless for proper control of application.

CRITERIA FOR THE SELECTION OF AN APPROPRIATE COMPOSITE RESIN

Besides considering factors such as packaging, shelf life, ease of mixing, color-matching ability, viscosity and the degree of translucency, the selection of an appropriate composite resin restorative material should be based on biologic considerations and handling characteristics.

Biologic Considerations

In the selection of a composite resin, biologic considerations are of special importance. The pulpal health of the tooth under repair is of prime concern. Marginal seal and preventive considerations are also important. Composites irritate dentin and pulpal tissue in a manner similar to silicate cement. The pulpal response may also be compared to that of conventional acrylic resin. Clinical experience has shown, however, that when teeth have been previously restored, or when sclerotic dentin has been formed from carious lesions, the pulp response to composite resin may be minimal. The potential for irritation also depends on the age of the patient and the thickness of remaining dentin.

Pulpal areas under all composite filling materials should be protected from contact with the resin by a base of calcium hydroxide, polycarboxylate cement or zinc oxide and eugenol (depending upon composite formulation). Calcium hydroxide is used in most instances and, of course, where a minute pulpal exposure exists or is suspected to exist; polycarboxylate cement where difficult placement is encountered and effective adherence is required; and zinc oxide and eugenol in the very deep, painful, overly sensitive or young tooth.

Where the palliative and sedative action of zinc oxide and eugenol cement is needed, the question arises: Will the composite resin material set adequately over this material? Of course, the unfilled acrylic resin will not polymerize in contact with zinc oxide and eugenol. However, most composites are so highly cross-linked that they should set hard over anything. It boils down to this: some composites harden perfectly over zinc oxide and eugenol, some less than perfectly, and some not at all. Quite a few composite materials available today state clearly in their printed directions for use that they

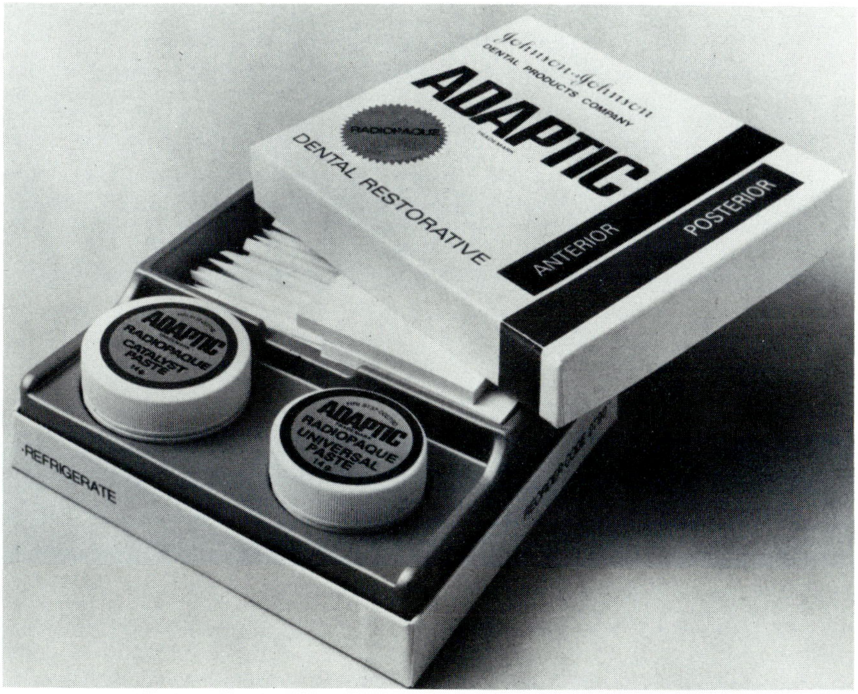

Figure 2–3 One of the composite resin restorative materials stated to be compatible with a hardened zinc oxide and eugenol base.

are compatible with zinc oxide and eugenol bases (Fig. 2–3). For example, Adaptic, Compolite,* Love and HL-72. In directions for use, some composite resin materials contain warnings against contact with zinc oxide and eugenol cement. For example, Blendant, Smile,** Exact,† and Concise.‡ However, a mixture of Concise will even set if placed in a thin mix of zinc oxide and eugenol.

Probably, the factors that influence hardening over zinc oxide and eugenol are as follows:

1. The degree of cross-linking
2. Paste/paste vs. powder and liquid
3. The presence of a tertiary amine

Recent research[7, 10] has shown that when unbased cavities are restored with composite resin, the contraction of the restoration results in a space between it and the tooth structure that usually contains a dense accumulation of bacteria. This has been pointed to as the cause of inflammation of the pulp. The bacteria may have been present on the walls before the restoration was placed, or they may have entered the space from the mouth through leakage after placement. An antibacterial cavity lining material, Tubulitec (Fig. 2–4), has been suggested to eliminate bacteria in the cavity prior to placing a composite resin.[7] Tubulitec is a polystyrene liner that is inert and provides protection to dentin under zinc phosphate cement, amalgam, silicate, and composite resin. This lining should cover the entire dentin surface. Not only does it provide good protection for the pulp but it may also prevent bacterial invasion. This may be because

---

*Rugby Laboratories, Inc., Inwood, L.I., N.Y. 11696.
**Kerr Manufacturing Company, Romulus, MI 48174.
†S. S. White Dental Products Division, Philadelphia, PA 19102.
‡3M Company, Dental Products, Saint Paul, MN 55101.

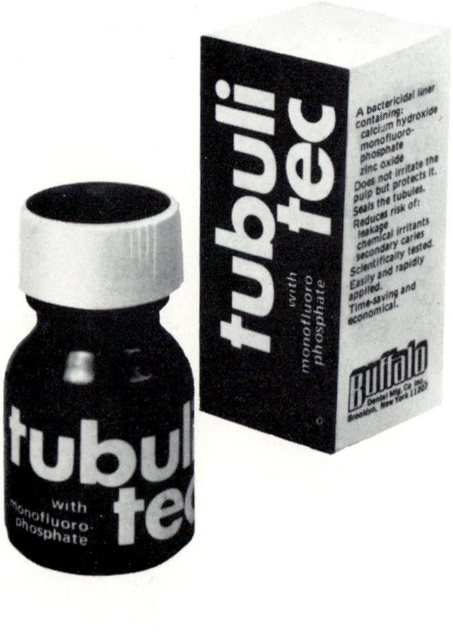

Figure 2–4 This liner has a bactericidal agent and a fluoride, and can provide reliable protection to the pulp under most restorative materials.

this liner adheres to the dentin rather than to the restorative material. Entrance of any leakage (fluid or bacteria) would be between the restoration and the lining rather than between the liner and tooth structure. Since this liner contains antibacterial components, bacteria already present may be rendered innocuous by the lining material.

Marginal Seal

The shrinkage of composite resins during setting is minimal. Expansion and contraction features are better than those of the unfilled resin. Yet, as far as microleakage is concerned, it has been pointed out that composite resins are probably not superior to the conventional resins. Adequate marginal sealing is a form of prevention. It is directed at eliminating recurrent caries. Acid etching may improve marginal seal.

Handling Characteristics of Composite Resins

Viscosity and Body for Placement

Composite resins offer very little resistance to the pressure of an instrument used to place them in position. No force can be used. However, some composite resins have more "body" than others and are almost granular before spatulation. The viscosity of a composite resin material may be decreased by adding a drop of a solution composed of isopropyl alcohol and phenyl carbinol.* This will allow for easier mixing, increased flow and a longer setting time. Placement instruments dipped into this solution will function more effectively without the adherence of a composite resin (Fig. 2–5).

* Ease, Transon Corporation, Granger, IN 46530.

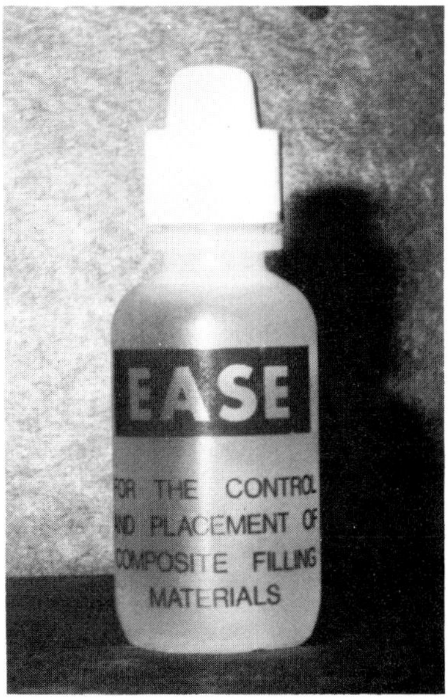

Figure 2–5 This solution, which contains isopropyl alcohol and benzyl alcohol (phenyl carbinol), will aid in the control and placement of composite resin restorative materials.

Instruments

Plastic instruments, jiffy tubes, disposable plastic syringes, and Teflon-covered metal instruments may be used to place the composite resin. Rubber interdental stimulators with the point cut off may also be used for adapting the composite to a preparation in a tooth. A Centrix* syringe is helpful in applying composite resins. It aids in obtaining void-free placement by filling from the inside out. The composite resin is mixed, placed in a disposable plastic tube, sealed with a plug, inserted into the barrel of the syringe, and injected (Fig. 2–6). In doing this, however, the dentist should work fast enough not to encroach on the working time of the composite resin. Also, 2 mm of the tip of the disposable plastic tube should be cut off routinely to speed up the flow of the material.

Working Time

The "working time" and "setting time" should be clearly defined. Working time is a very important consideration for the successful use of composite resin materials. It is the time clocked from the start of the mix until the material starts to thicken on its way to setting hard. It is the time allowed for the placement of the material. The viscosity of the mix should not increase during working time. Setting time is the time from the start of mixing to the time of hardening. The best adaptation of a composite resin material to tooth structure may be obtained when it is applied to the tooth *immediately after the completion of the mix.* Any packing, instrumentation, movement, or manipulation of any kind after the working time has elapsed (Fig. 2–7) may sabotage the integrity of the composite resin material.

*Centrix, Incorporated, Fairfield, CT 06430.

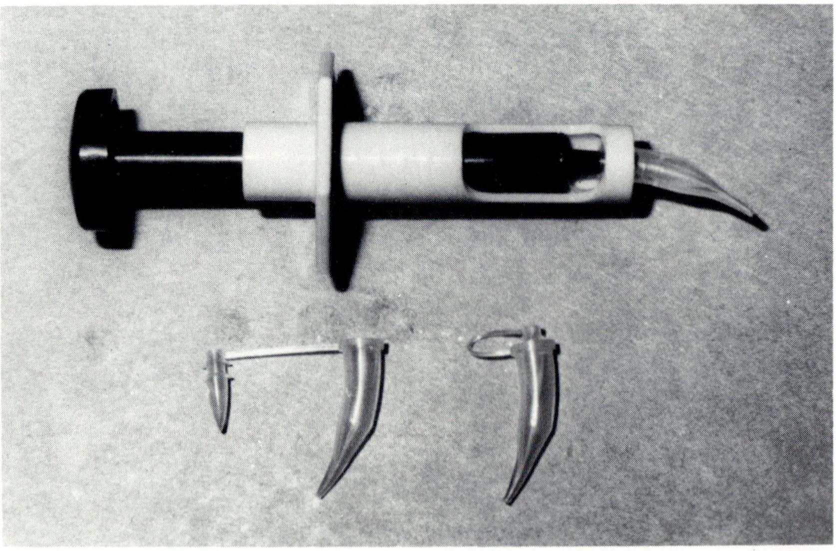

Figure 2–6 The Centrix syringe provides a neat, clean, and effective way to place resins or cements into a small area.

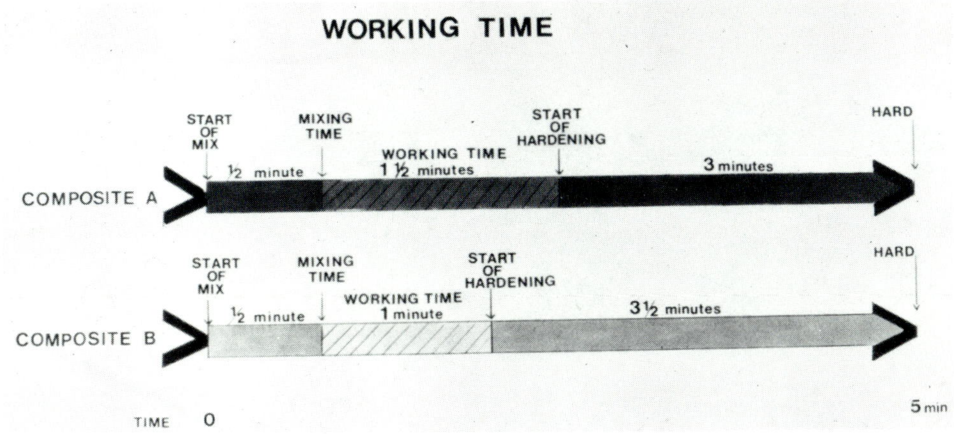

Figure 2–7 Composite resin A and composite resin B both set hard in the same amount of time. However, composite resin A should be preferred because it allows more working time before hardening starts.

Composite resins are very sensitive to failure just prior to setting. They are very weak at this time and may disintegrate, crumble, or develop cracklines if prematurely disturbed, or if the matrix is moved. A composite resin that continuously increases in viscosity during working time (the time for insertion) is an inadequate material.

Finishing

Finishing is the "weak link" in the chain of composite resin repair because composites are made up of hard particles scattered in a softer resin matrix. A truly adequate finishing procedure involves the cutting of glass as readily as that of the softer resin. This is difficult to accomplish. The gloss from the matrix is spoiled by finishing procedures, leaving a dull, rough surface of exposed filler particles, bonding matrix, and some voids where filler fragments have become dislodged. The surface, therefore, may look unattractive and feel rough to the tongue, the lips and cheeks. Rough surfaces tend to harbor germs and collect debris and plaque. A smooth surface facilitates impression making. It is best to wait 48 hours before finishing, for then there will be less discoloration.

Finishing may be accomplished with any of the following tools.

1. Twelve-bladed carbide burs (Emesco).

The fluted carbide burs are very effective for dry finishing. The cut composite resin stands out and is differentiated from the tooth structure when dry and can be trimmed with less chance of reducing tooth enamel.

2. White carborundum stones (Interstate Dental Company).

White stones, lightly coated with silicone grease, should be used at a slow speed with a light touch.

3. Tan rubber abrasive points (Dedeco).

These rubber abrasive points should be used wet and with reduced speed.

4. Finishing diamonds (Star Dental Company).
The fine diamond stones used should be of 300 mesh grit or less.

Polishing

After a smooth surface has been obtained, Adaptic Polishing Paste* on a felt instrument rotating at low speed with firm pressure will give a lustrous, well-polished surface.

ACID-ETCH BONDING

About 10 years ago, acid etching was introduced to improve the mechanical adhesion of acrylic resin to enamel. It has gained wide acceptance, and clinical observations indicate that it is highly successful (Fig. 2–8).

Acid etching is a giant step forward. It has application not only in restorative dentistry but in orthodontics, periodontics and preventive dentistry as well. For example, plastic adhesive bands in orthodontia, splinting in periodontia, and the sealing of pits and fissures. It is also used to improve marginal adaptation and seal, and for coating areas of tooth erosion.

---

* Johnson & Johnson Dental Products, East Windsor, NJ 08520.

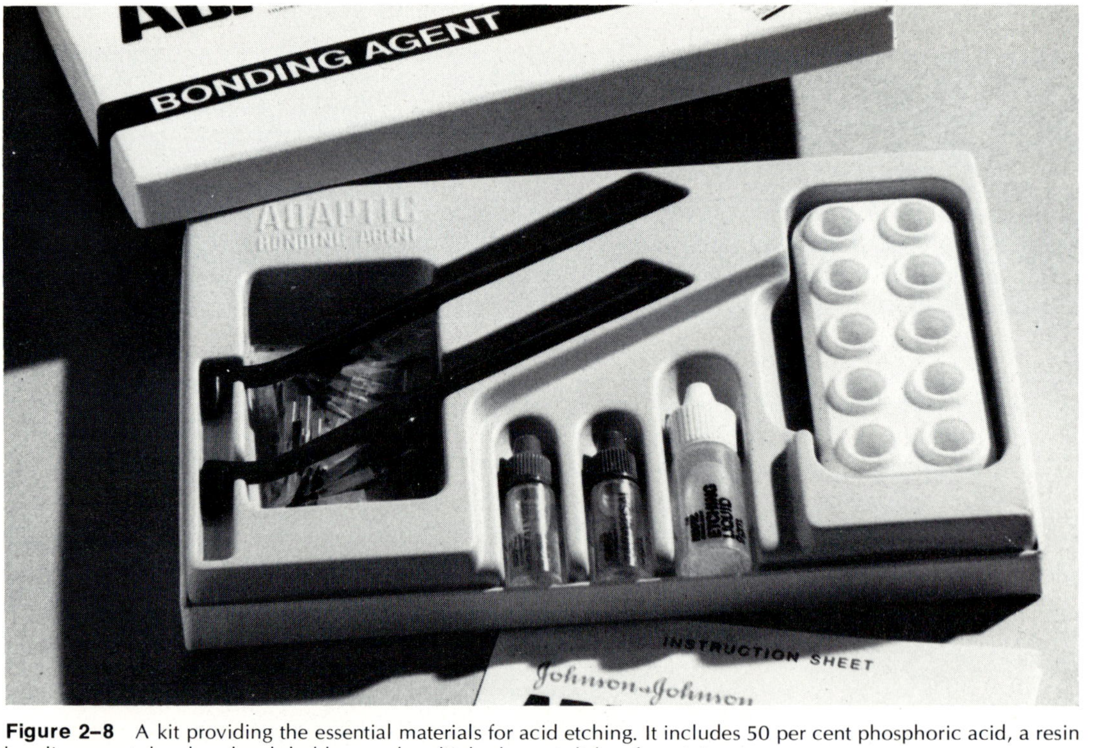

Figure 2–8 A kit providing the essential materials for acid etching. It includes 50 per cent phosphoric acid, a resin bonding agent, brushes, brush holders, and multiple dappen dishes for mixing.

Acid etching causes a temporary decalcification of the enamel surface. Retention depends on the ability of the resin to wet and adapt to the etched enamel surface, and also on tags of resin that extend into the enamel surface. The degree of adhesion is directly related to tag formation. For the first time in the history of dentistry, teeth may be repaired without the anesthesia, grinding, and discomfort involved in cavity preparation. Patients accept this type of treatment most willingly and feel very grateful for the service that has been performed.

Phosphoric acid of *25 or 50 per cent* concentration etches to a greater depth and will provide *more retention* than the 75 per cent phosphoric acid. Acid treatment removes surface debris, etches enamel, and makes surfaces more wettable.

Tag formation of various depths influence the degree of adhesion. Because of inadequate prism structure on the surface of deciduous teeth, etching does not produce the in-depth dissolution of the prism cores or the interprismatic areas necessary for resinous adhesion. Therefore, less mechanical retention results when resins are bonded to deciduous teeth than when they are bonded to permanent teeth.

In the mouth, remineralization, or the return to normal appearance, occurs in about 48 hours with no harmful side effects such as rapid plaque buildup. It occurs faster in the younger patients.

A base or liner should be placed prior to acid etching in deep cavities. The acid should be limited to the enamel walls of the cavity preparation. Phosphoric acid applied to the dentin is an irritant to the pulp.

It has been shown that treatment of a cavity with citric acid before insertion of a composite resin restoration can, within a month, result in a massive bacterial invasion of most dentinal tubules. This may also be true with phosphoric acid. Therefore, it is questionable whether citric acid is suitable for cleaning dentin before cementation with a resin cement or the placement of a resin filling.

Practical Considerations for Acid Etching

Prior to etching, the teeth should be cleaned with dry pumice and water, but not with prepared mixes that may contain glycerin or fluoride. Exposed dentin should be protected with calcium hydroxide before etching. The application of the acid should be confined to the area to be restored. However, it is not harmful to other surfaces since remineralization occurs in 24 to 48 hours. Etch one to two minutes with 30 to 50 per cent phosphoric acid. After the acid etch solution is washed off, the patient's tongue should not be allowed to touch the etched area.

Teeth with fluoride need a longer etching time for success. The etched area of the tooth should look frosty. If not, repeat the etching procedure. Moisture exclusion is important to bond strength. The ability of the acid etch to change the enamel surface varies from patient to patient, tooth to tooth and area to area. There is a great variation in enamel surfaces and in the way in which they react to phosphoric acid. Repair of a fractured incisor using this technique is contraindicated when the occlusion is unfavorable.

Some Essentials for Success

1. The surface must be completely dry, before and after the acid etch is applied.
2. Rinse well. Phosphoric acid must be thoroughly washed off the tooth with water.
3. Care must be taken to prevent contaminating the treated tooth surface with saliva prior to adding the restorative material.
4. A definite frosty or decalcified appearance must be present for adequate retention. If the tooth surface does not appear chalky, the acid should be reapplied.
5. Longer than usual etching times may produce a more adherent bond and a longer lasting seal.

OTHER USES OF COMPOSITE RESIN IN CROWN AND BRIDGE THERAPY

The endodontically treated tooth may be successfully reinforced for use as an abutment in various ways. Posts, pins, and cores coupled with amalgam and cement are often utilized. Cements have always been weak and soluble, and amalgam has always taken too long to harden to suit the operator. Various methods using composite resins for cores and reinforcement of endodontically treated teeth have been presented in the dental literature.[33,34] A core made of a composite resin material has a surface texture that is especially conducive to a retentive bond with a dental cement.

Epoxylite CBA #9080 is a composite resin material that has been modified to be a dental cement.* It is probably the strongest dental cement available, but problems with film thickness and biocompatibility limit its widespread utilization. It may be the ideal luting agent where retention is a problem and the abutment teeth have been treated endodontically.

SUMMARY

Composite resin may be used in crown and bridge therapy for repair of prepared abutment teeth, for core and pin techniques, and, in selected cases, as a final cementing material. It is also the best tooth-colored filling material available. It has shortcomings, nevertheless, and these should be recognized by the dentist. In selecting an appropriate composite, he should especially consider the following:

1. Ability to set hard over zinc oxide and eugenol cement
2. Ability to set without the exclusion of air and moisture

*Lee Pharmaceuticals, South El Monte, CA 91733.

3. Ample working time
4. Acid-etch effectiveness
5. Ease of finishing and polishing
6. Ability to bond to itself

PROTECTION OF THE ABUTMENT PREPARATION

With the best of care and consideration, and despite all precaution some dental pulps die after the preparation of tooth structure. A tooth prepared for a crown may have a minute or microscopic pulp exposure as a result of the preparation or from a previously existing carious lesion. In many instances these do not bleed and are not painful. However, at some future date, perhaps more than a year later, the pulp may die with or without pain.

Pulps may not recover completely from the effects of abutment preparation. Chronic inflammation may persist for a long period, ultimately leading to partial, and then total necrosis of the pulp. Nevertheless, treatment may appear to be satisfactory when evaluated by the absence of pain, the patient's comfort and lack of radiographic evidence. Many teeth with irreversible pulp damage survive for years, provided infection does not occur. This may mislead some dentists to believe that the crown and bridge therapy was successful. Stanley[35] so aptly notes, "If nature would let every pulp die within 30 days after we did something wrong, many of our questions and controversies would be resolved much quicker."

Every effort should be made to protect the abutment tooth and to reverse pulpal damage. The pendulum of survival swings in response to the following:

1. Application of calcium hydroxide to the very deep areas of the remaining tooth structure or to those areas suspected of minute exposure.
2. Well-fitting acrylic resin protective coverage with all margins smooth and rounded; that is, no sharp edges.
3. Temporary cementation of the protective coverage with a zinc oxide and eugenol cement (powder and liquid, not paste form) to soothe and sedate, and possibly reverse any pulpal damage.
4. Avoidance of medicaments and drugs. No phenol, alcohol, silver nitrate, hydrogen peroxide, corticosteroids, or antibiotics.
5. Drying with a pledget of cotton and a little warm air in the gingival crevice. Do not overdry with continuous blasts of air.
6. Repair of retentive form and contour with a nonirritating material such as polycarboxylate cement or composite resin with a protective liner.
7. Careful adjustment of occlusal relationships.
8. Careful tempering of hot impression materials prior to application. Overheating a prepared tooth with hot impression compound may increase hyperemia of a pulp enough to hasten its demise.

9. Coupling of well-fitting temporary coverage with a preparation of proper retentive form to avoid loosening between visits. *It is also important to select the proper temporary cement according to the biophysical factors involved.*

10. Completion of the fixed prosthesis without delay. The sooner a prepared tooth receives the permanent restoration, the healthier it is for the pulp. Therapy should not stretch out for many months before completion.

TEMPORARY CROWNS AND BRIDGES

Immediately after preparation, temporary crowns and bridges are necessary to accomplish the following:

Protection

Protection of the prepared abutment teeth from physical, thermal and chemical irritation.

Therapy

Temporary coverage may be considered a "bandage" for wounded teeth. It applies an anodyne temporary cement that obtunds pain and provides *therapy* to soothe and sedate dentinal and pulpal tissues that have been traumatized by preparation.

Function

Maintenance of occlusal function and the providing of contacts to stabilize positional relationships until the permanent restorations are completed.

Esthetics

Esthetics should be provided to obtain a reasonable amount of good looks during crown and bridge therapy. In many instances a dramatic initial esthetic improvement provides the impetus for continued successful restorative treatment.

Tissue Control

Soft tissue management and conditioning may be accomplished with adequately contoured crowns, with margins that are smooth, rounded, and neither overextended or underextended, and with properly designed and placed pontics. The gingival tissues are often abused by the trauma of subgingival preparation. Even preparations accomplished with the greatest care may damage the sulcular epithelium of the free marginal gingiva. The temporary crowns should promote the healing of this tissue and contribute to an environmental relationship that will sustain the health of the tissue until the final restoration has been cemented.

Psychologic Considerations

Temporary crowns and bridges are usually fabricated and installed in a patient's mouth at a time of critical concern in the patient's psychological makeup. Although the patient is marking time and looking forward to the completion of the final restoration, the provisional restorations, if not esthetically acceptable, can produce a severe psychological impact.

Occasionally, the temporary crown or bridge initiates a substantial esthetic improvement which satisfies the esthetic demands of the patient so completely that the permanent restoration may be rejected. The changeover from tooth-colored occlusal surfaces to gold occlusal surfaces often cause patient dissatisfaction. Also, the arrangement, form, and bulk of some of the newly installed final teeth may meet with objection after the patient becomes accustomed to the slimmer, easily modified temporary restorations. The dentist should explain these inevitable changes before treatment is started. Unfortunately, and too often, the patient is preoccupied with glowing and unrealistic hopes of flawless esthetics, and the dentist's explanations are forgotten—especially if the course of therapy covered an extended period of time. If problems such as these are anticipated they may be handled as follows:

1. Have the patient read and initial notations on his record that the occlusal surfaces of the final restorations will be visible as gold; that opposing teeth hit harder on contact with gold or porcelain than on contact with the temporary resin; that abutment crowns may have slightly more bulk; and that pontic design may be modified for efficiency.

2. Present visual aids such as stone casts with wax-ups of the final restorations, and paint the surfaces that will be gold with a gold material,* or a silver material* may be used to show lingual gingival collars of porcelain-over-metal crowns. These gold- and silver-colored solutions may be painted on diagnostic casts over wax, stone or acrylic to show the design of crowns, inlays, bridges, amalgam restorations, and partial dentures. They are easily removed with a thinner.

Methods for Temporary Protective Coverage

Temporary protective coverage for multiple crowns or bridge units may be effectively fabricated by any one of a number of direct and indirect methods.[36, 37] Methods utilizing the vacuum-formed plastic matrix, the elastic impression matrix, and the processed heat-cured acrylic resin restoration are well known. However, temporary coverage for the single crown preparation with the generally used polycarbonate (or other resin) pre-formed crown and the celluloid crown form leaves much to be desired. These are difficult to fit accurately at the gingival margin, are usually over-contoured, and pose problems in adjusting and polishing. For the sake of gingival health

* TRU-FIT, George Taub Products, Jersey City, NJ 07306.

they should be avoided. An ideal esthetic single temporary crown that may be easily adjusted to any contour, width, or length, fits well, has well-adapted gingival margins, and is easily polished may be obtained with an aluminum shell and acrylic resin. This combination is applicable to anterior or posterior preparations. Similar to a copper band impression, the festooned and toed-in aluminum shell carries the acrylic resin to a thin, well-fitting contact at the gingival area of a posterior preparation, and *slightly* below the gingival margin of an anterior preparation. Unlike the old aluminum shell filled with cement that had improper contour and was not adjustable, the aluminum now is stripped away, leaving acrylic resin that may be shaped properly and adjusted as needed to the necessary contact and occlusion.

Abutment Protection for an Individual Tooth

For a single prepared abutment tooth the following procedure provides adequate protective coverage:

1. Select an aluminum shell with an opening two sizes larger than the diameter of the prepared abutment tooth.
2. Festoon and trim the edges with a small scissors to match the gingival curvature of the tooth.
3. Smooth all rough edges with a small stone in a straight handpiece.
4. Crimp and toe in the festooned edges with pliers.
5. Identify labial or buccal positions by marking with a stone.
6. Select and mix the required shade of acrylic in a dappen dish.
7. Pour this liquid mix immediately into the aluminum shell avoiding air bubbles.
8. Seat in correct position on the abutment tooth after the gloss of the acrylic monomer has disappeared (Fig. 2–9). There are two reasons for this:
    a. It prevents excess monomer from irritating the dental tubules.
    b. It shortens the time that the shell must be held in position.

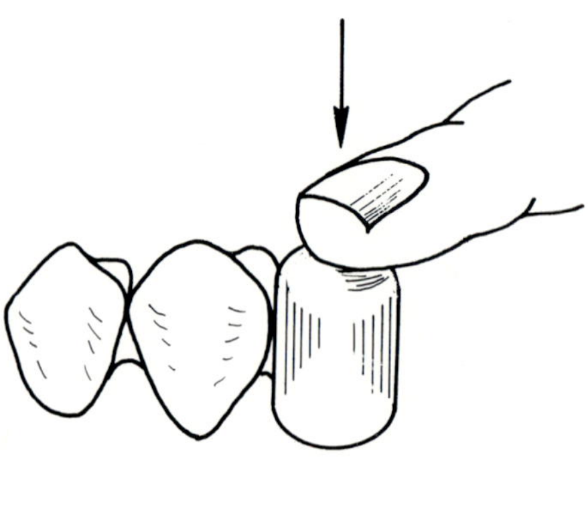

Figure 2–9 The festooned and crimped aluminum shell with acrylic resin is seated on a prepared abutment tooth. It may extend slightly into the gingival crevice.

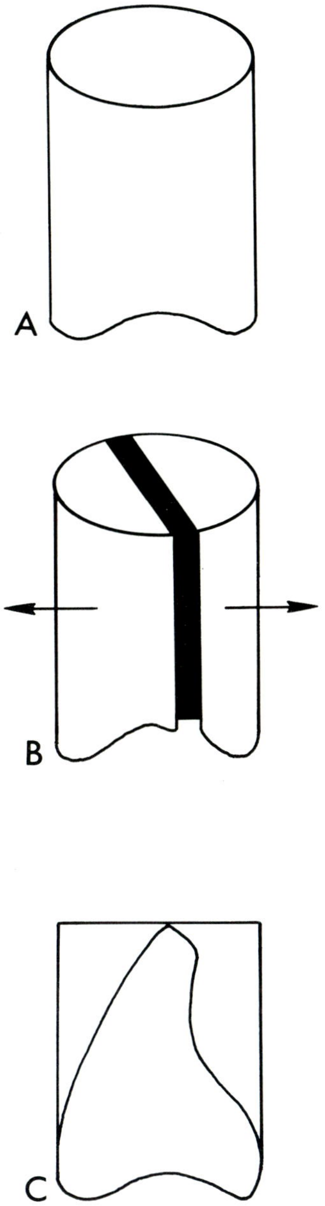

Figure 2–10 *A,* The prepared aluminum shell; *B,* the aluminum shell after slitting and removing the acrylic resin; *C,* the cylinder of acrylic resin is sculptured into the required tooth form.

The aluminum shell should carry the acrylic resin slightly into the gingival crevice.

9. Remove from the mouth in approximately one minute, before the acrylic hardens.
10. Dip in lukewarm water for one-half minute.
11. Replace in correct position on the abutment tooth.
12. Remove and allow to harden completely under water.
13. With a carborundum disk, slit the aluminum shell on a vertical wall and across its occlusal surface (Fig. 2–10).

14. Peel off the aluminum shell and discard. This leaves a cylinder of acrylic that fits the abutment tooth.

15. With stones and disks, shape the acrylic cylinder into proper tooth form and occlusion.

16. Add contact points with a paint-on brush technique and replace in the mouth before hardening occurs, to prevent over-contact.

17. Adjust occlusion.

18. Polish the acrylic crown with a rubber wheel,* flour of pumice and Lustershine.**

19. Cement with a powder and liquid type zinc oxide and eugenol cement.

Resins for Abutment Protection

Self-curing acrylic resin crowns, bridges, and splints provide the most adequate provisional coverage to protect prepared abutment teeth, prevent abutment malalignment, preserve gingival health, and maintain patient comfort. An unfilled acrylic resin *filling* material will provide a better temporary restoration than one of the cheaper bulk resins because it has better handling characteristics and is more *color stable,* owing to cross-linking. This is important in order to

* Burlew, J. F. Jelenko & Company, Incorporated, New Rochelle, NY 10801.
** Accurate Set, Incorporated, Paterson, NJ 07501.

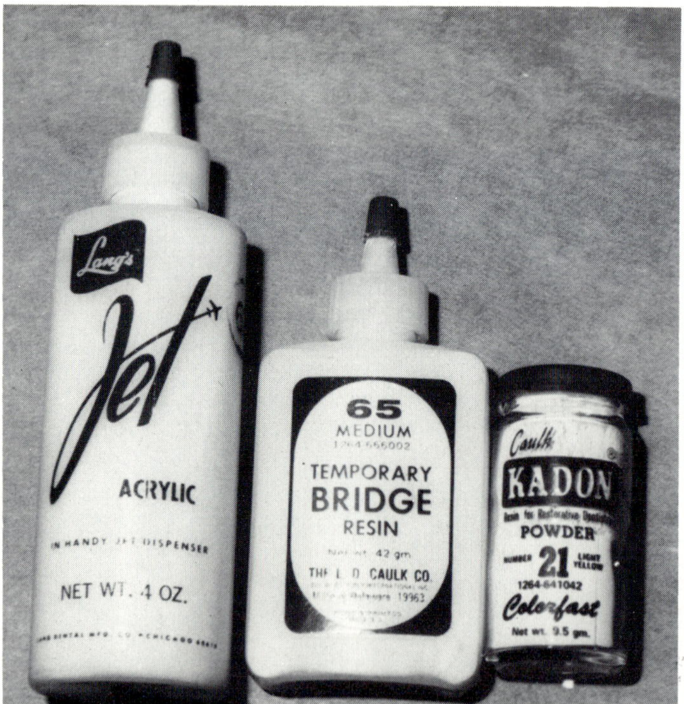

Figure 2–11 Examples of self-curing acrylic resin for temporary crowns and bridges. Kadon is a cross-linked, colorfast filling material that may be used for temporary protective coverage that is destined for extended oral service.

provide the patient with adequate esthetics for a longer period of time, and especially if the course of therapy is unduly delayed for one reason or another. At best, acrylic resin is prone to change color. But it will do so sooner with the non-cross-linked bulk resin. Chapter 6 expounds on the wide variety of reasons for discoloration of acrylic resin veneers. The same reasons are applicable to the self-curing acrylic resin materials. Examples of self-curing acrylic resin for temporary crowns and bridges are Jet Acrylic,* Temporary Bridge Resin,** and Kadon** (Fig. 2–11).

Temporary protective coverage may also be accomplished through the utilization of resins other than acrylic. Trim† is an ethyl methacrylate polymer and monomer that may be used effectively as a temporary restorative material over a short period of time. *It is not color stable* or fluorescent. However, it provides ample working time and causes less heat and chemical irritation to the pulp and gingival tissues than does polymethyl methacrylate. Another relatively new type of polymeric material intended as an alternative for acrylic resin for curing temporary protective crowns and bridges on the prepared tooth is Scutan.‡ This self-curing ethylene imine material is supplied as a base paste in a tube with a bottle containing the cross-linking agent, the catalyst. Scutan has a few advantages over acrylic resin. The setting reaction is less exothermic, and there is no free

*Lang Dental Manufacturing Company, Chicago, IL 60610.
**L. D. Caulk Company, Milford, Delaware 19963.
†H. J. Bosworth Company, Chicago, IL 60605.
‡Premier Dental Products Company, Norristown, PA 19401.

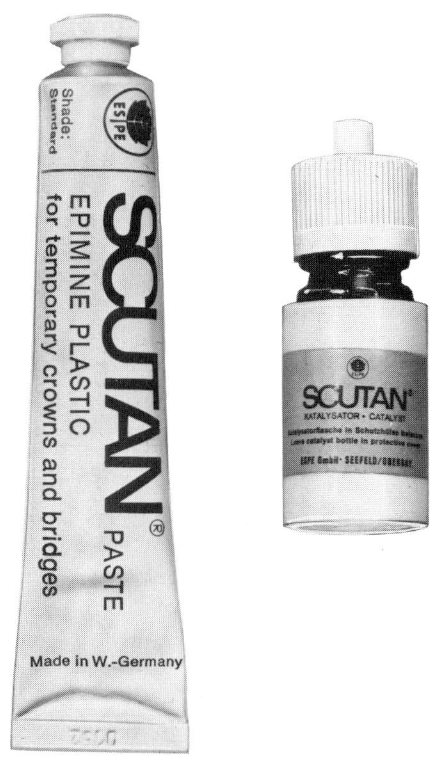

Figure 2–12 A self-curing ethylene imine material for temporary crowns and bridges. There is no free monomer. Scutan hardens readily over zinc oxide and eugenol.

monomer.[38] However, it also has a few disadvantages. Properties such as impact strength and tensile strength are inferior to acrylic resin.[38] Also, it lacks fluidity when poured, has limited esthetic shade values, and costs twice as much as any other temporary resin material. To make additions to Scutan to modify contours or contacts, a new mix of the material is required. The color of Scutan is modified by the thickness of the material formed: a thin film has a lighter color than a thicker film of this material (Fig. 2–12).

Temporary Cementation of Temporary Protective Coverage

Acrylic resin, heat-cured or self-cured, is a resilient material and may be easily deformed under the functional pressures of mastication. Also, its coefficient of expansion and contraction is greater than those of tooth structure and other restorative materials. Therefore, the marginal seal between the temporarily cemented acrylic resin crown or bridge and the prepared abutment tooth may be readily broken. The resulting seepage of saliva and bacteria may cause hypersensitivity, pulpal damage, or caries if allowed to exist over an extended period of time. However, these untoward sequelae are opposed and minimized by the presence of a film of anodyne cement with upgraded antibacterial activity. An ideal material for this purpose is a zinc oxide and eugenol cement such as Temrex Cement* combined with an antibacterial additive such as Opotow Crown and Bridge Paraben** (Fig. 2–13).

No material known to the dental profession is more capable of sedating a painful vital tooth than a mixture of zinc oxide and eugenol. This cementitious material is an obtundent to dental pain and provides a continuous anodyne action.

Because of its unique ability to sedate tooth structure and its excellent initial adaptation and sealing effectiveness, zinc oxide and eugenol is the most ideal material for the temporary cementation of acrylic fixed restorations. It provides crown and bridge therapy!

Temporary acrylic resin coverage is usually cemented on the prepared abutment tooth with a selection from a large assortment of commercial zinc oxide and eugenol cements. The powder and liquid type is better and more effective than the paste type that is supplied in two collapsible tubes. It allows for a thinner mix, lower surface tension, and a slower setting time. Also, the powder and liquid type is more readily modified by the unique and beneficial action that paraben additives have on zinc oxide and eugenol mixes.[39]

Parabens are listed in *Accepted Dental Therapeutics*.[40] They are chemical powders that, as additives, enhance the antibacterial and

*Interstate Dental Company, Incorporated, New Hyde Park, NY 11040.
**Teledyne Dental, Elk Grove Village, IL 60007.

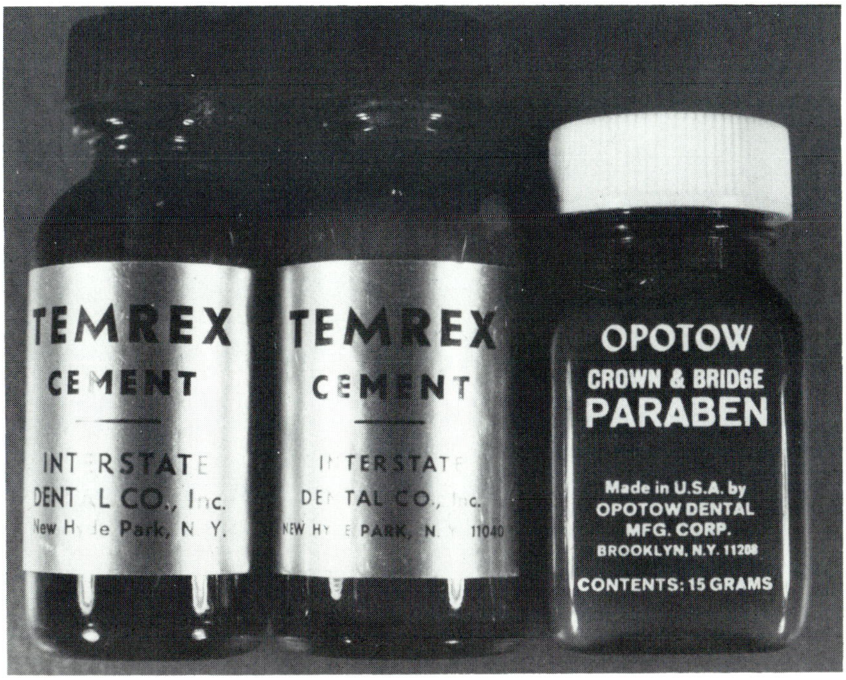

Figure 2–13 This powder and liquid type zinc oxide and eugenol cement sets hard and fast and teams up with the paraben additive for effective therapy to prepared tooth structure.

physical properties of zinc oxide and eugenol temporary cements. Crown and bridge parabens are composed of a mixture of methylparaben and propylparaben. A small percentage added to the mix of zinc oxide and eugenol cement will lower the surface tension of the mix and increase its fluidity, flow, and penetrability. It also *slows down the setting time.* All this allows for easier and more complete seating of acrylic crowns and bridges.

The acrylic resins utilized for complete and partial dentures, or in fixed prosthodontics, temporary or permanent, are similar in their ability to dry out or to absorb water. Drying takes time. Acrylic resin, *although it looks dry,* may still represent a *water system,* and the inherent moisture therein speeds the set of zinc oxide and eugenol on contact. Water, in fact, moisture of any kind, accelerates the setting of zinc oxide and eugenol cement. In many instances the temporary cement in the temporary acrylic crown sets too fast *because it contacts moisture in the resin.* If full seating is not accomplished without a moment's delay, the cement may thicken enough to cause incomplete seating. Now the occlusion is high and requires grinding to accommodate closure. Now, also, the margins are less precise. This problem is minimized by adding crown and bridge paraben (Opotow Crown and Bridge Paraben*) to the zinc oxide and eugenol mixture. The paraben improves the antibacterial activity of the cement and eliminates bad odors on removal of the temporary restoration. It also increases the ultimate compressive strength of the

*Teledyne Dental, Elk Grove Village, IL 60007.

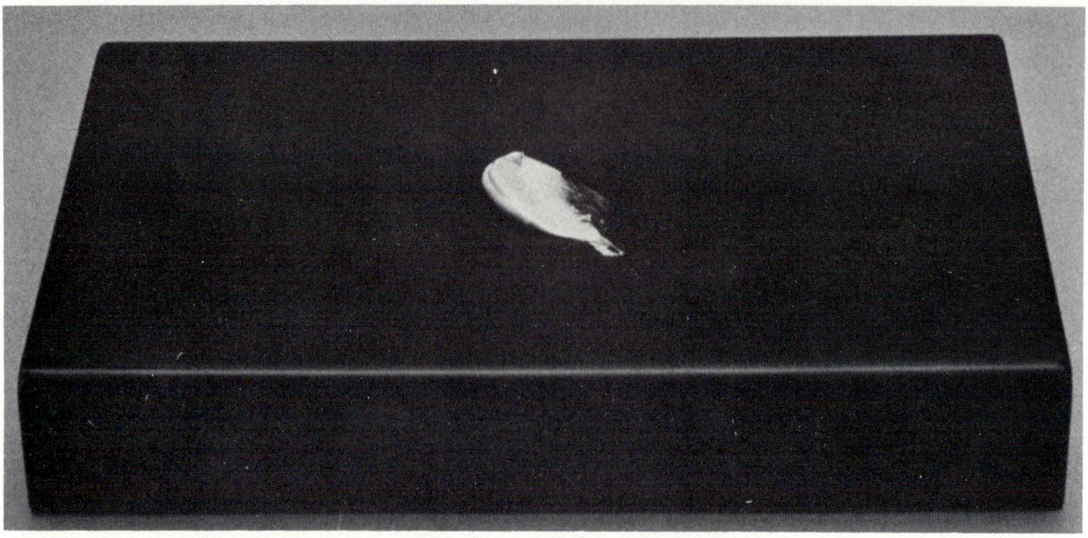

Figure 2–14 A mixture of zinc oxide and eugenol of medium consistency.

cement. Its prime virtue, however, is its ability to slow down the fast set engendered by the moisture in the acrylic that makes up the temporary protective coverage. This allows for more complete seating and better marginal adaptation. (Figs. 2–14 to 2–17).

Methylparaben, U.S.P., and Propylparaben, U.S.P., are the neutral esters of parahydroxybenzoic acid. They are white, fine powders that show marked bacteriostatic and fungistatic activity at low concentrations against a wide variety of microorganisms. The parabens are non-toxic, are soluble in eugenol, and are classified in Group A by the Council on Dental Therapeutics of the American Dental Asso-

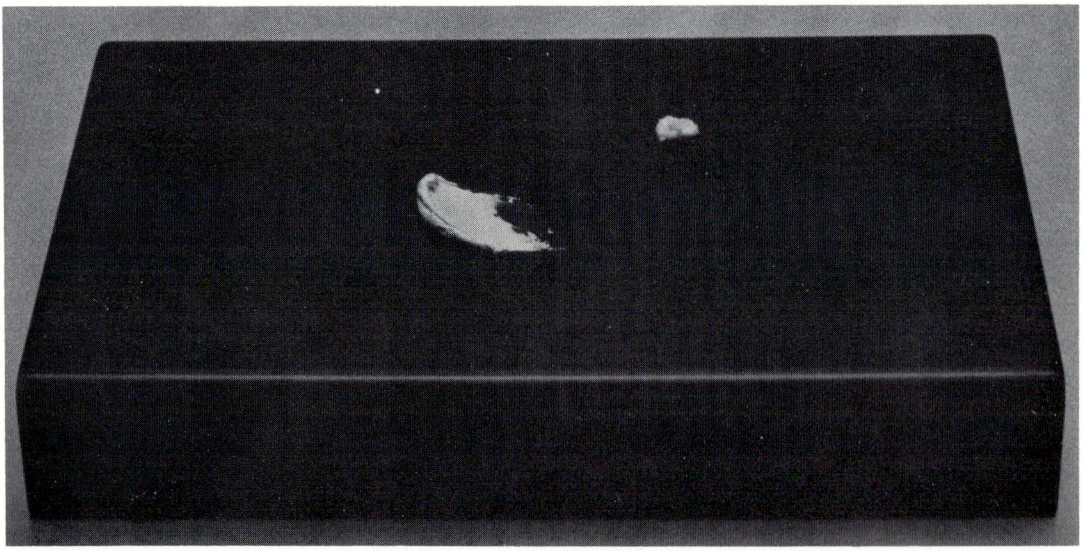

Figure 2–15 The same mixture with crown and bridge paraben placed on the slab.

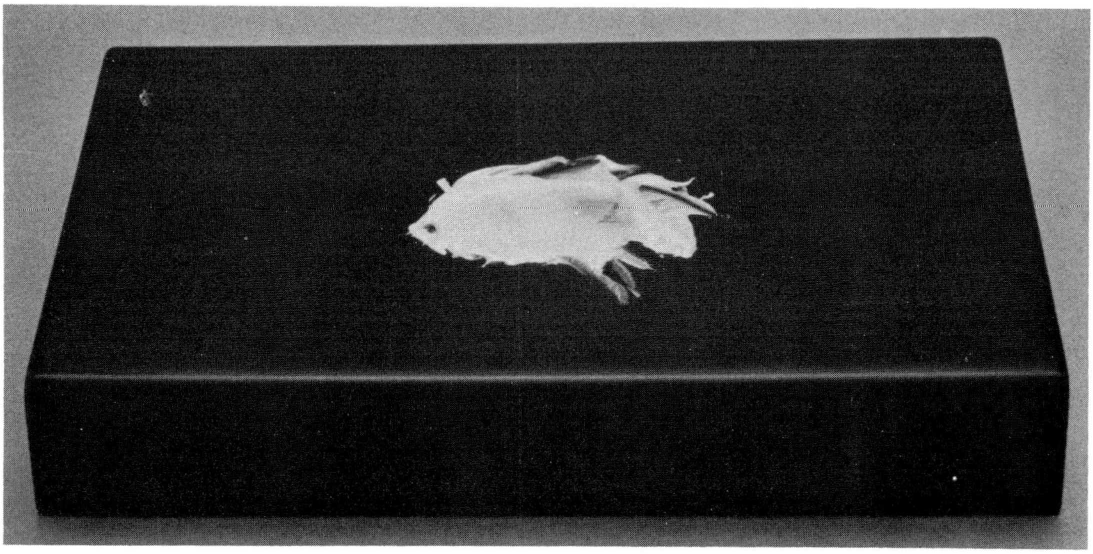

Figure 2–16 After spatulating the paraben into the zinc oxide and eugenol, the mixture becomes more fluid and of a thinner consistency.

ciation.[41] Since the use of an antibacterial agent may cause the surface of the dentin to be an unsuitable locale for bacterial proliferation when exposed to seepage of saliva, the parabens are added to enhance this property of the eugenol. This is important in the light of

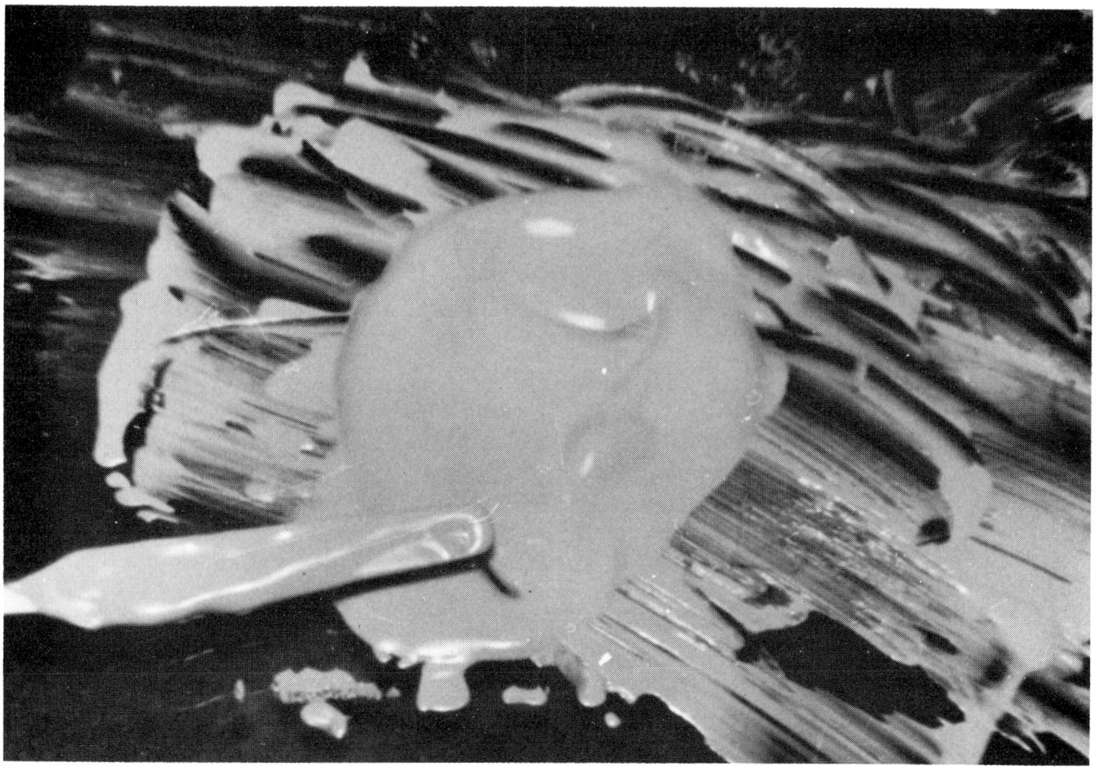

Figure 2–17 A close-up view of the increased fluidity.

current research showing that all restorations have some degree of leakage under oral conditions.

A small percentage of Methylparaben or Propylparaben (approximately 1 per cent) added to the usual mix of zinc oxide and eugenol employed in temporary cementation will increase the plasticity of the mix and upgrade its physical properties and antibacterial values. Although the parabens work well with most zinc oxide and eugenol mixtures, they are especially effective with Temrex Cement.*[39] The extent of their action on a zinc oxide and eugenol mixture is influenced by the following: the amount of zinc acetate in the mixture, the presence of rosin, the type of rosin, the method of compounding, the type of zinc oxide and its mode of manufacture, the presence of acquired moisture, and the shelf life of the materials. The parabens also influence other zinc oxide and eugenol cements, such as ZOE 2200,** ZOE B&T** and After Prep.† It is interesting to note that the mechanical effect produced by the paraben on the zinc oxide and eugenol may also be obtained by incorporating powdered aspirin or saccharin into the mix. However, these materials do not have the antibacterial value of the parabens.

Incorporating a small amount of crown and bridge paraben into a mix of zinc oxide and eugenol will contribute to a decrease in consistency, viscosity, and surface tension, and an increase in fluidity, plasticity, and flow. To summarize, the benefits to be derived from the additive action of parabens in an appropriate zinc oxide and eugenol mixture are as follows:

1. More working time
2. Decreased film thickness and increased flow
3. Easier and more complete seating of temporary crowns
4. Elimination of offensive odors on removal of restorations
5. Improved antibacterial activity
6. Increased ultimate compressive strength of the cement

In contrast to the powder/liquid type of zinc oxide and eugenol cement, the commercial zinc oxide and eugenol products supplied in two collapsible tubes may be too heavy bodied for complete seating of temporary protective coverage that has been polymerized to intimate contact with an abutment preparation. However, they may be utilized with final prostheses that have been fabricated with internal room for the cement. Also, tube cements are loaded with plasticizers, fillers, and thickening agents that could detract from the efficacy of therapy that pure zinc oxide and eugenol provides. Non-eugenol cements do not obtund pain and do not provide the desired continuous anodyne action.

---

*Interstate Dental Company, Incorporated, New Hyde Park, NY 11040.
**L. D. Caulk Company, Milford, DE 19963.
†Teledyne Dental, Elk Grove Village, IL 60007.

To Dry or Not To Dry

Prepared tooth structure should be dry to benefit from contact with zinc oxide and eugenol temporary cements. The sedative and anodyne action of these cements is enhanced when applied to a *dry* prepared abutment tooth. A dry preparation upgrades retention in both temporary and final cementation.

Ask 10 dentists to dry a prepared abutment tooth and you will probably have 10 teeth of different degrees of dryness. Each dentist may have a different interpretation of what is meant by a dry tooth. Since there are no well established criteria, and no yardstick to measure by, the drying of a tooth is a nebulous thing. There is inherent moisture built right into every tooth. Air-dried primary dentin becomes moist as tissue fluid ebbs up from the cut tubules. Teeth differ with regard to moisture content, depending on age, extent of repair, and vitality. Some general clinical guidelines have evolved.

1. To begin with, don't *overdry* or *dehydrate* a prepared abutment tooth.
2. A dry tooth may be defined as one that exhibits no visible signs of moisture.
3. The inherent dryness of a non-vital tooth contributes to cementing efficiency.
4. Drying an abutment tooth is accomplished by patting with pledgets of cotton and then applying a few gentle blasts of warm air in the gingival crevice until there are no visible signs of moisture.

CLASSIFICATION OF TEMPORARY CEMENTS FOR TEMPORARY PROTECTIVE COVERAGE

Many of the available commercial brands of zinc oxide and eugenol cement differ in their physical setting as far as hardness is concerned, some setting to a relatively soft state and some setting hard. Add to these the very-hard-setting final zinc oxide and eugenol cements and the classification is as follows:

1. Soft-setting cements, such as Moyco ZRE Cement,* After-Prep,** and ZOE 2200.†
2. Hard-setting cements, such as Temrex Cement,‡ and ZOE B&T.†
3. Very-hard-setting cements, such as Opotow Alumina EBA,** Fynal,† and Zebacem.†

Note the listing of final cements such as Alumina EBA, Fynal, and Zebacem. A cement that is adequate for the final cementation of a rigid metal casting may also be utilized with a flexible, easily

---

*J. B. Moyer Company, Incorporated, Philadelphia, PA 19132.
**Teledyne Dental, Elk Grove Village, IL 60007.
†L. D. Caulk Company, Milford, DE 19963.
‡Interstate Dental Company, Incorporated, New Hyde Park, NY 11040.

deformed temporary acrylic crown as a temporary cement. The holding ability of a temporary cement depends on its compressive strength, hardness, film thickness, dryness, *and what it is holding:* hard metal, or soft resin. Couple these considerations with the biophysical factors that govern retention (Chapter 7), and it becomes quite evident that the selection of a temporary cement for a given temporary restoration is similar to the selection of a particular casting gold for a given type of restoration. If abutment preparations are long and walls are parallel, and if there is little or no span, temporary cementation with a hard-setting cement may make subsequent removal difficult, and even hazardous if teeth are fragile and old. A soft-setting cement should be selected. On the other hand, if retentive form is questionable, preparations short, and span long, a soft-setting cement may not be retentive enough, and premature loosening may occur. A hard-setting cement should be selected. There are also instances with challenging conditions of retention, such as the temporary acrylic cantilever bridge, unfavorable occlusion, noxious habits of clenching and bruxing, and the overly long-span bridge. Successful retentive temporary cementation for these conditions may only be accomplished by selecting a very-hard-setting cement. Actually in this case a final cement is used as a temporary cement, and removal may be easily accomplished because of the heroic conditions and the ability of the acrylic resin to spring (deform). A schematic illustration of the selection of an appropriate cement influenced by the biophysical consideration of abutment height is shown in Figure 2–18. Note that decreasing height requires cement of increasing hardness. For example, from right to left, ZOE 2200, Temrex Cement, ZOE B&T, Fynal and Alumina EBA.

All of the cements classified, regardless of physical properties, are non-irritating, pain-relieving luting agents that will seal and sedate prepared abutment teeth and retain acrylic resin protective coverage during the course of fixed restorative procedures.

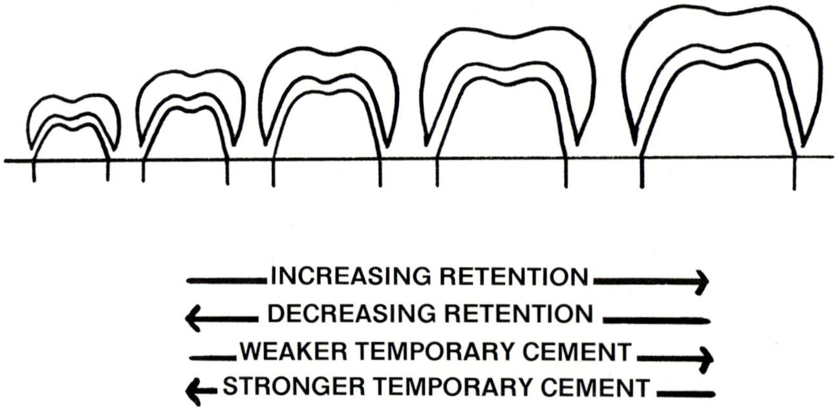

Figure 2–18 The smaller the preparation, the stronger the zinc oxide and eugenol cement necessary to effectively retain a temporary acrylic resin crown.

Practical Considerations

1. The liquid (eugenol component) and the powder have an unlimited shelf life. The liquid is usable and just as effective if its *color has changed to dark yellow or brown.*

2. No aspect of spatulation is critical. The powder may be added to the liquid at any rate of speed, utilizing any size of increment. In fact, all the powder may be incorporated into the liquid at once.

3. A thick mix sets faster. A thin mix sets slowly. Any mix will set faster in a warm or humid room.

4. Don't fill crowns with cement, just line the inside walls.

5. *CAUTION:* Be sure the acrylic restorations are *dry.* Abutment preparations should be lightly dried to show no visible signs of moisture. Do not dehydrate. A *properly dried* abutment preparation allows better retention and a more positive palliative action. Immediately after cementation, dryness need not be maintained. Water and saliva will not interfere with the set. A warm water rinse will accelerate the set.

6. Excess cement should be wiped away from the external surfaces of the acrylic restorations as soon as possible after insertion with cotton rolls or gauze squares. This will minimize or prevent any untoward action of the eugenol component of the cement on the acrylic resin. The potential of eugenol for harming acrylic depends on *time*—the time they are in contact. Therefore, the cement should not be allowed to harden on the resin prior to removal. It should be wiped away immediately. This small problem, which is so easily resolved, has been the basis of a lot of misunderstanding. Poor technique that allows delayed removal of the cement or hardening of the cement prior to removal from the external surfaces of the resin will increase the potential for discoloration. But poor technique may cause failure anywhere. Dentists have been overly and erroneously warned against using zinc oxide and eugenol cement with acrylic resin crowns and bridges. Nevertheless, countless thousands of temporary crowns and bridges are cemented with zinc oxide and eugenol quite successfully. It is a simple matter of recognizing certain pertinent considerations:

   a. The resin may be protected externally by a film of silicone grease, or by simply wiping the cement away immediately.
   b. Internally, the cement attacks the walls chemically, *but to a limited depth.* This is of no significance with a crown of normal thickness, but with a very thin crown there may be a problem. Actually the chemical attack causes a bonding or adhesive attachment to the inside of the crown that may benefit retention.
   c. The biologic benefits of zinc oxide and eugenol are more important than other considerations.

Removal of Temporary Protective Coverage

Temporary acrylic resin crowns and bridges may be removed at certain intervals after the initial temporary cementation to allow for

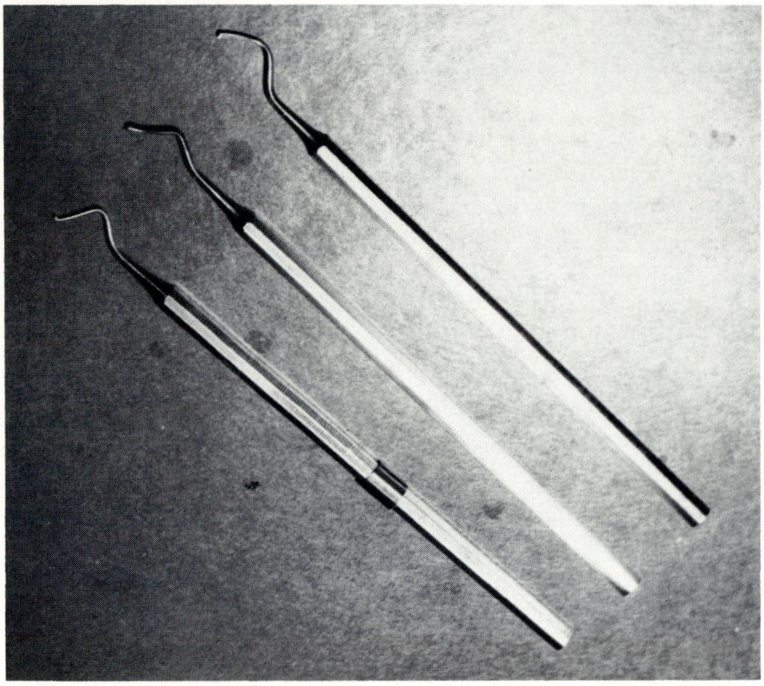

Figure 2–19 Orban type hoe scalers used to remove acrylic resin crowns and bridges. They reach under the buccal or lingual margin of a crown and lift it off the tooth.

various restorative procedures. Removal accomplished with hand instruments is more desirable than with the reverse mallet. Dulled hoe scalers (Orban type) No. 5 and No. 6 are very effective for the removal of acrylic crowns or bridges (Fig. 2–19). The appropriate instrument is applied at the gingival margin of the buccal or lingual surface, and the crown is lifted off. Just enough pressure may be necessary to slightly spring or deform the crown. It may be necessary to apply the instrument first to the buccal surface and then to the lingual surface a number of times before the acrylic resin deforms and lifts off. Also, it may be necessary to alternate the application of the instrument from one end of a bridge to the other until loosening occurs.

Multiple unit splints, and bridges with many abutments, may be difficult to remove with hand instruments. Retention of these crowns is especially enhanced by the multiplicity of their tenso-frictional grip. *Gentle taps* with a reverse mallet at each end and in the middle may be necessary for removal.

The operator should be intensely aware of the potential for fracture of an abutment tooth when a reverse mallet is used forcefully.

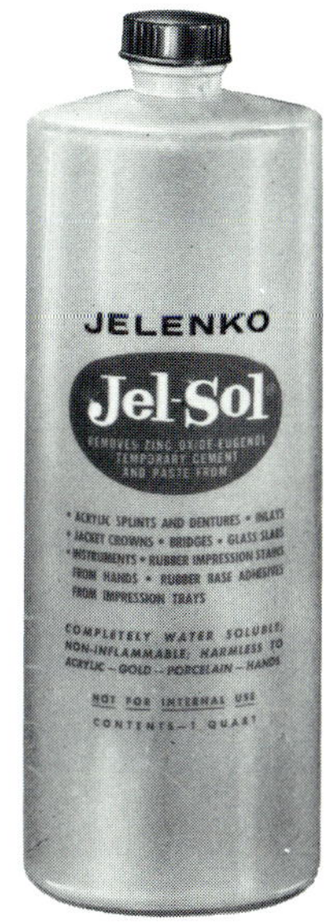

Figure 2–20 A solution used to remove zinc oxide and eugenol cement from crowns and bridges.

Acrylic resin crowns retain the film of temporary cement when removed from the mouth. The old, adherent cement must be removed to allow for a new film of cement that will not disrupt the existing fit and occlusion. It is wrong to try to apply a new film of cement without removing the old, no matter how thinly the new cement is mixed. The occlusion will be high, and margins will be open. New cement does not flow out well over old cement. *It is absolutely necessary to remove the old zinc oxide and eugenol cement.* This is accomplished very effectively with Jel-Sol,* a solution designed specifically to remove zinc oxide and eugenol type temporary cements from acrylic resin prostheses. The restorations are placed in a wooden handled porcelain casserole dish containing Jel-Sol solution (Fig. 2–20). The dish is placed over a Bunsen burner, the solution is brought to a boil, and the flame is turned off. After 10 minutes in the solution, the restorations are removed and all of the cement is washed and brushed out in tap water. They may now be dried, adjusted if necessary, polished, and recemented.

Factors that Influence Pain and Comfort

Pain may be defined as an unpleasant sensation, an extreme of sensory perception. It is a subjective sensation felt by the patient regardless of whether it is of organic or psychic origin. Pain belongs completely to the individual. The extent, intensity, duration, and nature of the pain can only be described by the person who experiences it. The reaction to pain varies greatly from one individual to another and may be altered or modified by the emotional status of the individual and by his previous experience with pain.

*J. F. Jelenko & Company, Incorporated, New Rochelle, NY 10801.

Treatment and control of pain require recognition of the physiological and psychological perception of pain. Why the patient feels the unpleasant sensation is of practical clinical significance. Dental therapy, although it may not reduce the fear of pain, should nevertheless be directed toward alleviating it by suppressing or eliminating its source. Inadequate protection and treatment of prepared abutment teeth may cause unnecessary pain. In dental therapy it is the minutiae that count! It has been said in jest that a faulty margin may lead to death. The progression begins with a tiny flaw in the margin that allows recurrent decay; this progresses to an abscess followed by infected heart tissue and possible death. This sequence and other more likely ones may just be the result of carelessness. Much of truth is said in jest. The dentist should be concerned with all of the small details that prevent or diminish pain.

Prepared abutment teeth have been stripped of the natural covering that nature supplied to protect them from pain. Chemical, thermal, and physical irritation may elicit pain from the denuded tooth structure. The "bandage" of protective covering is medicated with zinc oxide and eugenol temporary cement. Acrylic resin temporary crowns cemented with an anodyne temporary cement play a major role in controlling discomfort and pain in abutment teeth. However, other factors may also influence the presence or absence of pain.

Pain may be caused by *leakage of protective coverage.* If temporary crowns or bridges loosen prematurely, the patient will present very sensitive and painful abutment preparations. Conversely, if the temporary restorations are difficult to remove, and have been effective in preventing leakage, prepared teeth will be comfortable.

Regardless of the efficacy of protective coverage, and the use of an anodyne cement, prepared teeth may become painful from the hydraulic pressures engendered in the process of cementa-

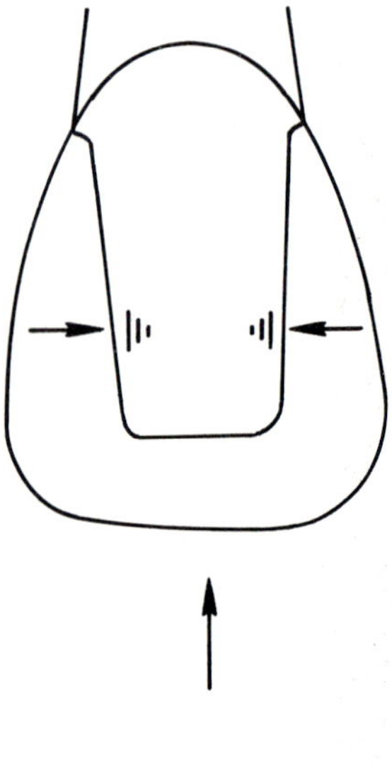

Figure 2–21 A schematic illustration of the hydraulic pressure engendered against the walls of the prepared abutment tooth in the process of cementation.

tion. The fluid cement is confined between the internal walls of the casting and the related tooth structure. Pressure is transmitted against the thin remaining walls of the prepared tooth (Fig. 2–21). Some overly prepared abutment teeth may have only paper-thin dentin remaining between the pulp and the outside world. These thin walls are pressed or dented slightly toward the pulp chamber by the pressure exerted by the cement. When the temporary cement hardens, the constrictions are perpetuated. Pain may ensue and remain until the pulp accommodates the annoyance, and perhaps thereafter. A thin mix of temporary cement will minimize hydraulic pressure. A zinc oxide and eugenol cement modified by paraben will provide a temporary luting agent of low viscosity and surface tension that will not inaugurate hydrodynamic phenomena.

High occlusion may predispose an abutment preparation to sensitivity. A premature contact with an opposing cusp may cause pain or perhaps loosen the temporary restoration and compound the injury. The occlusal relationships of temporary fixed restorations should be adjusted with meticulous care and maintained by precise cementation with a thin, slow-setting zinc oxide and eugenol cement.

The elimination of pain is of vital importance to successful crown and bridge therapy. The patient suffers a parade of insults that may bring pain and discomfort. First, because the grinding for preparation causes friction pain, this should be accomplished slowly and with warm water. Second, hot or irritating impression materials may contribute to pain. If a crown or bridge falls off during the waiting period between appointments required for laboratory procedures, pain is almost certain. In fact, just a small amount of loosening will allow leakage that causes pain.

Suggestions to Eliminate Pain

1. Properly constructed, well-fitting temporary acrylic resin restorations.

2. Cementation with a thin mix of an anodyne cement (zinc oxide and eugenol).

3. A small percentage of paraben added to the cement mix will lower the surface tension and film thickness, and increase the flow, setting time and antibacterial activity.[39, 42]

4. To prevent premature loosening with short tapered or retentively poor preparations, use a much stronger zinc oxide and eugenol cement such as Fynal Cement or Opotow Alumina EBA Cement. In a challenging situation, even an intermediate filling material may be utilized for positive retention. The acrylic resin crowns may be removed, nevertheless, despite the stronger cements, since the resin is easily deformed by the pressure of a removal instrument, and since the preparations are not too retentive.

5. Dry abutment teeth gently with cotton before cementation.

6. As soon as the cement is placed into the temporary resin restoration (haste is essential) seat the restoration on the abutment teeth without delay. There is no need to completely fill a resin crown with temporary cement. Temporary crowns are usually well-fitting, and not shimmed to make room for cement as the final crowns are. A small amount of temporary cement applied to the internal walls should suffice. Excess cement should be removed as soon as possible and as completely as possible.

7. Don't use non-eugenol temporary cements. They are analogous to rubble between the prepared abutment teeth and the temporary restoration. They do not provide a sedative effect on pulpal pain, stimulate the formation of reparative dentin, or provide antibacterial activity.

Temporary protective coverage may be effectively accomplished through the utilization of acrylic resin crowns and bridges fabricated by any one of a number of direct and indirect methods. Temporary restorations contribute largely to the success of the final fixed reparative therapy, and to the comfort and satisfaction of the patient. Esthetic, well-fitting and retentive temporary coverage that does not loosen between the various procedures leading to completion of the final restoration is an essential requirement for effective crown and bridge therapy. Also, good temporary coverage that does not loosen during construction phases contributes greatly to the control of pain.

Loosening aborts therapy.

Complete loosening or partial marginal leakage will usually cause pain, discomfort, and an unpleasant odor. Temporary coverage that maintains a good marginal seal, also provides for a comfortable, non-sensitive abutment when impressions and occlusal relationships are made.

In a nutshell, if temporary coverage is successful, a painless, comfortable and healthy abutment tooth is evident. If temporary coverage is inadequate and fails, an overly sensitive abutment tooth must be dealt with, and the possibility of irreversible pulp damage exists. Therefore, the dentist should keep in mind that well-fitting temporary restorations, cemented efficiently to retentive-shaped preparations, provide biologic and preventive benefits.

SUMMARY

Abutment teeth are the pillars that support the fixed therapeutic device. Most of them have been ground down, disked, sprayed, and subjected to thermal change, pressure, and chemical irritation. Every effort should be made to preserve the health and vitality of abutment teeth if they are to successfully withstand the bondage they will incur while carrying substitute teeth in a "piggy-back fashion."

For preventive restorative dentistry, and for successful crown and bridge therapy, the prepared abutment tooth deserves the following biologic and preventive considerations prior to final cementation.

1. Protection and insulation from saliva, irritating fluids and thermal and galvanic change
2. Effective marginal seal and sedation
3. Repair of contour with composites and polycarboxylates
4. Adequate pain control
5. Protection from irritating medicaments and drugs
6. Protection from overdrying
7. Temporary cementation with a powder and liquid type of zinc oxide and eugenol cement

REFERENCES

1. Englander, H. R., James, V. E., and Massler, M., Histologic effects of silver nitrate on human dentin and pulp. J.A.D.A., *57*:621, 1958.
2. Massler, M., Sterilization of dentin. J. Tennessee State D.A., *35*:375, 1955.
3. Zander, H. A., and Smith, H. W., Penetration of silver nitrate into dentin. J. Dent. Res., *24*:121, 1945.
4. Seltzer, S., and Bender, I. B., The Dental Pulp. Philadelphia, J. B. Lippincott Co., 1965, p. 145.
5. Seltzer, S., and Bender, I. B., The Dental Pulp. Philadelphia, J. B. Lippincott Co., 1965, p. 148.
6. Langeland, K., Response of the adult tooth to injury. *In* Finn, S. B. (ed.): *Biology of the Dental Pulp Organ: a Symposium,* Birmingham: University of Alabama Press, 1968, pp. 169–187.
7. Brännström, M., and Nyborg, H.: Cavity treatment with a microbicidal fluoride solution: Growth of bacteria and effect on the pulp. J. Prosthet. Dent. *30*:303, 1973.
8. Brännström, M., and Nyborg, H.: The presence of bacteria in cavities filled with silicate cement and composite resin materials. Swed. Dent. J. *64*:149, 1971.
9. Brännström, M., and Nyborg, H.: Pulpal reaction to composite resin restorations. J. Prosthet. Dent. *27*:181, 1972.
10. Vojinovic, O., Nyborg, H., and Brännström, M.: Acid treatment of cavities under resin fillings: Bacterial growth in dentinal tubules and pulpal reactions. J. Dent. Res. *52*:1189, 1973.
11. Brännström, M., and Nyborg, H.: Bacterial growth and pulpal changes under inlays cemented with zinc phosphate cement and Epoxylite CBA 9080. J. Prosthet. Dent. *31*:556, 1974.
12. Brännström, M., and Johnson, G.: Effects of various conditioners and cleaning agents on prepared dentin surfaces: A scanning electron microscopic investigation. J. Prosthet. Dent. *31*:422, 1974.
13. Brännström, M.: A new approach to insulation. Dent. Pract., *19*:417, 1969.
14. Johnson, G., and Brännström, M.: Dehydration of dentin by some restorative materials. J. Prosthet. Dent. *26*:307, 1971.
15. Brännström, M., and Nyborg, H.: Pulpal protection by a cavity liner applied as a thin film beneath deep silicate restorations. J. Dent. Res. *50*:90–95, 1971.
16. Brännström, M., and Nyborg, H.: The protective effect of a liner applied as a thin film beneath deep composite fillings. Odontol. Revy *24*:235–242, 1973.

17. Eriksen, H. M.: Pulpal responses to "composite" dental materials lined with Tubulitec or Dropsin. Scand. J. Dent. Res. *81*:285–291, 1973.
18. Miller, C. J.: Inlays, Crowns and Bridges. Philadelphia, W. B. Saunders Co., 1962, p. 250.
19. Kornfeld, M.: Mouth Rehabilitation. St. Louis, The C. V. Mosby Company, 1967, p. 320.
20. Klotz, M. D., Gerstein, H., and Bahn, A. N.: Bacteremia after topical use of prednisolone in infected pulps. J.A.D.A. *71*:871, 1965.
21. Langeland, K.: Biologic considerations in operative dentistry. Dent. Clin. North Am., March, 1967, p. 140.
22. Sinkford, J. C., and Harris, S. C.: The case against topical use of adrenocorticosteroids in dentistry. J.A.D.A. *68*:765, 1964.
23. Fox, J., and Moodnik, R. M.: Systemic reaction to polyantibiotic root canal dressing. N.Y. State Dent. J. *30*:282, 1964.
24. Barnes, G., and Langeland, K.: Antibody formation in primates following introduction of antigens into the root canal. J. Dent. Res. *45*:1111, 1966.
25. Kern, R. A.: Anaphylactic drug reactions. J.A.M.A., *179*:19, January 6, 1962.
26. American Dental Association: Accepted Dental Therapeutics. Ed. 35, 1973/74, p. 208.
27. Compton, D. E., and Mitchell, D. F.: Pharmacologic treatment of painful pulpitis: A five-year report. J. Dent. Res. *49*:183, 1970.
28. Langeland, K.: Prevention of pulp damage. Dent. Clin. North Am. October, 1972, p. 709.
29. Harris, S. C.: The use of adrenol steroids in dental practice. Dent. Clin. North Am. October, 1970. p. 845.
30. El-Kafrawy, A. H., et al.: Pulp reaction to polycarboxylate cements in monkeys. J. Dent. Res. *53*:15, 1974.
31. Bhaskar, S. N., et al.: Pulp capping with isobutyl cyanoacrylate. J.A.D.A. *79*:640, 1969.
32. American Dental Association: Accepted Dental Therapeutics. Ed. 35, 1973–74, p. 309–310.
33. Steele, G. D.: Reinforced composite resin foundations for endodontically treated teeth. J. Prosthet. Dent. *30*:816, 1973.
34. Stahl, G. J., and O'Neal, R. B.: The composite resin dowel and core. J. Prosthet. Dent. *33*:642, 1975.
35. Stanley, H. R.: Pulpal response to dental techniques and materials. Dent. Clin. North Am., January, 1971, p. 115.
36. Weinberg, L. A.: Atlas of Crown and Bridge Prosthodontics. St. Louis, The C. V. Mosby Co., 1965, p. 26.
37. Fiasconaro, J. E., and Sherman, H.: Vacuum-formed prostheses. A temporary fixed bridge or splint. J.A.D.A. *76*:74, 1968.
38. Braden, M., Causton, B., and Clarke, R. L.: An ethylene imine derivative as a temporary crown and bridge material. J. Dent. Res. *50*:536, May-June, 1971.
39. Horn, H. R.: Improved cementation. J.A.D.A. *63*:813, 1961.
40. American Dental Association: Accepted Dental Therapeutics. Ed. 35, 1973/74, p. 274.
41. American Dental Association: Council announces classification of additional products. J.A.D.A. *72*:1495, 1966.
42. Horn, H. R.: The cementation of crowns and fixed partial dentures. Dent. Clin. North Am. March 1965, p. 78.
43. Brännström, M., and Nyborg, H.: Pulp reaction to a temporary zinc oxide/eugenol cement. J. Prosthet. Dent. *35*:185, 1976.

three
Impression Making

In all things, success depends on previous preparation and without such preparation there is sure to be failure.

Confucius

BIOLOGIC CONSIDERATIONS IN MAKING IMPRESSIONS

In the course of crown and bridge therapy, fixed restorations are fabricated in the dental laboratory to fit accurate reproductions of the hard and soft tissues. The reproductions are obtained from impressions made after all necessary abutment preparations are accomplished. Impression making is a highly technical endeavor with almost total concern for accuracy and, unfortunately, not enough concern for biologic considerations. In making impressions, heat, pressure, and chemical agents may be applied to the intimate insides of tooth structure, in many instances, with little awareness of the potential for pulp damage. An abutment tooth after preparation is a most vulnerable target. Its outside protective covering has been stripped off. It presents walls of cut dentinal tubules that may be sensitive to thermal change, pressure, drying, bacteria, or chemical agents. To aid in the preservation of pulpal health the dentist should minimize any annoyance to prepared tooth structure during impression making and balance any necessary physical, thermal, or chemical trauma against biologic considerations.

Impression techniques should be recognized as biologic as well as mechanical procedures. It would be biologically beneficial if impressions of prepared abutment teeth could be made without heat, pressure, or chemical irritation, and with a material that would soothe and sedate tooth structure. The only available material that could meet these requirements would be an appropriate formulation of zinc oxide and eugenol. After all, impression pastes of zinc oxide and eugenol have proved to be reliable and accurate in the fabrication of complete dentures. They are also used as temporary liners or stabilizers in dentures and occlusion rims, for recording jaw relationships, and for cementing gnathological clutches.[1] Utilized in a copper band, zinc oxide and eugenol would not only fulfill the aforementioned biologic criteria but may also be readily copper-plated. Also, because of its dimensional stability, impressions need not be electroplated and poured immediately.

However, regardless of potentials for therapy, it is important to focus down on the untoward effects of impression procedures. Impression making itself may be harmful to dental health in the following ways:

Heat

It has been shown that heat applied to dentin has a harmful effect on the human pulp, and recovery may not be complete.[2] Impression compound or hydrocolloid that is too hot may cause thermal shock to the pulp of a prepared tooth. Obviously, repeated attempts to make an acceptable impression with either of these hot materials will contribute to additional sensitivity. Hot stick compound is apt to cause a pulpal reaction because it tends to adhere to the dentin. An impression material that does not adhere to the dentin transfers less heat to the tooth surface. The heat from a hydrocolloid impression material is not as damaging as that of impression compound. Impression compound *should not go from the Bunsen flame directly to the tooth* without tempering in water of about 130° F. After seating a copper band filled with heated impression compound, *it should be chilled as soon as possible;*[3] otherwise, the pulp chamber remains at a high temperature for more than three minutes if the impression is allowed to cool on its own.[3] Several copper bands should not be seated in sequence without chilling. When three or four copper-band impressions of nonadjacent abutment teeth are being made with hot impression compound, it is best to chill each one as soon as it is seated; otherwise, if the cooling is delayed until all the bands are seated, the teeth are exposed to injury from heat for a longer time than necessary. It should be remembered that during chilling, the impression material and the facing tooth structure cool off first; last to cool is the pulp chamber, which is at a greater distance from the water coolant.

Pressure

Pressure on the preparation during impression making may force bacteria through tubules into the pulp. If the pulp is already chronically inflamed, the microorganisms forced into it through the dentin may cause an infection of the pulp. Pressure may also squeeze thin, remaining dentinal walls inward and thereby contribute to pulpal damage. Hydrodynamics is involved in many instances as fluid impression material is progressively entrapped against the walls of the tooth by the confines of its carrier. Seltzer and Bender[4] investigated the effects of pressure on the dental pulp in the making of a copper-band impression of a full crown preparation. Their examination of histologic sections revealed that pressure alone caused edema, hemorrhage, and displacement of odontoblastic nuclei. But pressure and heat in combination caused an even greater inflammatory reaction in the pulp.

Dryness

Drying prepared tooth structure prior to impression making may be harmful if overdone. Air blasting of dentin with compressed air or an air syringe may dehydrate the tooth structure and cause injury to the odontoblasts.[5] Langeland has shown that even 10 seconds of air blasting is enough to produce odontoblastic displacement.[5] Obviously, for pulpal health, air drying should be minimized. Where drying is required, cotton rolls and pellets should be applied to the tooth structure. However, air may be used as sparingly as possible to dry the gingival crevice. The use of desiccating drugs such as alcohol and chloroform is contraindicated.

Other Harm

Impression-making procedures may also have the potential for chemical irritation, soft tissue trauma and abrasion, and the fracture of tooth structure.

Preventive restorative dentistry is dependent on the accuracy of impressions that are used for fabrication of well-fitting prostheses. Well-fitting crowns and bridges made from accurate imprints of teeth and soft tissues will contribute to the prevention of caries, premature loosening, and periodontal problems.

Copper band impressions are not always perfect. Regardless of the impression material of choice, modeling compound, polysulfide rubber, silicone elastomer, or even zinc oxide and eugenol, sometimes it is necessary to repeat the impression procedure because of some shortcoming in the end-result. These efforts should be kept to a minimum. Repeated impression making should be avoided! Keep in mind that it may cause thermal shock to the tooth, or it may traumatize the soft tissue and cut the periodontal membrane attachment.

Gingival recession may also result from the injury caused by the impression technique. The extent of this recession depends on the following:

1. Care and protection of teeth and gingiva during subsequent procedures (protective temporary coverage)
2. Occlusion
3. Fit and contour of restorations
4. Home care

COPING WITH COPINGS

A great deal of the accuracy of crown and bridge therapy depends on the little details related to the effective utilization of transfer copings. Transfer copings are crowns of special design made to fit the dies obtained from the impression procedure. They are used in certain master impression procedures (plaster of Paris, silicone putty, or combinations of the two) to obtain accurate positioning and alignment of dies to each other and to remaining teeth and edentulous areas. Although low-fusing metal transfer copings and acrylic resin copings may be used, it is generally accepted that well-cast metal transfer copings provide more accurate seating of the dies. The transfer castings can be made of gold, silver, or a technique metal. Some dentists use transfer copings to establish a desirable occlusal relationship. This is accomplished by extending the copings occlusally and incisally to make contact with opposing teeth, thereby maintaining the required vertical dimension of occlusion.

Despite the fact that transfer copings provide a valuable and critical linkage to the accuracy of crown and bridge therapy, there has been little or no attempt to focus on the significant details involved in their utilization. Transfer copings are recognized as simply a means of positioning dies in a master impression. However, there are other benefits to be derived from transfer copings. These, and considerations for more effective use, are as follows:

1. Transfer copings supply the first proof of the chain of accuracy linking the abutment impression, the die fabrication, and the cast coping. If the transfer coping does not fit the prepared abutment in the mouth, a new impression must be made.

2. Transfer copings are useful in determining the extent of over- or underextension of the crown margins. The transfer coping may act as a blueprint or pattern for the subsequent crown. The margins of a coping may be shortened if overextended. Since short margins cannot be lengthened, a notation is made to accomplish this in the final cast crown.

3. Transfer copings may be bonded together with a self-curing acrylic resin, DuraLay,* prior to the master impression for security of alignment. The self-curing acrylic resin (Fig. 3–1) utilized may also

*Reliance Dental Manufacturing Company, Chicago, IL 60643.

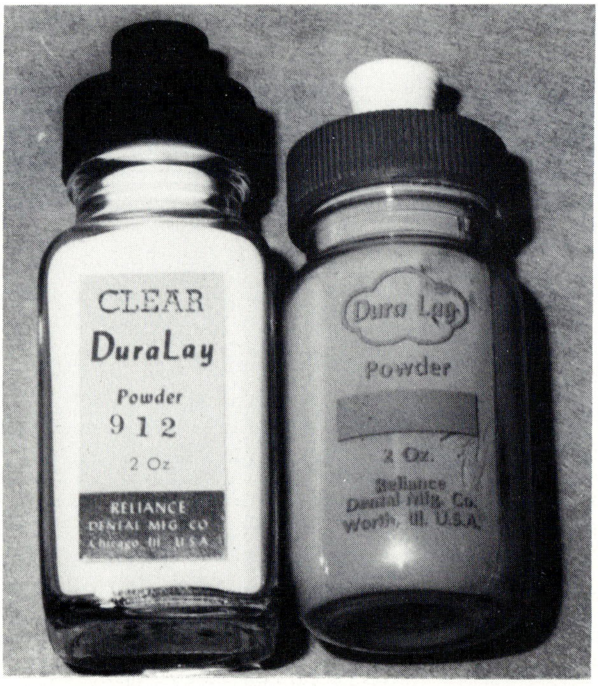

Figure 3–1 This non-tooth-colored self-curing resin has improved dimensional stability and may be used to bond transfer copings or castings together into an accurate and stable relationship.

be indented occlusally or incisally by the teeth of the opposing arch to establish a positional occlusal relationship. The DuraLay powder and liquid is applied with a brush-on technique between and around the transfer copings. Then a mix of the resin, which has polymerized to a point at which it may be picked up as dough, is pressed along the mesial-distal extent of the copings and edentulous areas and is bonded to the resin between and around the transfer copings. On closure, the opposing teeth indent this mass of resin to register an occlusal relationship. If the opposing teeth contain any acrylic resin fillings or facings, a thin film of silicone grease should be applied to them before closure to prevent adherence to the DuraLay. Just prior to the final hardening of the resin the patient should be instructed to open about a half inch and close immediately to insure that the jaws are not bonded together because of contact with opposing resins or invasion of undercuts.

Characteristics of an Effective Transfer Coping

1. The coping should have a non-binding positive fit to both the die and the abutment tooth.

2. Precise coverage and contact of margins are prime requirements.

3. A planned opening (hole) is helpful to visually assess the extent of seating. A transfer coping that fits well with proper gingival margin contact and coverage, and with visual determination (through opening) of complete seating, provides good proof of impression-making accuracy. The planned opening should not be placed too close to a removal extension, for it would then limit the enlarging of the opening if needed. The opening should be placed on the labial surface of anteriors near the incisal edge, and on the mesial-buccal aspect of posteriors near the occlusal surface (Fig. 3–2).

4. Buccal (or labial) and lingual removal extensions should be designed to facilitate removal of the transfer coping within the final master impression material. Unfortunately, too many so-called "removal buttons" are half-round, rounded, irregular in shape, or too small and do not suit the purpose. They are not designed to facilitate removal. To be useful for this purpose they should extend horizontally 1 to 1½ mm from both the buccal and lingual surfaces and have *a flattened surface facing the gingival tissues* (Fig. 3–3). The flattened surface is a positive bearing area for contact with the impression material. This will aid in its removal and in maintenance of an accurate position. The extensions should also be 1 to 1½ mm wide. If the transfer coping is not removed from the mouth with the overall impression, the properly designed extension with the flattened underside provides the means for precise repositioning in the master impression. The extension that is too small and rounded cannot be relied upon to insure proper removal and positioning. Removal extensions may be smaller and less exacting when copings are bound together and related to each other with self-curing acrylic resin. However, this technique, although acceptable, depends upon the ac-

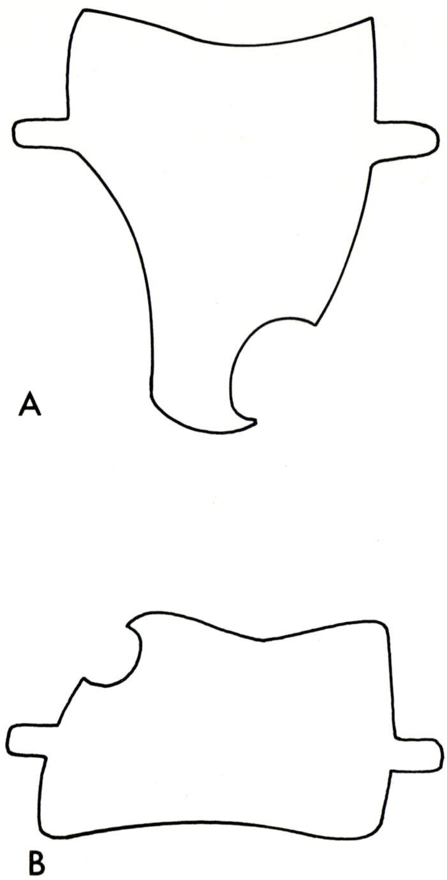

Figure 3–2 The correct outline form of anterior *(A)* and posterior *(B)* transfer copings showing the location of the planned opening. The opening should be large enough for adequate visual assessment of complete seating.

curacy of the acrylic resin for splinting, and occasionally for reproduction of the pontic area. It should be noted that plaster of Paris will flow better and is more accurate and kinder to the tissues of a pontic area than self-curing acrylic resin. This is indeed a biologic consideration.

The removal extensions should not be positioned on the coping too close to the gingival margin. This would limit the bulk of impression material under the flattened surface and lessen the chances for successful removal within the master impression. Of course, placement too close to the occlusal aspect may interfere with occlusal relationships. Transfer copings for short posterior teeth should have removal extensions that are larger (broader and longer), since there is less body of the transfer coping to be enclosed and gripped by the master impression material. For the same reason, but conversely, a long abutment coping may have smaller removal extensions.

5. The external contour of the transfer coping should have an asymmetric shape to resist rotation. One or more proximal surfaces should be flattened to enhance the accuracy of reseating in the master impression if this should be necessary.

6. Transfer copings should be seated on the abutment teeth with mallet force.[6] No matter how well a hand placed coping seems to fit

an abutment tooth, a few light taps with a mallet and a small wooden bite stick* will refine the accuracy of seating. However, biting pressure to seat cast copings should be avoided.

7. Transfer copings may be used to indicate the extent of the subgingival placement of the labiogingival margins of anterior crowns. With the transfer coping seated on the preparation in the mouth, a line is scratched on the coping with a sharp instrument to show the extent of subgingival coverage on the labial surface. This cervical line is a guide to the amount of gingival collar that may be used in the design of the boxing for an acrylic resin veneer. It allows control of the amount of metal that will be displayed in the area critical to esthetics.

8. Transfer copings should not be discarded after the working cast has been constructed. It may be necessary to compare their fit and coverage with those of the final crowns, or perhaps to reuse them if necessary.

9. The final impression should be examined closely. If plaster of Paris or silicone putty impression material has flowed inside the transfer coping through the planned opening it indicates that the coping has moved out of position during placement of the impression tray and a new final impression should be made.

---

*Aidaco Bite Sticks, Interstate Dental Company, Incorporated, New Hyde Park, NY 11040.

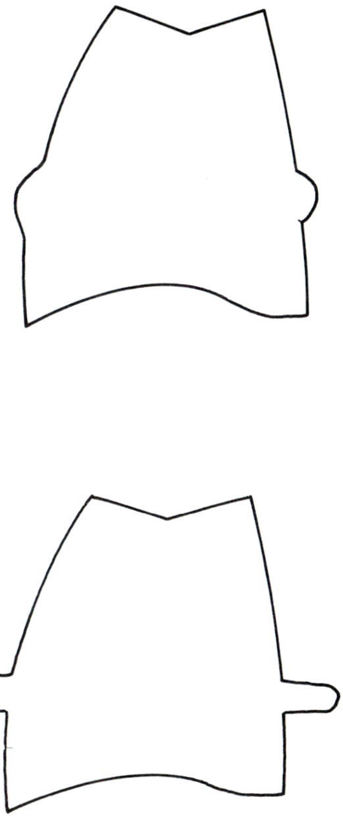

A

B

Figure 3–3 *A,* The rounded, so-called "removal buttons" usually seen on transfer copings are not shaped to facilitate removal in the master impression. *B,* The flattened extensions promote removal and accurate positioning.

SUMMARY

Transfer copings are useful to appraise the fit and the extent of coverage of proposed castings. They may also indicate the extent of occlusal clearance required for porcelain coverage. The copings establish and secure the relative position of the abutment teeth, and may be utilized to register occlusal relationships. However, it is important that they be designed with the necessary details for effective utilization.

The Story of Silicone Dental Materials

One of the world's first silicone products was developed during World War II. It had the consistency of petroleum jelly and was used to coat spark plugs and other electrical junctions in aircraft as a means of preventing electrical fires. Shortly thereafter it was determined that by control of structure and chemical behavior, fluids and rubber-like materials with unusual combinations of physical properties could be obtained.

The basic ingredient of silicone is the element silicon. It is derived from common quartz and sand. Only oxygen is more abundant on earth than silicon. Converting sand to silicone is a complex process requiring the tailoring of atoms; however, the end product can be almost as liquid as water or as solid as rubber. Thus there are *silicone fluids* of various viscosities, *silicone grease,* and finally *silicone rubber.*

Restorative dentistry, taking advantage of this advance in chemical research, has found practical uses for silicone grease and silicone rubber. Silicone fluids are also used in dentistry, for the disinfection of dental instruments by heat.

SILICONE GREASE

Silicone grease is made by thickening a silicone fluid with an inert silica filler. It has excellent insulating properties, water repellency, and oxidation resistance. It is an inert, nontoxic, and highly stable material. Silicone grease is noncorrosive to metals and is inert to most plastics. It is an excellent lubricant. The high water repellency of silicone grease makes it especially valuable as a sealing agent. Also, it is insoluble in mouth fluids or monomer, is not affected by heat, and is tasteless and odorless. With properties like these, it is easy to understand why silicone grease has been found so useful as an adjunctive material in dentistry.

Dental applications and advantages are as follows:

1. Applied to acrylic resin it protects against excess zinc oxide and eugenol cement during trial or final cementation.[7]
2. It protects resin fillings or facings in the mouth during the subsequent application of self-curing resin to adjacent areas.

3. It protects silicate fillings after insertion.
4. Combined with a zinc oxide and eugenol mixture it makes a non-setting trial cement for fixed bridges.
5. Applied to external surfaces of crowns and bridges prior to final cementation it facilitates the removal of excess cement.
6. It protects dentin during polymerization of self-curing acrylic resin protective crowns.
7. Applied to occlusal surfaces of opposing teeth, it prevents sticking after closure to obtain an occlusal registration with a self-curing resin material.

Examples of dental silicone grease are Opotow Dental Silicone (Teledyne Dental Products), R. M. Silicone Grease (Rocky Mountain Products), and Masque (H. J. Bosworth Co.).

SILICONE RUBBER

These silicone products are room-temperature vulcanizing rubber compounds of liquid and paste-like consistency specifically designed for use in formulating dental impression materials. When a curing catalyst is added they will vulcanize to form firm, flexible silicone rubber with precise reproduction of surface details.

In uncured form, current silicone compounds exhibit shelf stability greatly exceeding that of previous silicone materials. Shelf life may be increased even further by use of refrigerated storage.

Examples of dental silicone rubber impression material are Jelcone (L. D. Caulk), Xantopren (Unitek Corp.), and Stalite Silicone (Stalite, Inc.).

A New Era of Silicone Imprinting

Rubber impression materials, also termed elastomer polymers, have been popular in restorative dentistry because they have better dimensional stability and greater strength than hydrocolloids. Polysulfides set slowly, smell bad, and are messy to handle; on the other hand, silicones are less messy to handle, have no undesirable odor, and are cleaner to work with. The early silicones showed less dimensional stability than polysulfides, were distorted by electroplating, and had a catalyst system with limited stability. Indeed, the first silicone impression materials used in dentistry had a variety of problems, not the least of which was poor shelf life. Despite the neat, clean characteristics of these materials, they seemed destined to be forsaken for polysulfide rubber materials. However, improvements in shelf life and the advent of the putty-like, thick-bodied silicone material, often referred to as "silicone putty," has caused new interest in silicone impression material. At first, the catalysts for some of these new products were faulty and exhibited erratic behavior. Impressions did not set completely unless the catalyst was fresh. Manufacturers ultimately learned how to stabilize the catalyst, and today silicone putty impression material is dependable and has a number of uses in restorative dentistry.

SILICONE PUTTY

Silicone putty may be used instead of plaster of Paris for a master impression of a full arch involving transfer copings. Plaster of Paris is the conventional material used for making impressions into which dies may be accurately positioned for the construction of crowns and bridges. Plaster is messy and difficult to use, and may be unpleasant for patients because of the heat generated by the setting reaction. Although undercuts around adjacent teeth may be blocked out with materials such as Cavit* or Kwikseal,** it is usually necessary to fracture a plaster impression to remove it from the mouth, leaving the dentist with a jigsaw puzzle to contend with. Also, during removal efforts the potential for the fracture of a fragile abutment tooth must be recognized. Therefore, although plaster may be an effective impression material in some situations, its use is now minimized by the substitution of silicone putty. This material, which sets harder than the regular silicone impression material, is strong enough to remove transfer copings in the master impression and to allow firm seating of dies. Silicone putty allows for a complete impression without the breakage common to plaster of Paris. It provides for more precise contact with adjacent natural teeth, and lessens the chance of fracturing a fragile abutment tooth on removal.

Silicone putty may be used in a stock tray to make a custom tray after an intraoral imprint. Relief for the final wash impression with a thinner silicone material is provided by using a spacer between the impression material and the oral structures or by cutting away some of the silicone putty tray.

Bite relationships may be obtained by using silicone putty instead of wax. Hard, quick-setting materials such as baseplate wax require greater closing forces of a shorter duration than do the softer, slow-setting silicone putty materials.[8] Also, a more accurate maxillomandibular registration is obtained with a resilient material because it is not distorted by undercuts.

Imput,† Optosil,‡ and Citricon,§ are examples of silicone putty impression material (Fig. 3–4). They have the same dough-like consistency before and immediately after mixing. Because silicone putty is lower in the usual silicone content and higher in filler content than other types of silicone, polymerization shrinkage and thermal contraction of these putty-like materials is lower.[9] The manipulation of silicone putty materials is the key to their effectiveness. If not kneaded or mixed sufficiently they will have a prolonged setting time. If they are overmanipulated, they may begin to set before placement is accomplished. The dentist may be puzzled and trapped in the middle of these time schedules. If he takes too long in preparing the material, he may lose some of the working time needed to load the tray and seat it in the mouth. As a result, the next time he may not take as

---

*Premier Dental Products Company, Philadelphia, PA 19107.
**Interstate Dental Company, New Hyde Park, NY 11040.
†Buffalo Dental Manufacturing Company, Brooklyn, NY 11207.
‡Unitek, Monrovia, CA 91016
§Kerr, Sybron Corporation, Romulus, MI 48174

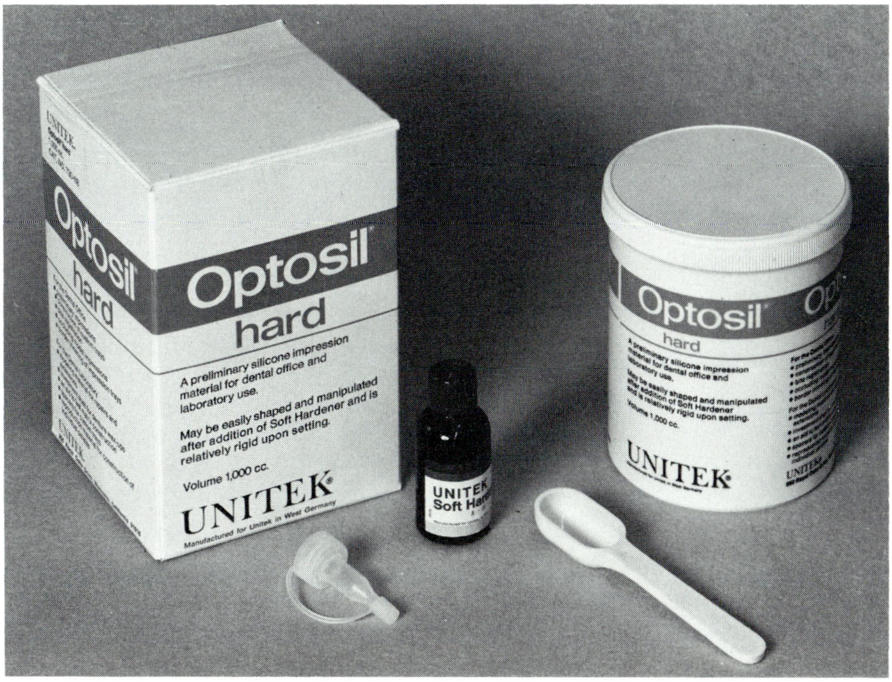

Figure 3–4 A Silicone putty impression material. Optosil is white in color, and has a moldable, non-sticky consistency.

much time to mix. To insure enough working time he may mix too briefly and ineffectively, and the impression material may set very slowly or not at all. Therefore, when mixing these materials the manufacturer's suggested manipulation time should be carefully noted and the timing should be precisely controlled by a timing device. However, when temperature and humidity fluctuate, the mixing time should be modified. For example, slightly less mixing time is necessary when the temperature and humidity are high, and slightly more when the temperature and humidity are low.

Reisbick and Matyas[10] used a specific test to determine the accuracy of the highly filled silicone impression materials. They proved to be as accurate as the other standard impression materials tested.

After using a metal spatula for the initial incorporation of the liquid accelerator into the stiff base material, the mixing of a silicone putty impression material is usually continued by hand kneading. It is recommended that the hands be moist during this mixing stage. One small but frustrating problem that has not been easy to solve is the difficulty in removing the impression material from the fingers and fingernails after the kneading. Multiple washings with soap and water are ineffective. Sometimes the odor and minute particles of the impression material persist on the dentist's hands unless a strong solvent is used. However, a new moisturizing preparation called Non-Tac* applied before kneading will prevent the silicone putty impression material from adhering to the fingers. It forms a light film that

*Accurate Set Incorporated, Paterson, NJ 07501.

acts as a protective "glove" on the hand, and has no adverse effect on materials or tissues. It is tasteless, colorless, and mildly scented, and may be rinsed away with water.

The New Polyether Impression Materials

Polyether impression materials are the newest types of elastomers used in dentistry. They have a pleasant taste and odor and are easy to mix and clean up. They set fast, have unexcelled accuracy[11, 12] and dimensional stability, and may be used with either stock or custom trays. Regardless of other properties, appearance, smell, and taste are important factors to be considered in selecting an impression material for use in the human mouth. Polyether impression materials are supplied in two collapsible tubes. One tube contains the base, which is a low molecular weight polyether containing ethylene imine terminal groups. The other tube contains the accelerator (aromatic sulfonic acid ester). Equal lengths are mixed on a paper pad in the same manner as are the other rubber impression materials.

Examples of a polyether impression material are Impregum* (Fig. 3–5) and Polyjel.** These impression materials are especially recommended for crown and bridge impressions. Both stock trays and custom trays are suggested for use with these materials. One polyether material, Ramitec* is supplied specifically as a bite registration material.

In a comparison[13] of elastic impression materials the polyether material compared favorably with the others in mixing time, working

---

*Espe, Seefeld, Oberbayern, Ger. Premier Dental Products.
**L. D. Caulk Company, Milford, DE 19963.

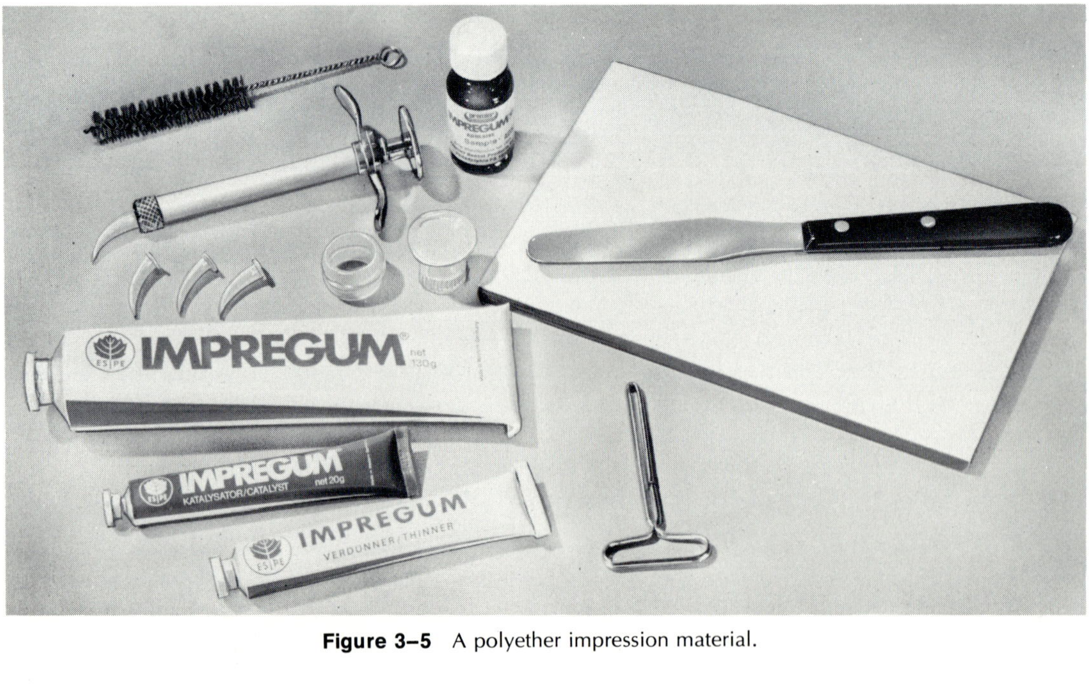

Figure 3–5 A polyether impression material.

time, and consistency, and was the most stable of all the materials. The working time of the polyether materials, however, is less than that of polysulfide or silicone rubber.

Since the polyether impression materials have a high affinity for water, it is necessary to avoid prolonged contact with water. Impressions should be dried soon after they are made to avoid dimensional change.

Physical contact with the accelerator should be avoided during mixing, for the aromatic sulfonic acid ester may cause a skin irritation.[14] Also, to avoid any possible irritation to the mouth tissues, the two components should be very thoroughly mixed.

Some manufacturers advertise that their impression material will "make perfect impressions every time." It should be remembered that it is not the impression material that makes the impression, it is the dentist. In fact, using an impression material with the most perfect physical properties and handling characteristics, a dentist with careless procedure may make an unsatisfactory impression. A good impression results from good handling of a good material. The "perfect impression" can only be approached by a knowledgeable and competent operator, using an impression material that meets the required ADA specification, with skill and concern for the biologic and preventive considerations.

Biologic and Psychologic Considerations

Recognition of the biologic considerations involved in making impressions should guide the dentist in his attempts to obtain an accurate duplication of the oral structures. During the impression procedures the operator should be cognizant of the injury that drying, heat, and pressure may inflict on the prepared teeth. He should also be concerned with avoiding fracture of a prepared abutment tooth when a hardened impression material is being removed from the mouth. Also, every effort should be made to avoid injury to the gingival tissues with the edges of a copper band. Periodontal attachments should not be cut.

Impression techniques should be refined and carefully accomplished in recognition of the importance of obtaining a good impression at the first attempt. Repeated impression making compounds the biologic harm to the hard and soft structures of the mouth. At the same time, it should be emphasized that impressions should be remade without hesitation if they are faulty. Herein lies an important psychological complexity. Some dentists, young dentists especially, feel that it is a measure of their competency to be able to obtain a perfect impression on the first attempt. They fear that perhaps the patient will think less of their ability if the impression has to be repeated. This fear, based on their psychological conditioning of what constitutes a "good dentist," may cause them to accept a less than adequate impression. Any rationalization and attempt to "make do" with a less than adequate impression at this time will be reflected in additional problems of adjustment, in patient discomfort, and in the probability of a need to remake the prosthesis at the time of installation. Instead, the dentist should be eager to repeat the making of an impression. He should inform the patient that it is necessary to repeat and improve the impression to a certain level of acceptability, no matter how many times it takes. This is the art and science of dentistry—not pushbutton mechanics. The dentist's integrity is not measured by the failure of an impression procedure but by his willingness to subjugate his own psychologic make-up and professional image to the ultimate goal of an accurate impression.

The selection of impression materials should be influenced by biologic considerations. For example, some impression materials do not require heat or the drying of prepared teeth. Some impression materials transmit less pressure than others. Allergenic responses to an impression material should also be considered, especially when using polyether impression materials.

"Second-Hand" Restorations

A complete lack of accuracy and poor fit may be accommodated and tolerated in the human mouth. Unfortunately, it may even be

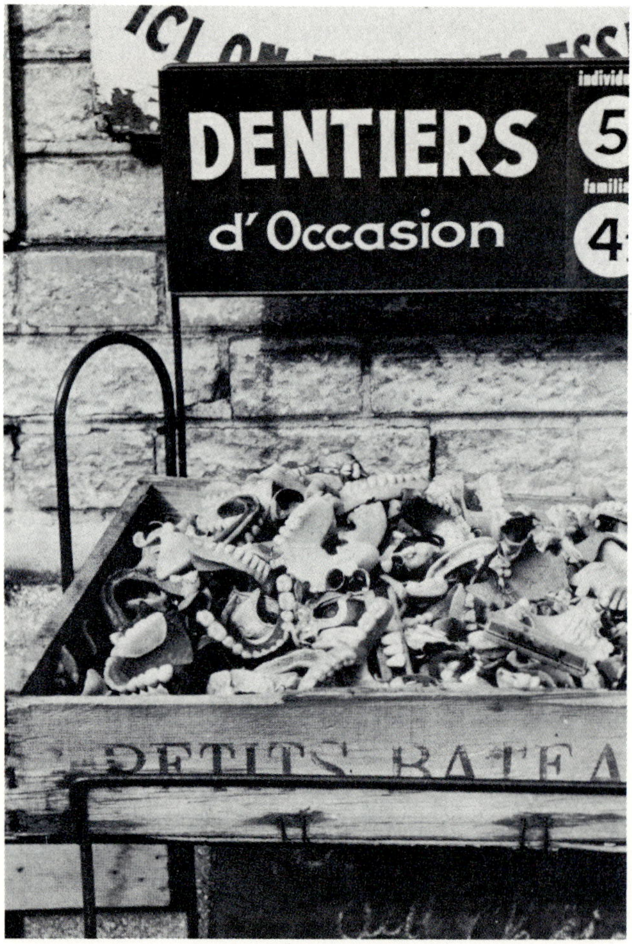

Figure 3–6 Restorations fitted "by trial and error" are in marked contrast to the meticulous techniques and the accuracy of fit required to justify crown and bridge therapy. (From Dent. Survey, October, 1970.)

searched for, welcomed, and eagerly paid for by those who, owing to economic factors, have no other alternative. The sale of old, "second-hand" dentures of unknown origin in the Paris Fleamarket is a dramatic example of the human ability to make positive use of negative values (Fig. 3–6). However, in crown and bridge therapy, as well as in all other areas of dentistry, meticulous techniques make for the best result.

It is important for the dentist to be visually and tactually sensitive to the anatomical relationship of the margins of crowns to the gingival sulcus, and to the inaccuracies that may exist in this area. Touching and feeling with an explorer may detect steps as low as 50 microns.

"Second-hand" restorations may be a compromise to fulfill a need, but not an ideal. The accuracy of fit and the infinite concern with minute details are the qualities that provide the ideal biologic and preventive values of restorative dentistry.

REFERENCES

1. Guide to Dental Materials and Devices. 6th ed, Chicago, American Dental Association, 1972–73, p. 68.
2. Seltzer, S., and Bender, I. B.: The Dental Pulp. Philadelphia, J. B. Lippincott Company, 1965, p. 129.
3. Grajower, R., et al.: Temperature of the pulp chamber during impression taking of full crown preparations with modelling compound. J. Dent. Res. *54*:212, 1975.
4. Seltzer, S., and Bender, I. B.: The Dental Pulp. Philadelphia, J. B. Lippincott Company, 1965, p. 137.
5. Langeland, K.: Tissue Changes in the Dental Pulp. Oslo, Norway, Oslo University Press, 1957, p. 74.
6. Weinberg, L. A., Atlas of Crown and Bridge Prosthodontics. St. Louis, C. V. Mosby Co., 1965, p. 51.
7. Horn, H. R.: The cementation of crowns and fixed partial dentures. Dent. Clin. N. Amer. March, 1965, p. 79.
8. Millstein, P. L., et al.: Differential accuracy of silicone-body interocclusal records and associated weight loss due to volatiles. J. Prosthet. Dent. 33:649, June, 1975.
9. Guide to Dental Materials and Devices. 6th ed, Chicago, American Dental Association, 1972–73, p. 76.
10. Resibick, M. H., and Matyas, J.: The accuracy of highly filled elastomeric impression materials. J. Prosthet. Dent. 33:67, January, 1975.
11. Sawyer, H. F., et al.: Accuracy of casts produced from seven rubber impression materials. J.A.D.A., 87:126, 1973.
12. Sawyer, H. F., et al.: Accuracy of casts produced from the three classes of elastomer impression materials. J.A.D.A., 89:644, September, 1974.
13. Stackhouse, J. A.: A comparison of elastic impression materials. J. Prosthet. Dent. *34*:305, September, 1975.
14. Craig, R. G., O'Brien, W. J., and Powers, J. M.: Dental Materials. St. Louis, C. V. Mosby Co., 1975, p. 151.

four

Esthetics in Crown and Bridge Therapy

I keep six honest serving men
(They taught me all I knew):
Their names are What and Why and When
and How and Where and Who.

Kipling

In a glossary of accepted terms[1] in all disciplines of dentistry, esthetics is defined as the qualities involved in the appearance of a given restoration. It includes the cosmetic effect produced by a restoration that affects the desirable beauty, charm, character, and dignity of the individual.

The esthetic considerations in crown and bridge therapy are increasingly recognized and appreciated in its overall evaluation. Mechanical perfection provides more valuable therapy if it also looks good. Discomfort and expense are more readily forgotten if the end results of fixed restorative dentistry contribute to an improved appearance. The general connotation of esthetics as related to dentistry is usually associated with the restorative phase. Crowns and bridges, complete and partial dentures, and tooth-colored filling materials all contribute to an improved appearance. Where indicated, oral surgery, orthodontics, and periodontics may also be of great value to esthetic improvement.

In past years, dentistry has modified its mechanical heritage, placing an increasing emphasis on biologic comprehension. And currently the profession has become more aware of the broader psychosomatic aspects to be considered in the treatment of patients, and has thereby further modified its technological image.

In fixed prosthodontics a patient's response to dental treatment often depends on the dentist's understanding of the patient's emotional needs. Meticulous mechanical repair and replacement of teeth are not enough! The dentist must appreciate that a mouth that is merely healthy without being attractive may be unsuited to the patient's psychological needs. And psychological welfare is equally as important as physiological comfort.

An attractive smile is essential to an esthetic appearance, and may also contribute to psychological well-being. An easy and gracious smile is a beautiful thing. As a means of communication, it speaks volumes without sound. A smile is one of the most common of all non-verbal signals, and can be used to indicate a variety of meanings, depending on its type and the context in which it occurs. A smile may be a sneer, a grin, or a smirk. It may reflect a response to humor, and can be described in particular situations as being happy, cynical, sarcastic, embarrassed, or reassuring.

All smiles involve some degree of widening of the mouth, and generally expose to view the upper or lower teeth, or both. There is also a smile that shows no teeth. However, in most cases this is considered either a grimace or an attempt to hide faulty, discolored, or missing teeth. The esthetics of a smile is strongly influenced by the condition and position of the teeth. Ugly teeth undermine poise and self-confidence in some people, and may cause irreparable damage to an individual's personality. Dentists are fortunate in having the unique responsibility of repairing the teeth of faulty smiles and in doing so repairing broken egos. How valuable a service to render! It contributes not only to physical health but to mental health as well.

However, much too often restorative dentistry produces false smiles. Crowns and bridges should look like real teeth, but seldom do. In many mouths an esthetic end result is difficult to obtain; while in others anything would be an improvement, and it is relatively easy. *Many factors influence the success or failure of dental esthetics.* It is important for the dentist to recognize as many of these as possible *before treatment begins* so that *the precise limitations* of the potential results may be discussed with the patient. Otherwise, if various problematic factors arise after therapy begins, recognition and discussion at this time may be construed as excuse-making.

FACTORS THAT INFLUENCE THE SUCCESS OR FAILURE OF DENTAL ESTHETICS

1. Individual tooth size, inclination and rotation.
2. Spacing of teeth.
3. Variations in the level of the gingival line.
4. Age of the patient.
5. Material selected to disguise metal (acrylic or porcelain).
6. Relationship of anterior teeth to upper lip.
7. Vertical dimension and interarch space.
8. Occlusal relationships.
9. Loss of translucency due to posts or metal understructure.
10. Tongue thrust.
11. Deviate swallowing.
12. Tissue tone and periodontal health.
13. Length of the span of missing teeth.
14. Splinting requirements.
15. Patient's wishes, fantasies, and educational level.
16. Color monotony.

17. Color: light or dark, young or mature.
18. Bruxism and clenching.

How does the dentist meet the challenge of creating a pleasing dental appearance? Actually, the dentist has only resin, metal, and pottery with which to reproduce the handiwork of Mother Nature. These are hardly enough to compete, and great frustration lies therein. Nevertheless, esthetic end results may be obtained in many cases when the following facts are recognized.

1. The dentist who has knowledge of various forms of art, such as sculpture, painting, and design, is better equipped to duplicate nature's handiwork.
2. It behooves the dentist to study natural dentitions more analytically and, in doing so, to recognize the subtleties that create dental beauty.
3. The dentist should place more emphasis on the details of individual tooth form, and coordinate the form and arrangement of collective teeth with their relationship to the face as well as to the oral environment.
4. Architects deal in symmetry. Nature rarely creates perfect symmetry. Dentists should not try.
5. Teeth should reflect the age, sex, and physical characteristics of the patient. There is only a nebulous relationship between teeth and personality.
6. "Beauty lies in the eyes of the beholder" is a much quoted truism. Therefore, the patient should be educated to comprehend the esthetic factors that contribute to an attractive smile.

This chapter will serve to help the dentist to meet the challenge of esthetic fixed restorative dentistry. The observations and guidelines should be beneficial to dentists seeking to obtain the most plausible good looks for their patients. Esthetics in dentistry is a provocative subject that may easily be clouded by a large assortment of theories and techniques. The presentation here will be simple and direct, with prime reference to the upper anterior teeth. Understandably, lower teeth, posterior teeth, gingival tissues, and the lips all may play a part in the creating of a pleasing smile; however, the upper anterior teeth are the star performers.

Factors that Influence a Smile

What makes a smile composed of natural teeth look attractive? In general, a uniform arrangement of upper anterior teeth with a few of nature's "built-in" irregularities, harmonious color and texture, and the proper relationship of all teeth to the lips, tongue, cheeks, and ridges—all in a framework of pink, healthy gingival tissues. It is exactly these considerations that make a repaired smile composed of crowns and bridges look attractive. However, as mentioned earlier, there are many obstacles to the reproduction of nature's handiwork.

Certain factors that are challenging to cope with contribute to the natural and true-to-life appearance of the prosthodontic smile. Indeed, as far as esthetic factors are concerned, much has been written and presented to the dental profession about the following:

1. Incisal guidance
2. Orientation of the occlusal plane
3. Full shoulder preparation
4. Electrosurgery
5. Minor tooth movement
6. Periodontal conditions
7. Color
8. Illusion

However, not enough guidance has been available to the dentist about the details of individual anterior tooth position, shape, and contour. A smile is strongly influenced by the manner in which the upper anterior teeth are manipulated for crowns and bridges. The details that contribute to an esthetic smile follow.

1. Upper Central Incisors

The maxillary central incisors are the first to catch the eye. They are dominant teeth, and they compose the first two basic elements of a smile and the principal components of an esthetic composition of upper anterior teeth. Both maxillary central incisors should be of the same size and form (Fig. 4–1). They should contact in a vertical line (median line) for at least a few millimeters. A small, narrow contact point at the median line near the incisal edge detracts from esthetics. It forms an overly large and shadowy interproximal area (Fig. 4–2). The incisal edges of the central incisors should not form a continuous straight line. One central incisor may be slightly longer than the other, and one may be positioned slightly more to the labial than the other. Gingival curvatures should be on the same horizontal level. The gingival curvature of a central incisor pontic and a central incisor abutment crown should be of similar form as well as on the same level (Fig. 4–3).

2. Upper Lateral Incisors

Lateral incisors should be distinctly smaller than centrals. They should be narrower and slightly shorter. The left and right upper lat-

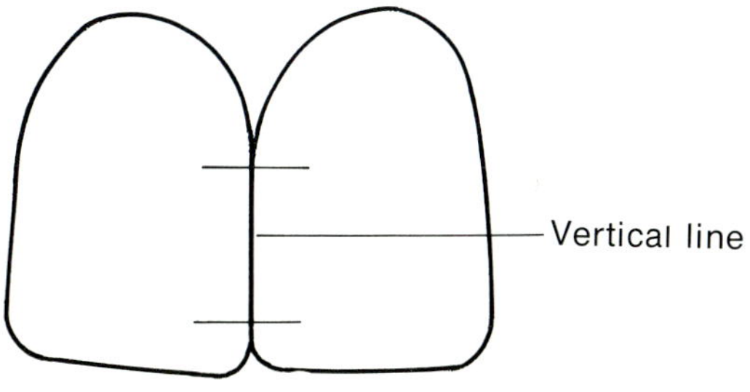

Figure 4–1 Upper central incisors should have the same mesial-distal width. The contact area of their mesial surfaces should form a vertical line.

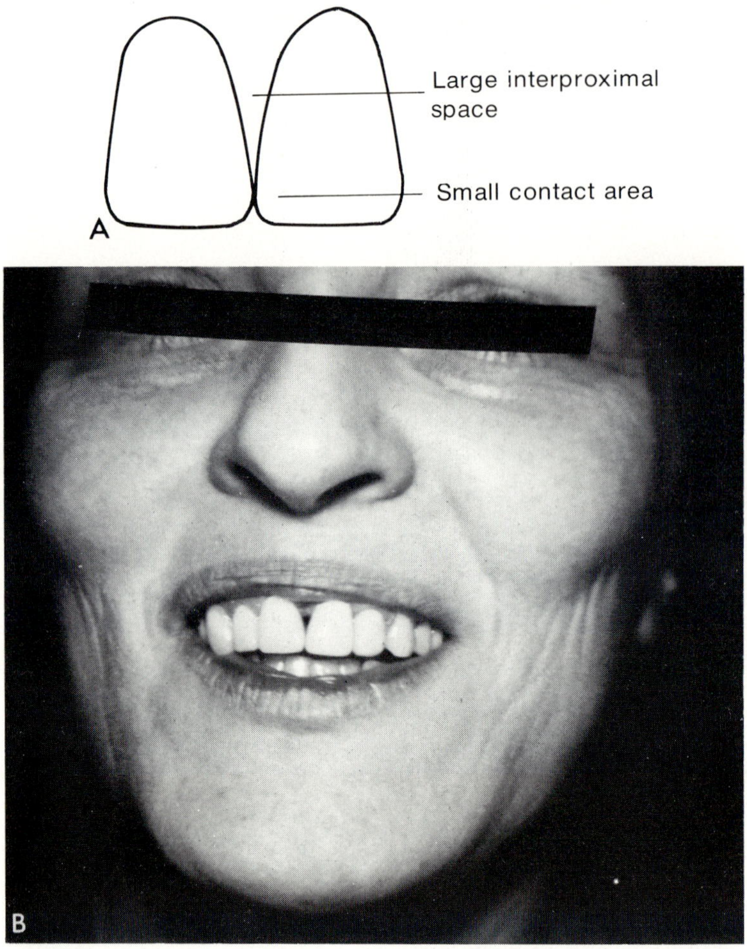

Figure 4–2 *A,* Upper central incisors that slant to the mesial, or have contact only at a point near their incisal edges, form an overly large interproximal area. *B,* An unesthetic smile with a large interproximal area between the central incisors.

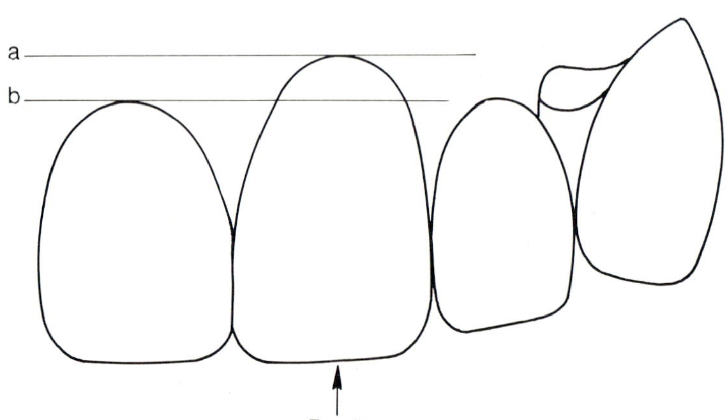

Figure 4–3 The gingival curvature of a central incisor pontic should be at the same horizontal level (b) as the central incisor abutment crown. If placed higher (a) on the edentulous area, the increased length of the tooth creates an unnatural appearance. Variations in length of central incisors are only appropriate when the incisal edges are modified and the gingival curvatures are on the same level. Central incisors should be almost twins.

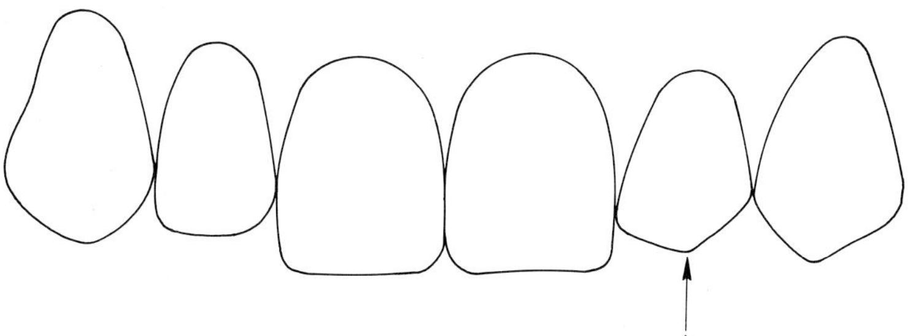

Figure 4–4 Upper lateral incisors may vary in size, form, and rotation. Making one lateral incisor slightly peg-shaped (A) may contribute to a natural appearance.

eral incisors need not match each other in form, length, or rotation; in fact, no other anterior tooth has more variations in form than the lateral incisor. On occasion, one lateral incisor may be slightly peg-shaped (Fig. 4–4). The appearance of femininity is increased by a labial rotation or overlap of the mesial surface; that of masculinity is accented by a lingual rotation of the mesial surface. Incisal edges may be in different alignment. Occasionally, slight lingual positioning of the lateral incisors breaks up the symmetry of the anterior arch and improves esthetics.

3. Upper Cuspids

Upper cuspids are slightly prominent, pointed, and *one shade darker*[2] than incisors and bicuspids. They are also rotated slightly vertically, so that their mesial surfaces face labially and their distal surfaces face posteriorly. *The mesial-incisal edge forms a large V-shaped angle of space with the distal wall of the lateral incisor.* This triangular area is essential to a natural look. Many crowns and bridges in existence today may be improved in appearance if the dentist would enlarge this triangular area with disks and stones (Fig. 4–5).

The upper cuspids are the cornerstones of the dental arch. The upper arch makes its turn around these teeth. A cuspid has two planes on the labial surface separated by the central bulge, and the arch bends around this tooth from buccal to labial, and from labial to buccal. Cuspids are very distinctive teeth. They are the most prominent ones in the dental arch. One of the most important single considerations in establishing an attractive, natural looking smile is the color of the cuspid teeth. If they are the same color as the central and lateral incisors the smile looks broad, monotonous, and unreal. This is the wide "wall of porcelain" that designates falseness. Cuspids should be slightly darker to interrupt and narrow the wall of porcelain.

4. Bicuspids

Bicuspids should harmonize with cuspids in length (slightly shorter), neckline, and mesial-distal width. The cosmetic effect of the

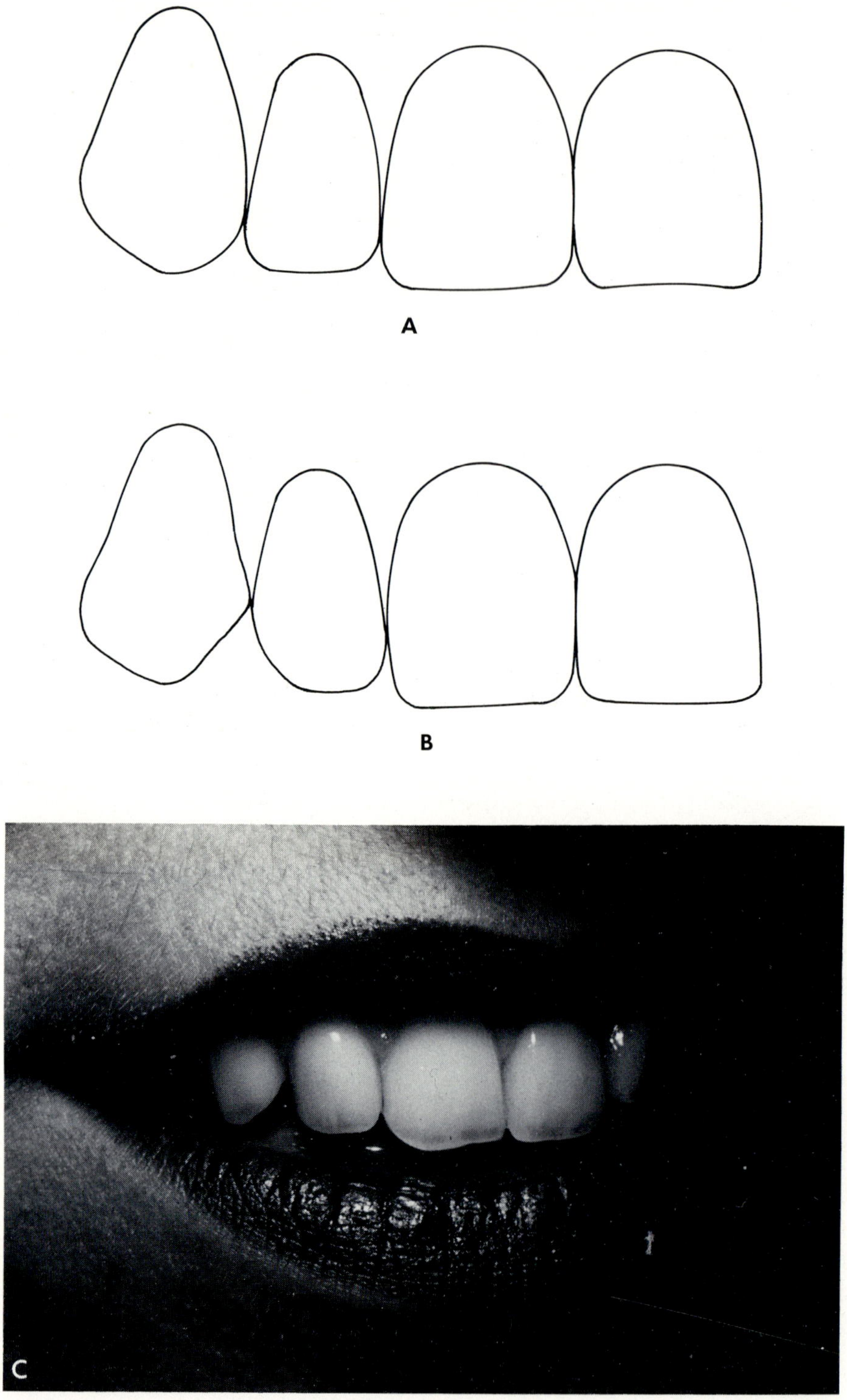

A

B

C

Figure 4–5 *A,* The cuspid-to-lateral contact point of crowns and bridges is often too close to the incisal edge. *B,* When the cuspid-to-lateral contact is modified so that the mesial-incisal edge of a cuspid and the distal of the lateral form a large V-shaped area, a more natural appearance results. *C,* The cuspid-to-lateral V-shaped space is one of the most important characteristics of a natural smile. When the dentist invades this space for a solder joint, or overlooks its anatomical necessity, an unesthetic appearance results.

smile is hampered when the first bicuspid is very much shorter than the cuspid. This often occurs in restorative dentistry with bridge and partial denture teeth. *The buccal cusp of the bicuspid should have a point similar to that of the cuspid.* The first and second bicuspids should be of the same shape, width, and length. Although maxillary incisors and cuspids are the more prominent teeth in a smile, the first and occasionally the second bicuspid are exposed to view during a wide smile at the angles of the mouth. Variations in the contour or the color of these teeth become very noticeable. Some large smiles may include the mesial half of the first molar, but this tooth plays a very minor role in the esthetics of the smile unless it is made of metal and reflects light. It may then detract from the appearance of the smile and cause the patient to look older. Conversely, the removal of a visible glint of metal on a molar (or bicuspid) will improve esthetics and cause a more youthful appearance. The first bicuspid links the anterior components of a smile with the posterior teeth by promoting a natural and gradual transition. In the very wide smile, the first bicuspid may be the turning point of the arch.

The Escape from Artificiality

It is easier to create an attractive smile with denture teeth set in denture base material than with fixed crowns and bridges. Complete dentures may be easily made to look natural by an artistically irregular arrangement of the anterior teeth. There is relative freedom for the positioning of each individual anterior tooth. In fixed bridgework, however, the dentist is not able to manipulate the individual anterior teeth as readily. The position of a crown is determined by the position of the abutment preparation and the pulp chamber. In fixed bridgework, the teeth may be arranged to bridge a gap or they may be single crowns splinted to each other. Here porcelain or resin is aligned to conceal the underlying metal structure. However, the metal blocks out the transmission of light and causes a "dead" and "different" appearance. Instead of looking like natural teeth, crowns and bridges usually look like what they are—artificial crowns and bridges! Anterior teeth composed of crowns, bridges, or splints are easily recognized as false; in fact, in many instances they scream their artificiality. The reasons for this are as follows:

1. Lack of translucency
2. Poor soft tissue relationships
3. Color monotony
4. Uniformity of arrangement
5. Failure to blend with the color of adjacent natural teeth
6. Failure to consider the factors that influence a smile

Lack of Translucency

The effect of the underlying metal in blocking out the transmission of light may be minimized by reducing sufficient tooth structure so that an adequate thickness of veneering material (porcelain or acrylic) may be used to disguise the metal. Proper opaquing of the metal is necessary. Incisal edges, if free of underlying metal, allow a small amount of translucency.

Soft Tissue Relationships

The margins of crowns should extend only slightly into the free gingival crevice. Gingival tissues respond poorly to a bulk of foreign material pressed against them, and to sharp edges of unpolished margins.

In the pontic area the relationship of an anterior tooth to the oral tissues plays a great part in establishing pleasing esthetics. A pontic may be too tight against underlying tissue and be framed by red or swollen tissues. Not infrequently a space exists between a pontic and visible tissue. This allows for an accumulation of debris and stain and forms an unattractive darkened area.

The tissues of elderly patients are more sensitive to pressure and take longer to recover from trauma than do those of young people.

Color Monotony

Nature is never monotonous in its artistic coloring of biologic things. Indeed, nature has a way of blending colors very subtly, as can be seen in trees, flowers, and people. So too does the color of different natural teeth vary in the same mouth. A smile that reveals an array of teeth of the exact same color looks monotonous and false. Upper anterior teeth should vary slightly in color, with the most appreciable variation in the cuspids. The dentist may cope with this problem easily and effectively by *simply making all cuspids (upper or lower) one shade darker* than the adjacent incisors and bicuspids. This gradation of color breaks up the monotony of the wall of artificial teeth and modifies its widening effect (Fig. 4–6).

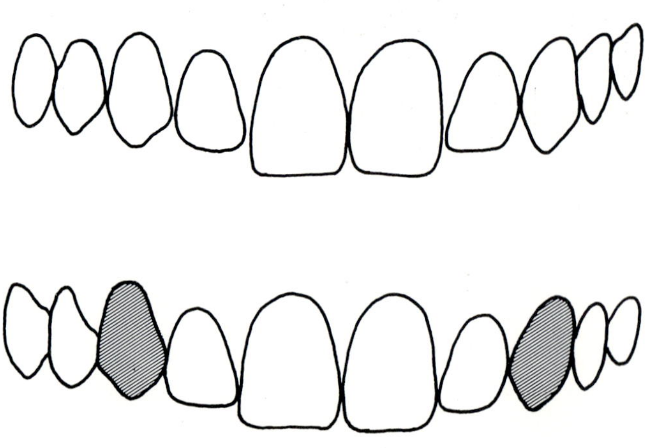

Figure 4–6 An arrangement of crowns or bridges looks more natural if cuspids are one shade darker. This breaks up the monotony of the wall of artificial teeth and modifies its widening effect.

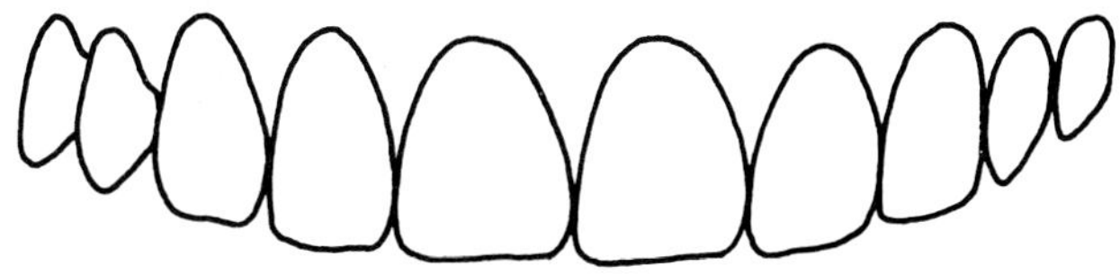

Figure 4–7 Crowns and bridges with incisal edges in a straight line look false. Even *natural teeth* look false when incisal edges appear to be "drawn with a ruler."

Uniformity of Arrangement

Upper anterior crowns and bridges do not look natural if they are too uniform in arrangement. The dentist should endeavor to break the monotony of a uniform tooth arrangement in any way possible. Asymmetry in arrangement may be achieved by subtle modifications in the rotation, angulation, and size of the upper central and lateral incisors. The size of a lateral on one side of the mouth may be reduced to make it appear smaller than the one on the opposite side. Also, an inward distal rotation of a lateral incisor will interrupt the uniformity of the arch and have a definite softening effect on the arrangement. Central incisors may also be rotated inward at the distal for the same purpose. The prominence or tilt of one cuspid may differ from that of the other.

An important rule: upper anterior teeth should never be arranged so that their common incisal edge looks as if it had been drawn with a ruler (Fig. 4–7).

Failure to Blend with the Color of Adjacent Natural Teeth

To obtain an esthetic end result, the color of a fixed restoration should match or harmonize with the color of adjacent natural teeth. The color-matching of artificial to natural teeth is very vexing to the dentist because in the determination of the proper color there are variables, such as lighting and color perception, that are difficult to control. When these variables differ between the dental office and the dental laboratory, prostheses with the wrong color may result. Lighting is a variable that a standardized light source can eliminate; however, critical color perception differs from one person to another.

The Color Dilemma. A dilemma exists with regard to color between the technician, the patient and the dentist. Each has an individualized impression of color and of what blends and looks attractive in the mouth. Here again, the issue is complicated by the truism that "beauty lies in the eyes of the beholder." The dentist wants to please the patient. The technician wants to please the dentist. But much too often no one is pleased at all, because the "common denominator" of color understanding is missing.

No patient wants a dark tooth. Most don't even want crowns and bridges to match their own remaining teeth; they want them to be lighter. They have a concept of tooth color based on nebulous values and fantasy. At times the dentist is guided by his own interpretation of an appropriate color, and the resulting restoration looks natural and blends with the remaining teeth; however, it may not be acceptable to the patient, who may say, "My own teeth have always been so gray. I want the new ones to look lighter and better," or "My teeth have always been too yellow. I don't want to spend all this time and money just to get another yellow smile." If the dentist acquiesces to the patient's desire for "white teeth" he may set off a chain of problems that are difficult to resolve. Unfortunately, when the patient gets exactly what he wants, he often rejects the fruits of his own desire. The teeth may look too light alongside the darker, mature teeth. They may look "ghastly white." Now the remark is, "It just doesn't look *natural*." Of course it doesn't. Young, light-colored teeth are *unnatural* in the mouth of a mature person. Consequently, a number of criticisms may ensue regarding fit, form, finish, angulation, surface texture, occlusion and speech. It is interesting to note that these criticisms are seldom heard from the patient who has allowed the dentist free rein to create a pleasing and acceptable appearance that harmonizes with his age and oral conditions.

Failure to Consider the Factors that Influence a Smile

The dentist should attempt to educate the patient to comprehend the esthetic factors that contribute to an attractive smile. In other words, "the eyes of the beholder" should be influenced to recognize and appreciate the same esthetic values that "the eyes of the dentist" recognize and appreciate. Actually, since many patients have vague and erroneous concepts of what constitutes an attractive smile, and think in terms of small, even, white teeth, the dentist must "brainwash" them to the true facts that govern esthetics. He should point out the benefits of planned irregularities, variations in color, rotations, angulations, and proper positioning. He should have the patient note the limitations to esthetics of interocclusal space, edentulous space, splinting requirements, opaqueness due to posts or metal substructure, and other problems pertinent to his oral condition. A collection of models, casts, and photographs showing esthetic factors is helpful in the education of the patient. However, one of the best methods of "brainwashing" and psychologically conditioning the patient to a successful esthetic end result is showing a collection of magazine covers portraying the smiling faces of well-known theatrical or political personalities with smiles that are generally accepted to be attractive. Here the details of esthetics, when pointed out, are bound to be remembered. Another aid is a collage of an assortment of attractive smiles (mouth and teeth only) cut out of magazines, newspapers, and dental advertisements. They are mounted (glued or taped) on a large page under a transparent acetate cover. These smiles may be selected to show various esthetic factors and perhaps include some obviously unattractive smiles for comparison (Fig. 4–8). The dentist should point out to the patient various details and pertinent features of an esthetic smile on the collage, such as the rel-

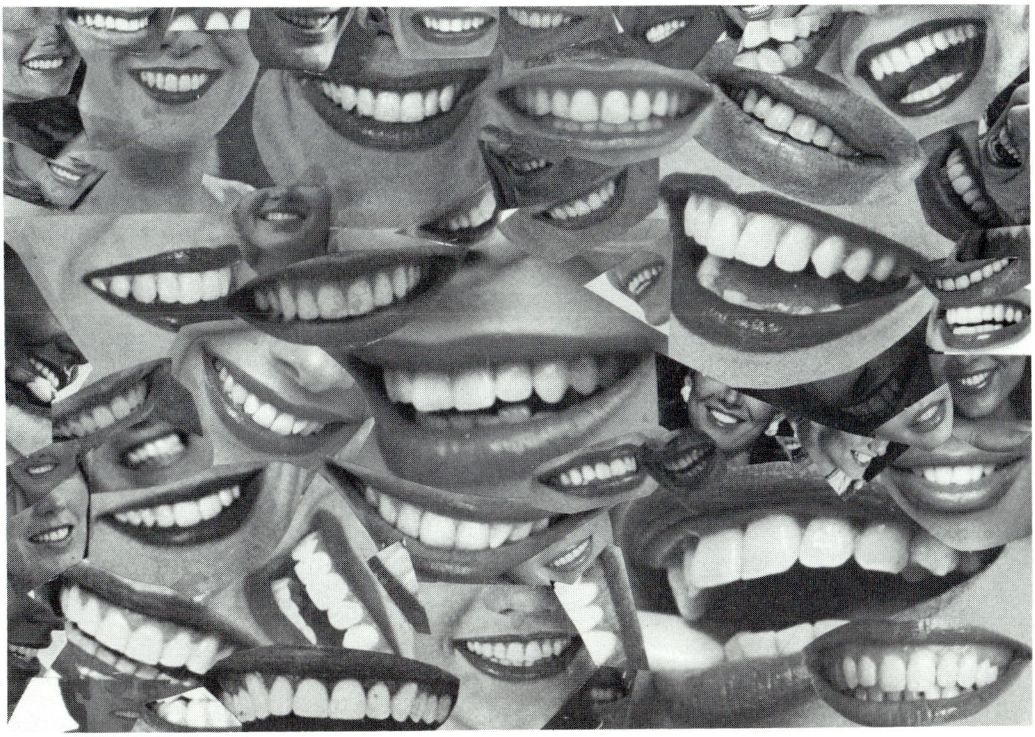

Figure 4–8 A collection of smiles make up a collage that can be used to educate the patient to esthetic factors.

ative sizes of the anterior teeth, irregularities, spaces, rotations, and color gradations.

Psychologic Considerations

Problems in esthetic dentistry result from the dichotomy between the dentist's concept of a satisfactory result and the patient's expectations. The dentist's training is necessarily concerned with rehabilitation and treatment that attempts to duplicate in form and contour the anatomic stereotype. However, it cannot be safely assumed that the patient has the same objective. Concepts of what is esthetic vary according to culture, temperament, and education. The dentist is often dismayed and surprised when a patient views "a successful esthetic result" as disappointing. Much too often there is a large gap between the dentist's concept of a satisfactory smile and that of the patient. Brainwashing and discussion prior to treatment could forestall such complications. Brainwashing entails educating the patient to the details of the esthetics to be derived in the case. This is accomplished readily with pictures and drawings. The desired end result is predicted. At the same time, the patient's views regarding esthetics are considered. The dentist should insist that the patient be as specific as possible about what he does or does not want. Of substantial importance to a good result, and to a good dentist-patient relationship, is a clear understanding of the patient's perception of this problem and what he expects dental therapy to achieve esthetically. Nevertheless, the esthetic judgment of the dentist is often modified by the taste or personal preference of the patient. Judgment is created by the knowledge that comes from information and experience. Taste, however, is biased, and personal preference is sometimes irresponsible to the principles of esthetics. Therefore, although esthetic judgment can be modified, modification should be kept to a minimum by educating the patient to the values comprising esthetics.

The dentist should recognize that many patients present themselves with well-established personality defects and neuroses. These patients may have the unrealistic dream that anterior crowns or fixed partial dentures will solve the problems of life. Examples of dreams that may never come true are as follows:

1. Teeth that are white and evenly arranged. The female patient who is saddened by the fading away of youth and attractiveness is motivated subconsciously to wish for the brilliant, white, flashing teeth of the beauty pageant contestant.
2. Restorations that are undetectable at close range.
3. Crowns and bridges that are durable and unbreakable, that last forever.
4. Esthetic restorative dentistry that removes facial folds and wrinkles.
5. Secret expectations that with a beautiful new smile will come an exciting new job or even sexual rejuvenation.

Sometimes the patient's esthetic demands are difficult to meet. Unreasonable expectations should alert the dentist to refuse the crown and bridge therapy until successful advances can be made in education and communication with the patient.

If

If the psychology of esthetics is ignored and the education of the patient is overlooked he may not revise his concept of his self-image that demands piano-key arrangements of ultra-white teeth.

If not informed otherwise, patients may not recognize that the restored smile with teeth that are white and even is not as attractive as the one with color gradations and rotated and slightly uneven teeth.

If the patient cannot understand the limitations involved after they are explained, restorative treatment should not be started.

If there is no understanding to begin with, how can there be any afterward?

The patient who is unreasonable prior to therapy could easily be more unreasonable after therapy.

Educating the Patient for Successful Crown and Bridge Therapy

In consideration of the aforementioned psychologic factors, the dentist should explain the following limitations and facts prior to treatment.

1. The limitations due to occlusal relationships, arch form, tooth alignment, and non-vital teeth.
2. The limitations of color and translucency.
3. The limitations due to asymmetries of the lips, alveolar bone, and gingival tissues. Sometimes the patient is not aware that there is a difference in the horizontal level of the gingival line around the necks of various teeth. After crowns and bridges are installed this difference may be even more noticeable. This should be pointed out to the patient before the teeth are prepared.
4. The plan of treatment, the time required for completion, and the need to avoid prolonging the treatment.
5. The shortcomings of various restorative materials. For example, gold is visible, acrylic resin wears and discolors, and porcelain may break. Porcelain jackets do not match porcelain-over-metal crowns, even though the shade of porcelain used is the same, because they have different light absorbing and reflecting qualities.
6. The need for cooperation in sanitation and other preventive measures.
7. Bruxism and clenching may destroy the restorative endeavor, and stress control therapy such as biofeedback may be necessary.
8. The anterior teeth that make up the smile are very dependent on the health, alignment, and occlusal relationships of the posterior teeth. Lack of restorative dentistry, or inadequate restorative dentistry in posterior quadrants, may allow a small decrease in vertical dimension that may contribute to the failure of the anterior restorations.
9. Teeth reflect age. Older people have darker and more discolored teeth than young people. Teeth also reflect age in other ways. Incisal edges that are rounded and smooth in young people may be worn, sharp, or chipped in older people.
10. The inevitable changeover from a temporary to a permanent restoration. Occasionally, the temporary restoration satisfies the esthetic requirements of the patient so completely that the permanent restoration is rejected as unacceptable. Explain the differences in bulk, contour, and surface hardness, and the reasons for gold occlusal surfaces.
11. Because of their underlying metal structure, permanent restorations may appear less vibrant and different in color from the translucent temporary restorations they replace.
12. The midline of the upper anterior teeth is not required to coincide with the midline of the lower anterior teeth, or with the midline of the nose.
13. The labial surfaces of anterior crowns and bridges are not necessarily smooth. They may have lifelike irregularities ground in

to reflect light. Simulated individual variations of natural teeth, such as enamel faults or striations, may be used to help duplicate the faults of nature.

14. No fixed restoration should be expected to last indefinitely. Nothing lasts forever. In some mouths the conditions allow a restoration to endure for many years; in other mouths wear, breakage, and discoloration occur in a comparatively short period of time. As time passes, the biologic relationship of the fixed prosthesis and the living tissues is modified. The changes that occur in the gingival tissues and the supporting bone structure may be cause for additional therapy. The longevity of fixed restorations strongly depends upon proper nutrition, oral hygiene, and the general health of the patient.

A Checklist for Common Esthetic Errors

Occasionally, the dentist as well as the patient may be unhappy with the appearance of new fixed anterior bridgework. The dentist will agree that something is wrong but cannot recognize exactly what it is. The following is a checklist for common errors that cause esthetic shortcomings.

1. Teeth too light in color.
2. Poor relationship of the labial surfaces of the anterior teeth to the upper lip.
3. Incisal edges that look as if they were drawn with a ruler.
4. Insufficient angle of space between the distal of the lateral and the mesial of the cuspid.
5. Faulty vertical relationship, overbite, and overjet.
6. Embrasures too large and presenting darkened areas.
7. Lateral incisors not shorter than central incisors.
8. Central incisors meeting in a small point contact instead of a vertical line.
9. Pontics far out of proportion in size to adjacent abutments.
10. Midline slanted and not vertical.
11. Cuspless bicuspids or molars. To be attractive, posterior teeth should have cusps. Flat teeth cause an unnatural straight-line appearance.
12. Short posterior teeth, which cause an abrupt breakup of the harmonious and gradual reduction in size that occurs in nature.

Methods to Improve the Esthetics of Anterior Restorations

To improve a smile composed of old or newly inserted crowns and bridges note the following suggestions.

1. Shorten lateral incisors until they are shorter than the central incisors and the incisal edge is broken into a definite step.
2. Enlarge V-shaped spaces between cuspids and laterals. This is *the single most effective way to improve the esthetics of any an-*

terior restorative composition, fixed or removable. Many fixed restorations are at fault in this contact area due to solder joint requirements and periodontal considerations. Nevertheless, this area always looks false unless the embrasure is deepened.

3. Open incisal embrasures between central and lateral incisors.
4. Round off the distal corners of the central incisors.
5. Change the incisal edge of one central incisor so that it does not match the other.
6. Grind small facets of wear on the incisal edges of the central incisors and the cuspids.
7. Accentuate the buccal cusp formation on bicuspids, and point up the cusp of cuspids when necessary.

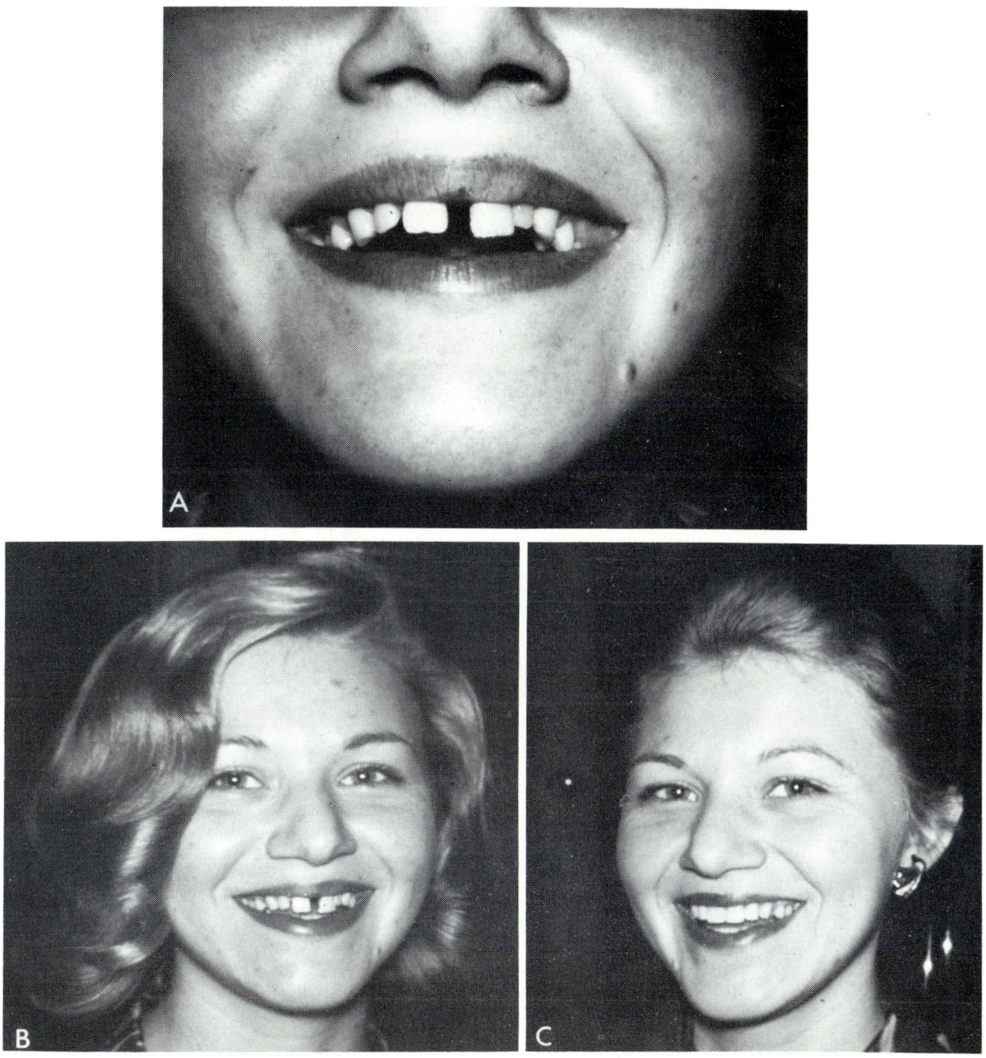

Figure 4–9 Psychologic as well as biologic considerations contribute to the crown and bridge therapy that transforms unattractive teeth (*A*) and associated personality (*B*) to an improved appearance (*C*) that reflects a restored inner confidence.

SUMMARY

Since crowns and bridges must be fitted to and coordinated with living tissues, they are actually therapeutic agents designed to function within the anatomic and physiologic limitations of a patient. However, they also supply therapy in the form of dental esthetics that must be accepted within the psychologic limitations of the patient. One of dentistry's greatest challenges is to eliminate the placing of unattractive, artificial-looking fixed restorations. Human vanity should not be underestimated. Few males, or females, walk past a mirror without a sly glance. Dental esthetics is of critical importance to the psychologic welfare of patients (Fig. 4–9).

REFERENCES

1. Boucher, C. O.: Current Clinical Dental Terminology. St. Louis, The C. V. Mosby Co., 1963, p. 132.
2. Martone, A. L.: Denture esthetics and its relation to facial esthetics, Dent. Clin. North Am. March 1967, p. 97.

five

A Method of Cosmetic Improvement

The gyrations of a fish caught on a hook look peculiar to other fish that do not understand the circumstances.

Unknown

In this age of beauty culture everyone is concerned with appearance to some degree. Something in the psychological makeup of the individual creates a strong desire to look attractive. A good appearance exercises a great influence on personality and attitude. Clothes may not make the man, or the woman; nevertheless, good clothing, coupled with a healthy complexion and a *sparkling smile*, are important factors in making a good first impression. No single feature of the face influences appearance more than the smile. Nothing is more charming than an attractive, slow-spreading smile; and how surprised we are to see a lovely mouth in an otherwise less than attractive face.

In today's dentistry the patient is treated as a total human being with his or her own individual personality. The dentist should be just as concerned with the patient's personal happiness, self-confidence, and state of mind as he is with routine dental problems. It has always been recognized that dental disorders or irregularities are capable of producing psychic manifestations that may contribute to mental illness. Improving the appearance of a smile can have a profound effect on a patient's self-esteem.

THE COSMETIC VENEER

Cosmetic contouring of natural teeth and "adhesive" resin bonding to fractured or whole teeth are practical and comparatively inexpensive alternatives to crowning of teeth. Another practical and inexpensive method of cosmetic improvement is accomplished with a cosmetic veneer that renders immediate first-aid to healthy upper anterior teeth that may be poorly spaced, twisted, discolored, broken, deeply striated, or subject to mottled enamel. The treatment consists of covering up defects in the upper anterior teeth with a thin layer of acrylic resin. This cover fits over the labial and incisal aspects of the upper anterior teeth like a "dental band-aid." It fits close to, but not in contact with, the gingival tissues and retains itself most adequately by a slight dove-tailing between the teeth. *The cosmetic veneer is removable, but while it is in position it simulates all the natural color and contour of an esthetic anterior tooth arrangement.* In other words, *it provides the patient with a more attractive smile by covering up all defects* (Fig. 5–1). Whether or not the patient can eat with the cosmetic veneer in position depends upon the nature of the bite. With care

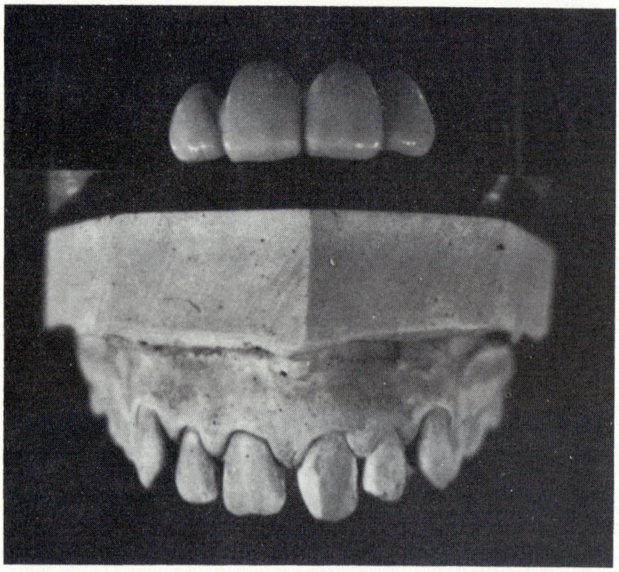

A

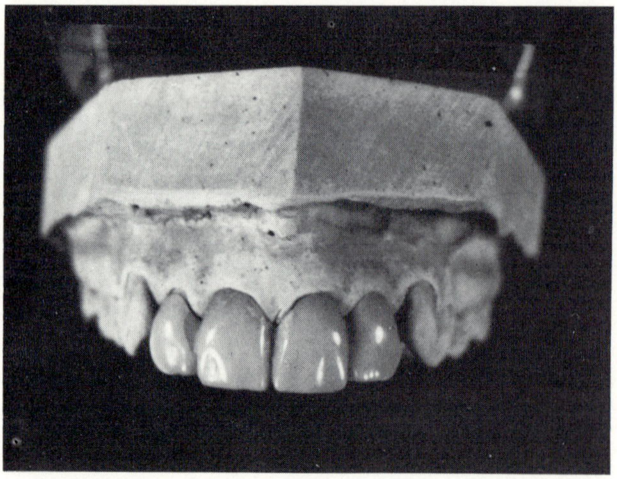

B

Figure 5–1 An example of a cosmetic veneer. *A,* Upper stone cast showing various defects in the anterior teeth and the cosmetic veneer (above). *B,* The cosmetic veneer in position on the stone cast covering up the defects in the anterior teeth.

and adaptation, many patients are able to do so, some with slightly less efficiency.

The cosmetic veneer is prescribed to improve a smile quickly by a simple, inexpensive, and painless procedure (Fig. 5–2). This usually brightens a patient's outlook toward dental treatment of a more permanent nature. It may also be utilized when financial conditions rule out or postpone necessary esthetic crown and bridge therapy, as they often do when multiple crowns are involved. Although both men and women may utilize the cosmetic veneer, this method of esthetic improvement is especially applicable to the young female seeking employment as an airline stewardess, model, or actress. It is usually pointed out that the improved smile will help the recipient to find a job, which may be helpful in coping with the costs of future dentistry. Of course, the "new smile" is a very effective ethical advertisement for subsequent dentistry of a more durable nature.

The Oral Psychiatrist

It is of great importance for any individual seeking placement in the business world to present a pleasing countenance. No matter how expensively or fashionably dressed a person may be, if he is afraid to smile and reveal unattractive teeth he is at a disadvantage, and may feel "disfigured." When the dentist provides a method to hide what may be construed psychologically as "disfiguring marks," a resultant improvement occurs in the person's general outlook on life. The dentist becomes an oral psychiatrist. With the aid of esthetic dentistry he transforms personalities and banishes inferiority complexes based on missing, crooked, or unattractive teeth.

The "Hollywood Bridge"

An acrylic resin device called the "Hollywood bridge" may be considered the forerunner of the cosmetic veneer. Unlike the cosmetic veneer, which is *made in the patient's mouth,* the Hollywood bridge is constructed in the dental laboratory from a cast of the mouth. It is made of *heat-cured acrylic resin* that is harder and more brittle than self-cured acrylic resin. It also tends to warp in thin sections, especially during polishing. Because of its harder, brittle nature, it tends to break more readily than the softer, less brittle self-curing resin. Also, extra thickness is generally required for ease of laboratory handling, and the potentials for retention are limited. Considering the laboratory costs and the time involved, the benefits of the self-curing, softer, more flexible, and inexpensive cosmetic veneer are apparent.

The Cosmetic Veneer Procedure

The actual fabrication of a cosmetic veneer is a simple procedure, similar to that of polymerizing self-curing acrylic resin in the

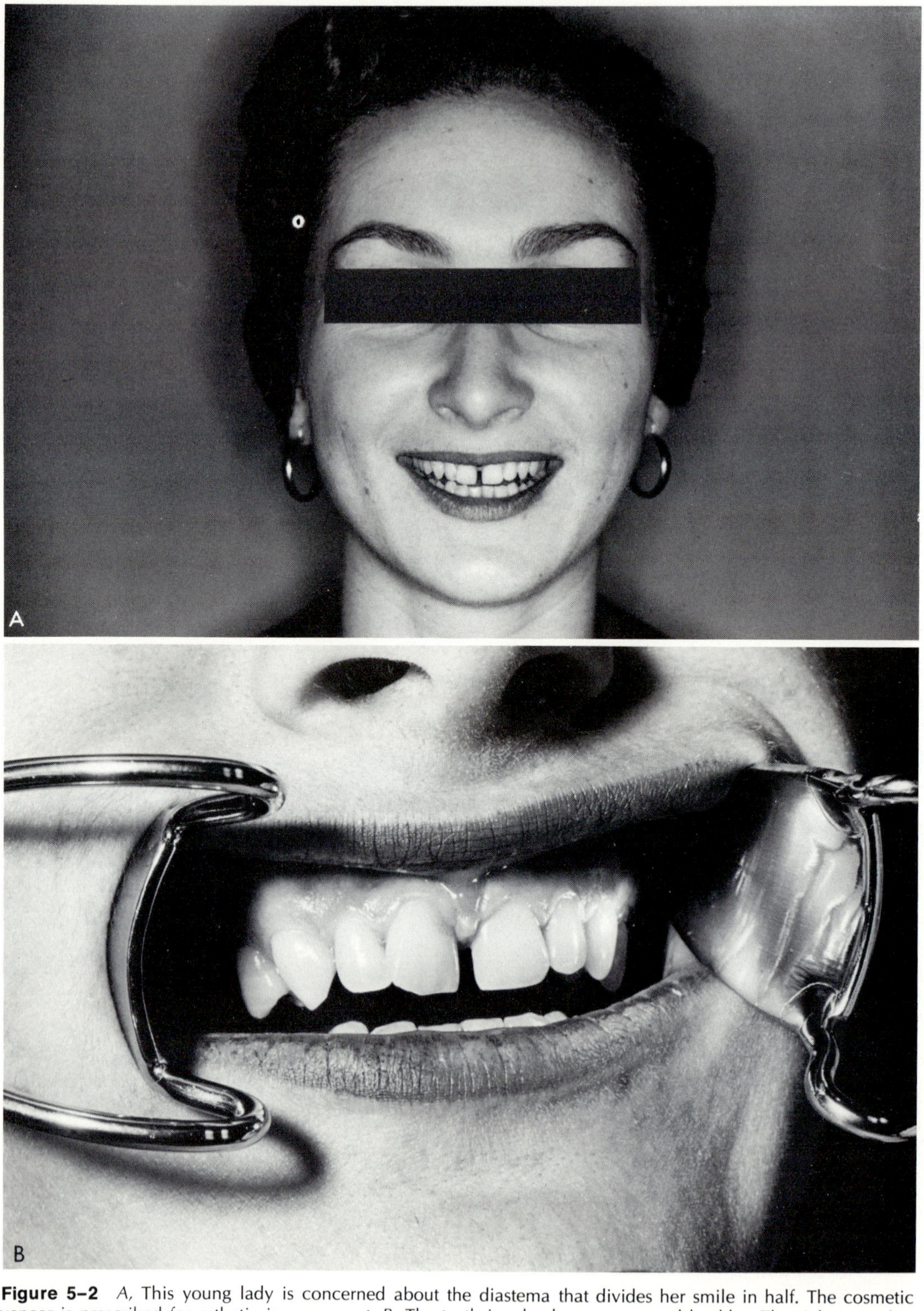

Figure 5–2 *A,* This young lady is concerned about the diastema that divides her smile in half. The cosmetic veneer is prescribed for esthetic improvement. *B,* The teeth involved are young and healthy. The right central is rotated and chipped.

mouth to obtain temporary crowns and bridges. A stone cast is poured from an alginate impression of the patient's maxillary arch (Fig. 5–3). When the stone cast is dry, ivory-colored inlay wax* is melted over the labial surfaces of the teeth to be covered with the cosmetic veneer (Fig. 5–4). Two to six anterior teeth may be involved. For each tooth, the ivory wax is applied from the gingival line to the incisal edge of the labial surface (approximately 1½ mm thick) and then extended to cover approximately 1 mm of the lingual surface (Fig. 5–5). The wax is carved and sculptured to the desired esthetic effect. The waxed cast is then placed into water until needed.

At the next dental appointment the patient's anterior teeth are examined closely and surveyed for deep interproximal undercuts and existing resin fillings or crown and bridge veneers. Large undercuts are blocked out with Cavit** and small undercuts with Rubber-Sep.† The Cavit is pressed into an undercut with a moistened instrument or finger. It sets hard enough and soon enough to prevent acrylic resin from flowing into an undercut. Later, after fabrication of the cosmetic veneer, when it has hardened completely the Cavit may be easily flicked away with a small instrument. The Rubber-Sep may be

*Kerr Manufacturing Company, Romulus, MI 48174.
**Premier Dental Products, Norristown, PA 19401.
†George Taub Products, Incorporated, Jersey City, NJ 07307.

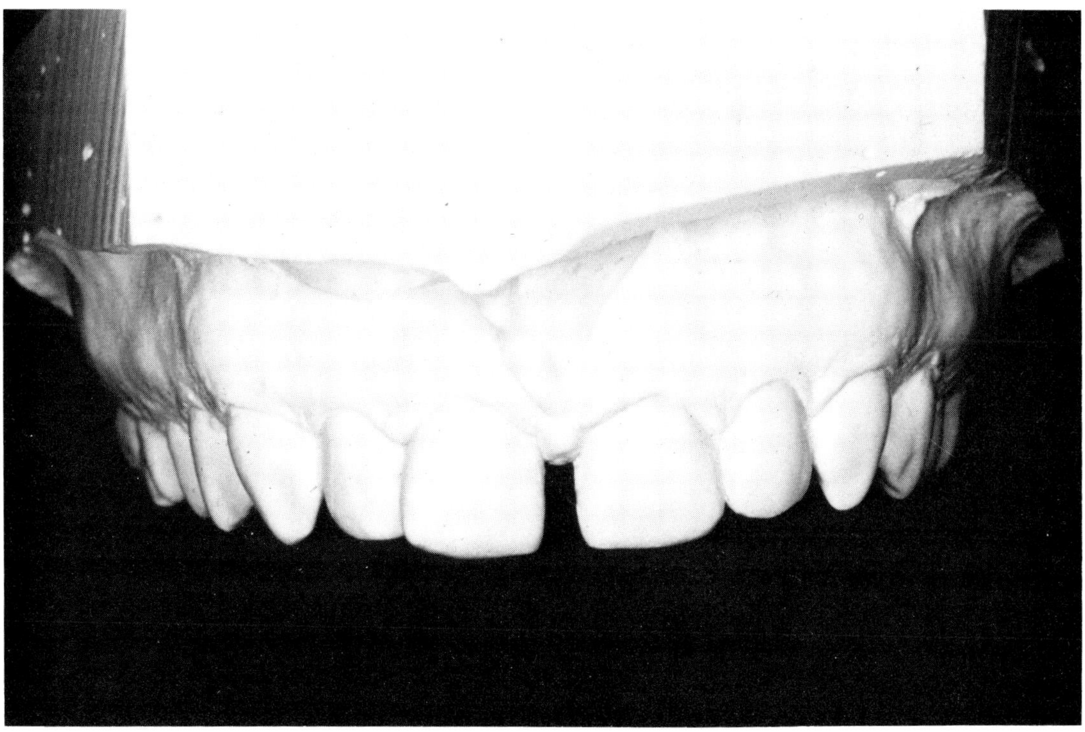

Figure 5–3 The stone cast obtained from an alginate impression.

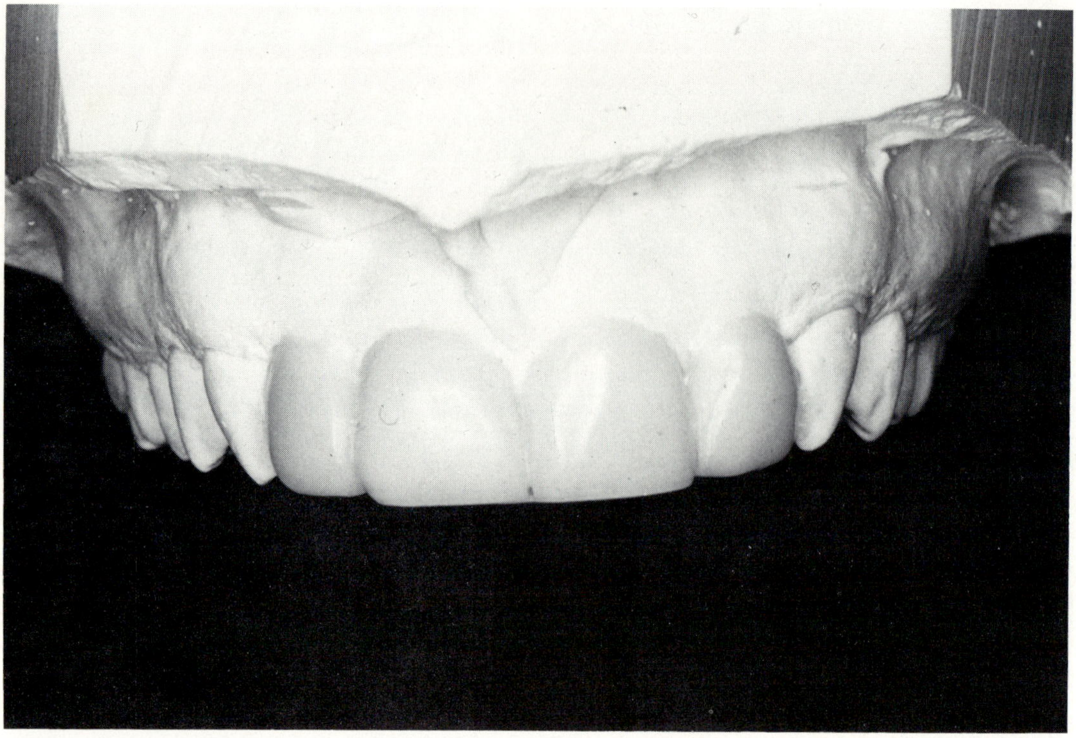

Figure 5–4 Ivory-colored wax is applied over the anterior teeth of the cast. It is carved and sculptured to the desired effect. An alginate impression of this wax-improved cast is obtained.

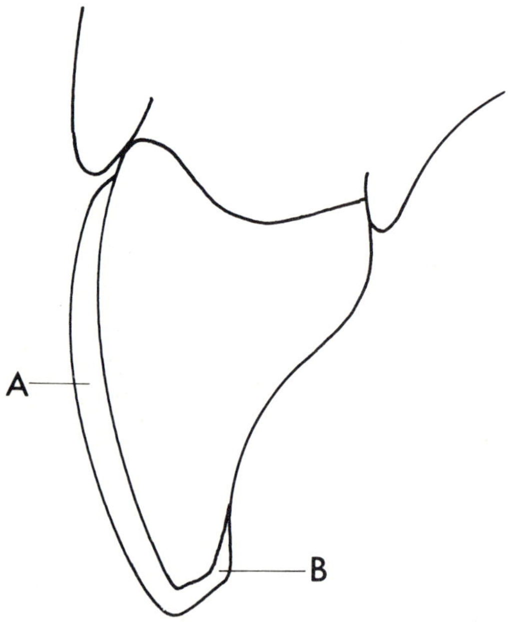

Figure 5–5 A, Cross section of an upper central incisor showing the area of the labial surface that is covered by the cosmetic veneer. B, The extent of the lingual coverage of the incisal edge.

painted into a small undercut, using a small sable brush or a pointed instrument. It dries in one minute to a rubbery consistency. It is a bright-red color, and the extent of its application may be easily visualized. After the procedure, it is peeled away from the teeth and the acrylic resin veneers. Acrylic or composite resin fillings and resin crown veneers in the vicinity are covered with a film of Rubber-Sep to prevent adhesion when the newly applied self-curing acrylic resin is polymerized. A thin film of dental silicone grease should be smeared on the labial and lingual surfaces of the teeth to be covered. The mouth should remain open, with a saliva ejector placed in position.

An alginate impression is made of the waxed stone cast (Fig. 5–6) that has been soaking in water. The selected shade of self-curing acrylic resin is mixed in a small dappen dish to a thin consistency and then flowed into the labial concavities of the teeth in the alginate impression that correspond to the teeth that have been waxed-up for the cosmetic veneer on the stone cast. The impression carrying the fluid mix of acrylic resin is seated in the patient's mouth (Fig. 5–7). The alginate impression serves as a matrix and molds the flowable resin over the patient's teeth. When the resin has hardened completely the alginate matrix is removed from the mouth. The heat of polymerization and the chemical irritation of the monomer are of little or no significance on the enamel of tooth structure, especially where dental silicone grease and undercut block-out agents have been applied.

Because of the intimacy of fit and the retention of hardened acrylic resin in the small irregularities on the tooth surface, the initial removal of the cosmetic veneer may be difficult. It may break if too much force is used to pry it loose. Excess flash material is peeled away, and the cosmetic veneer is removed slowly and carefully with the gentle tapping of a reverse mallet. It is trimmed to refine the proper gingival and labial contours, adjusted to rule out occlusal interference, and then smoothed with a rubber wheel, pumiced, and polished to a high luster* (Fig. 5–8). It should then be replaced on the teeth (Fig. 5–9) in the mouth and worn by the patient for a few hours to prevent warping while the polymerization becomes more stabilized (Fig. 5–10). A small container for moist storage will be necessary for subsequent removal of the cosmetic veneer.

Just as a denture wearer is educated to his obligation regarding home care, *the patient is instructed to remove and clean the cosmetic veneer* with due respect for the care and cleanliness of the underlying teeth and tissues.

The self-curing acrylic resin used for a cosmetic veneer should not be of the cheaper bulk-type material. It should be a high quality acrylic resin that is highly crosslinked. Unfilled acrylic resin filling materials such as Kadon** and Sevriton† are very suitable for cos-

---

* Lustershine, Accurate Set, Incorporated, Paterson, NJ 07501.

** L.D. Caulk Company, Milford, DE 19963.

† Amalgamated Dental Trade Distributors, Limited, London, England.

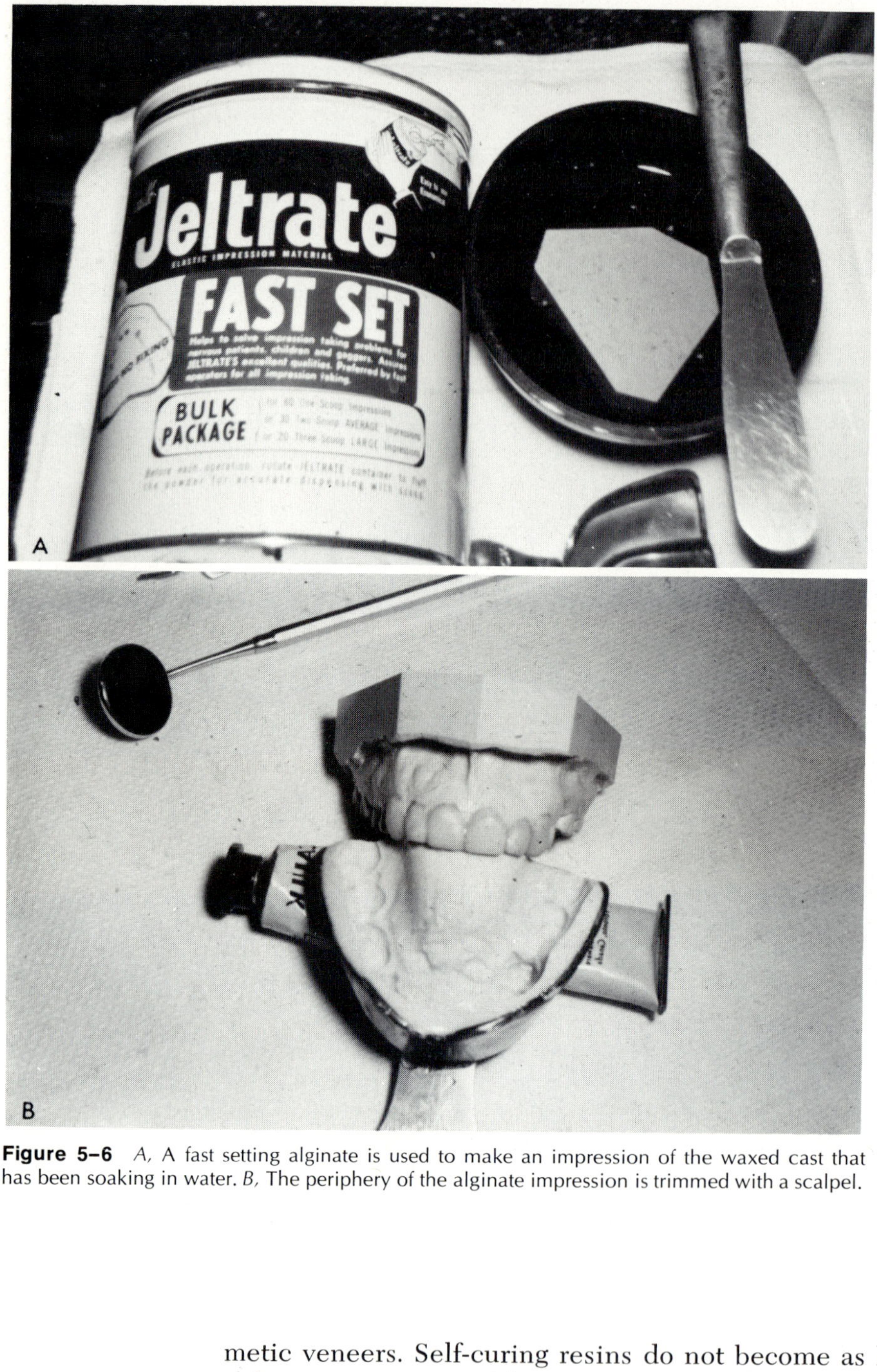

Figure 5–6 *A,* A fast setting alginate is used to make an impression of the waxed cast that has been soaking in water. *B,* The periphery of the alginate impression is trimmed with a scalpel.

metic veneers. Self-curing resins do not become as hard and brittle as heat-curing resins. They maintain a resiliency that allows for good retention in the small undercuts and interproximal spaces of the teeth that are covered for the cosmetic veneer. They are also less likely to break in handling, polishing, and insertion maneuvers than are the harder and more brittle heat-cured Hollywood bridges processed in the dental laboratory. They also fit more accurately, since they are polymerized to the teeth instead of a gypsum cast.

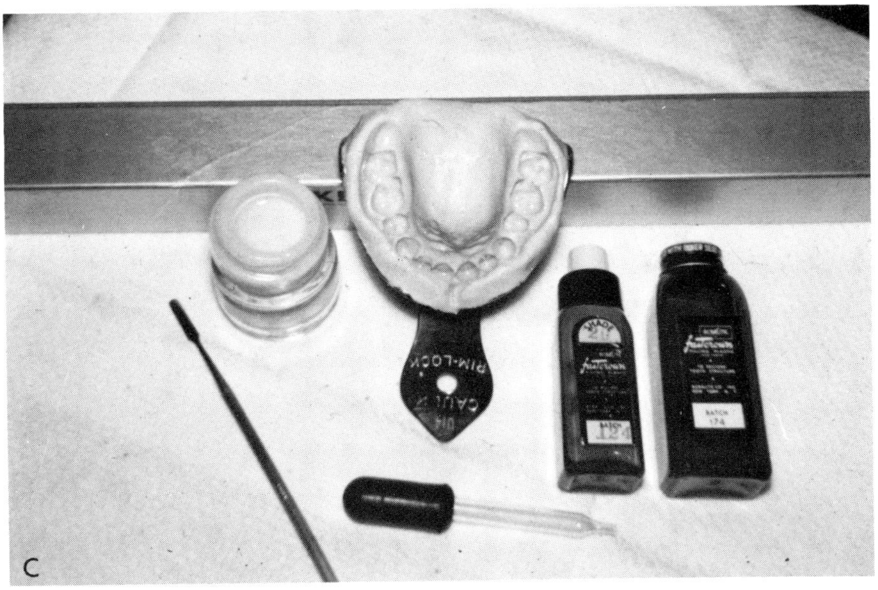

Figure 5–6 *Continued.* *C,* The self-curing resin is mixed in a dappen dish prior to placement in the alginate impression.

Limitations

The following limitations should be discussed with the patient prior to making a cosmetic veneer:

1. Cosmetic veneers always result in a smile composed of *larger teeth.* The patient should be informed that the cosmetic veneer not only will be longer but will extend around the incisal edges to a small portion of the lingual surface of each tooth. This will prevent food or debris from slipping between the cosmetic veneer and the

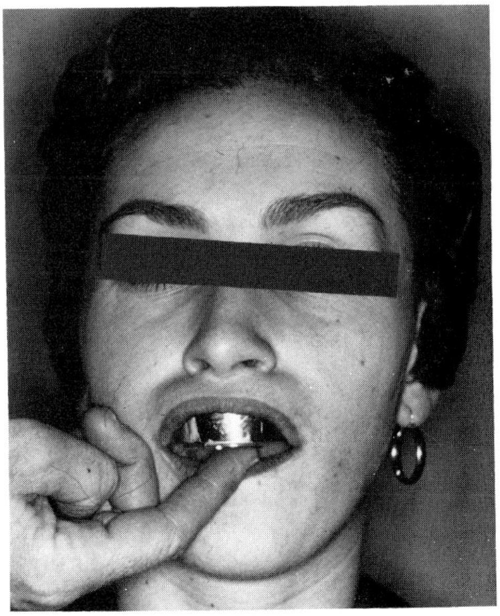

Figure 5–7 The alginate impression containing the fluid mix of acrylic resin is seated in the patient's mouth and held in position until the resin has hardened.

A

B

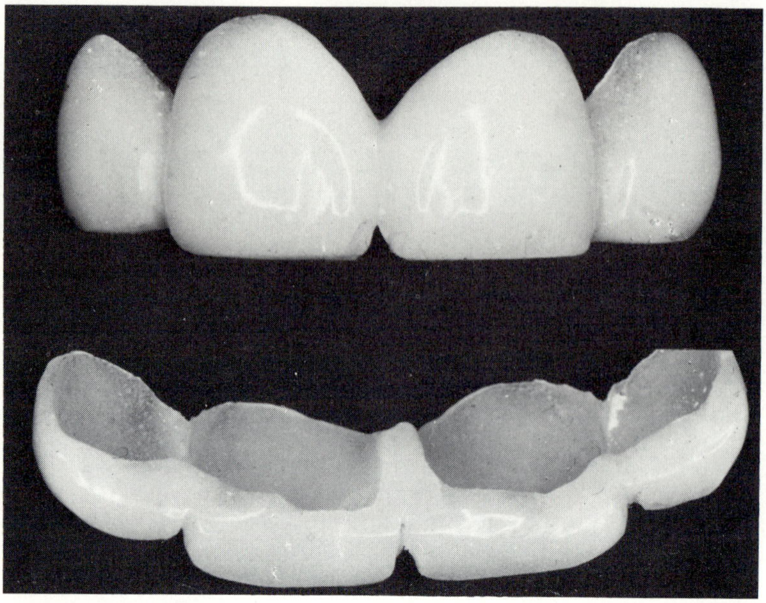

Figure 5–8 *A,* The cosmetic veneer after trimming and polishing. *B,* A lingual view of a cosmetic veneer.

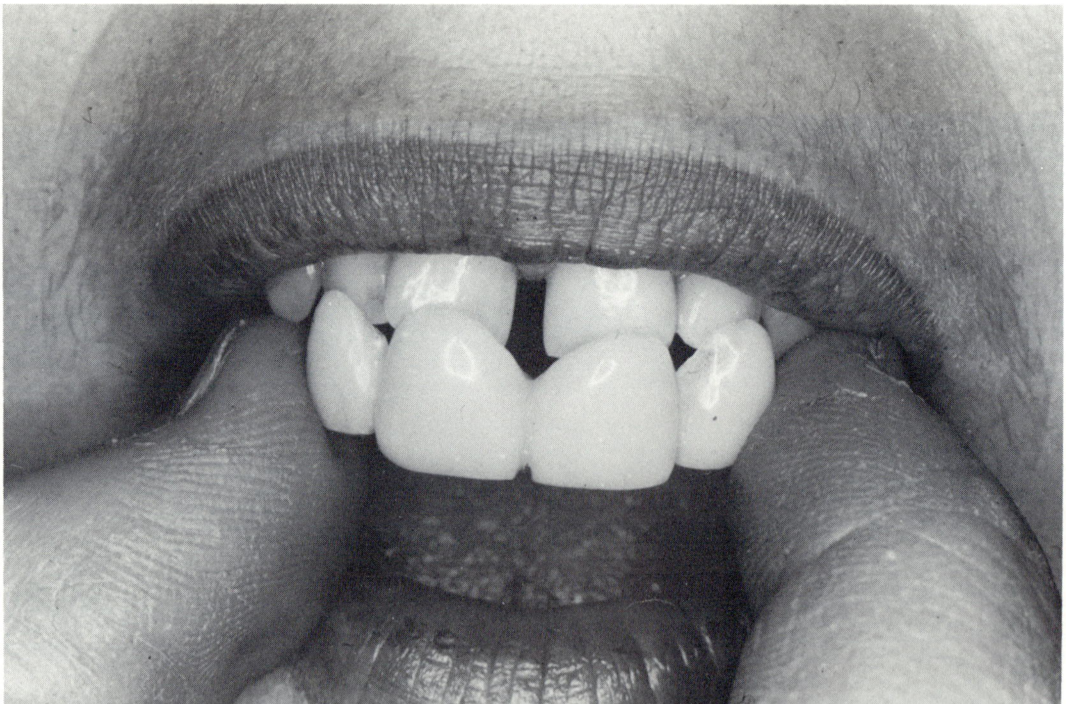

Figure 5–9 The cosmetic veneer is placed in position in the mouth. It should be worn for the first few hours after polymerization to prevent warping.

teeth. The layer of acrylic resin will be noticeable to the upper lip but this tactile sensation will diminish with time. It may also be pointed out that slightly larger teeth in many instances improve the appearance of a smile. A collection of magazine-cover smiles will verify the photogenicity of larger teeth.

2. Discoloration and wear may be considered shortcomings of the cosmetic veneer. However, it takes time for the manifestation of these effects, and very often cosmetic veneers have maintained adequate color and existed with little wear over a number of years.

3. Breakage is an occasional problem. This may occur during the initial removal of the cosmetic veneer after polymerization in the mouth or while inserting or removing or cleaning it at some future date. However, if this occurs despite due care, repair may easily be accomplished with the same acrylic resin material, using the powder, monomer, and a brush.

4. Gingival tissues may become irritated from the close proximity of the cosmetic veneer or from the chemical action of the monomer. It is best to avoid impinging upon the gingival tissues. However, any gingival irritation may easily be adjusted by a slight trimming and polishing of the acrylic material.

5. Actually, the cosmetic veneer is only a compromise method to improve appearance for limited periods of time. It should not be worn at all times. Continuous wear may be detrimental to the underlying teeth and tissues, and will cause accelerated wear and discoloration of the veneer. A cosmetic veneer may be inserted in the mouth just prior to a show, an interview, a photographic session, or a public appearance.

Indications for the Cosmetic Veneer

Esthetics is an important consideration in all phases of restorative dentistry. There are certain situations and problems in restorative dentistry that can only be resolved by utilizing a cosmetic veneer. It is indicated to cope with the following problems:

1. When *immediate cosmetic improvement* is necessary for business or professional purposes, such as for show people, photographers' models, airline stewardesses, or the individual preparing for a business interview (Fig. 5–11).

2. When jacket crown preparations are contraindicated, as they are for the very young person because of pulp chamber size. A cosmetic veneer may instill new confidence in one who is self-conscious because of an unattractive smile. A preview is given of what a more permanent type of prosthodontic endeavor may accomplish in the future (Fig. 5–12).

3. When the esthetic fault is minor or the upper anterior teeth are only slightly irregular, and the small amount of cosmetic improvement required would hardly warrant crown preparations on

Text continued on page 106

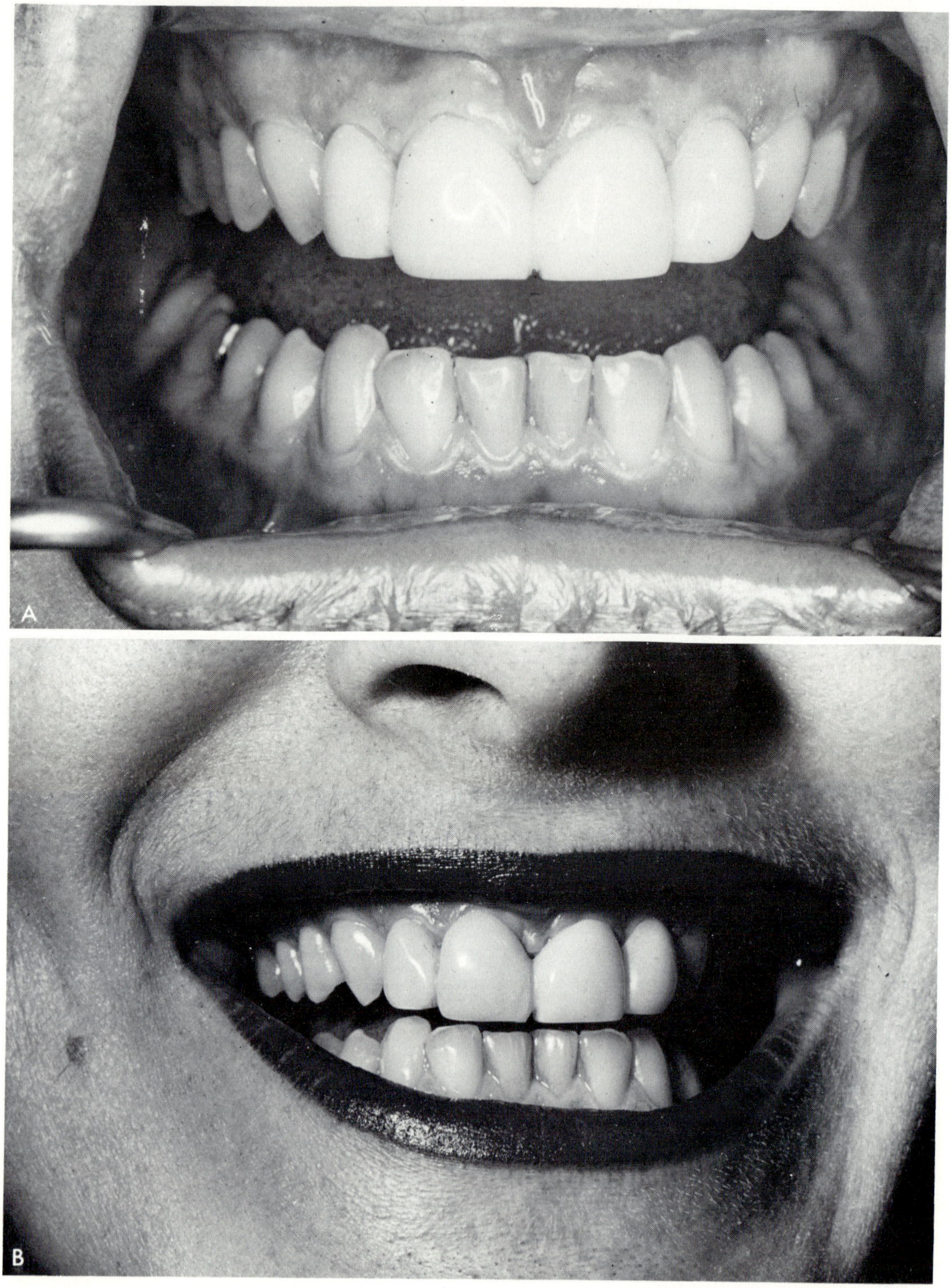

Figure 5–10 *A,* The cosmetic veneer in position covering four anterior teeth. *B,* The improved smile.

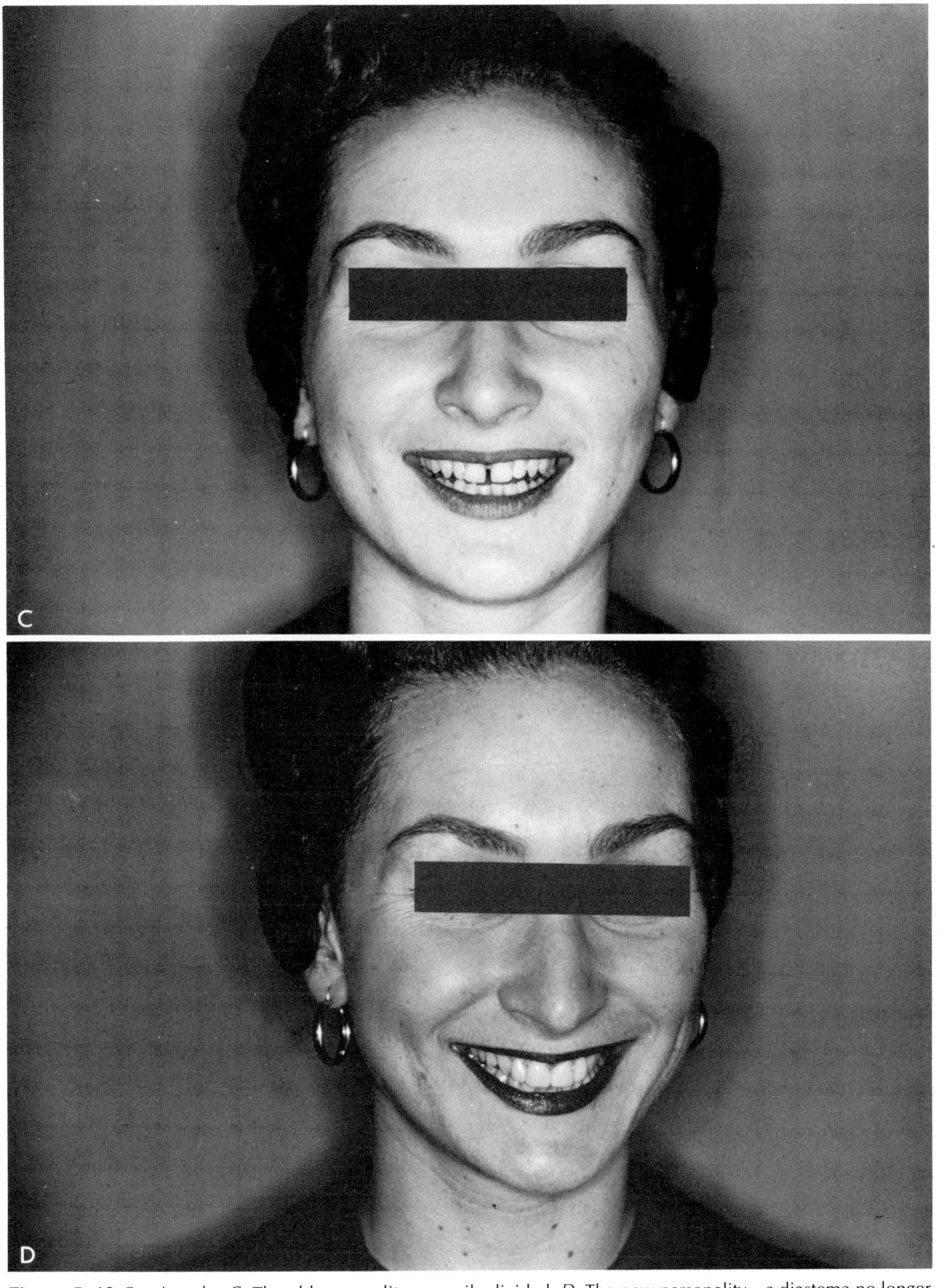

Figure 5–10 *Continued.* *C,* The old personality—a smile divided. *D,* The new personality—a diastema no longer cuts this smile in half.

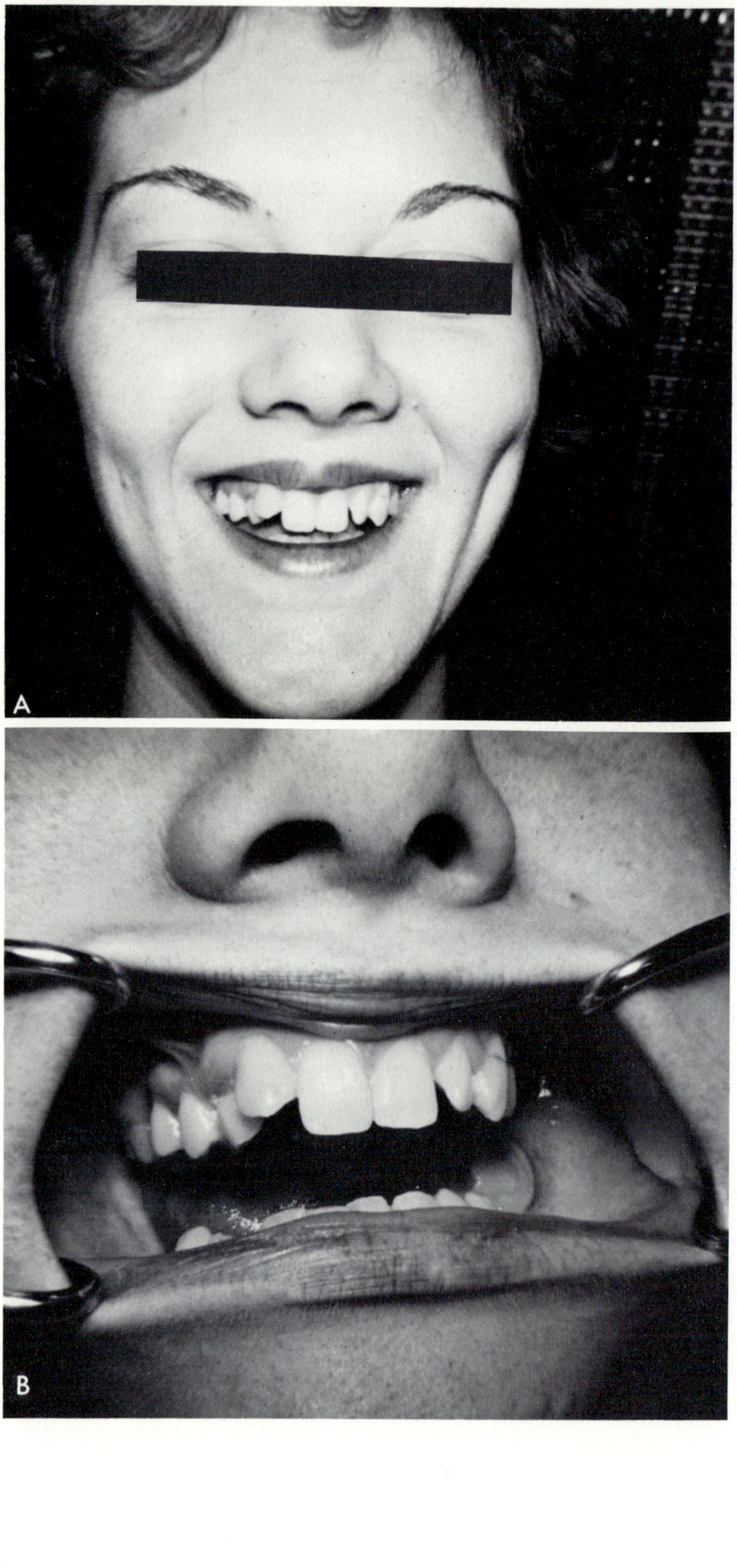

Figure 5–11 This young lady faces a business interview with a self-conscious smile (*A*) due to an unattractive anterior tooth development and arrangement (*B*).

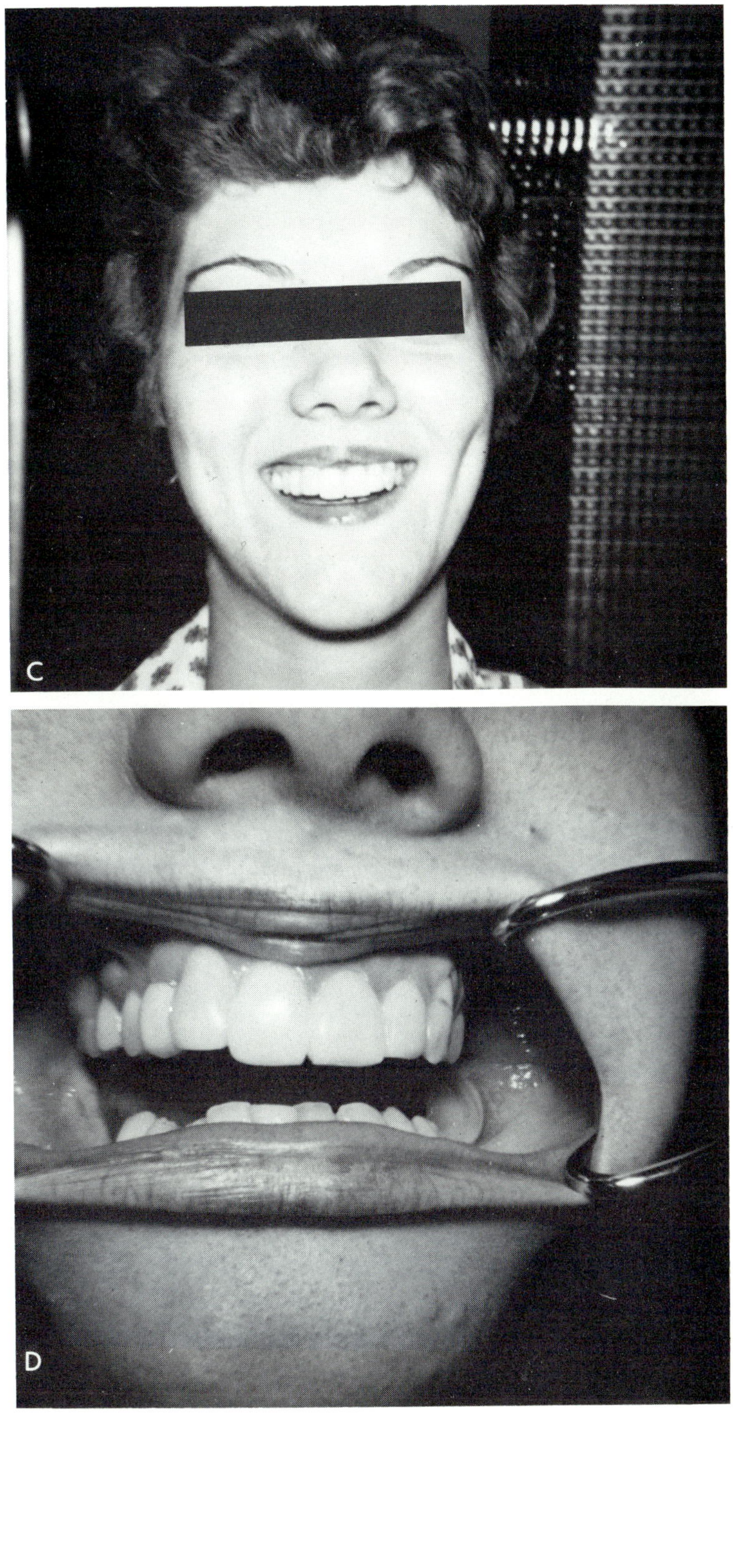

Figure 5–11 *Continued.* Her smile is changed to reflect self-confidence (*C*) after the insertion of a cosmetic veneer (*D*).

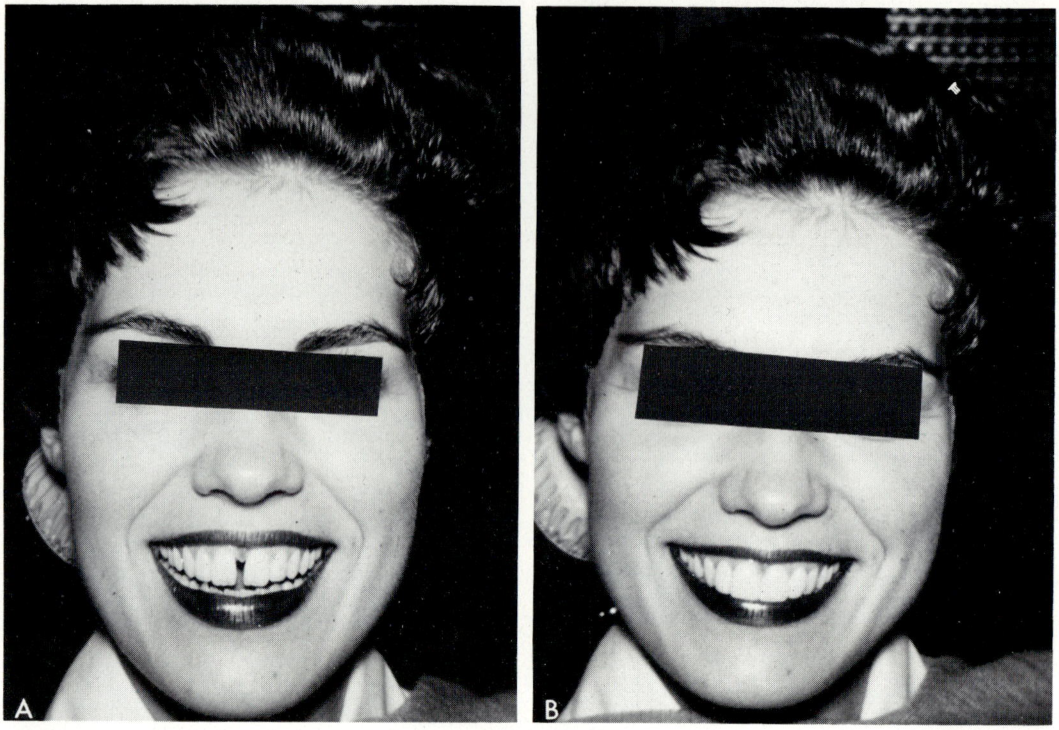

Figure 5–12 A very young lady with a very large gap (*A*) between very large central incisors. Despite concern for the extremely large acrylic resin central incisor covers necessary to close the diastema, the cosmetic veneer produced an attractive smile (*B*).

otherwise beautifully enameled tooth structure. The cosmetic veneer will provide the required esthetic effect.

4. An unusual problem of dental esthetics is presented by a mouth with a high lip line, which shows a lot of gingival tissue when smiling. Not every patient will accept electronic, or other, surgery to raise the necks of the anterior teeth so that longer crowns may be fabricated and the gingival area diminished. A cosmetic veneer may cover both the tooth and a few millimeters of the gingival area above the tooth. This is a periodontal compromise. Special care and consideration are necessary to maintain gingival health. The patient is informed of the problems to gingival health when the acrylic resin rests upon the gingival tissue (Fig. 5–13). If the margins are well polished there is usually a minimum of periodontal annoyance and the cosmetic veneer is very well tolerated by the patient for short periods of time.

5. When the physical or mental condition of a patient is so weak that it allows only a minimum amount of instrumentation, and cosmetic dental improvement is designated to be of therapeutic importance.

A mental patient in a New York City hospital was fitted with a cosmetic veneer as a therapeutic measure. It was prescribed by her psychiatrist after he traced the origin of her mental disorder to a loss of self-esteem resulting from broken upper anterior teeth. She showed remarkable improvement until one day she accidentally dropped the appliance down the washbowl drain. She suffered a severe mental collapse before it was recovered. This was a significant demonstration of the serious importance of a simple dental cosmetic service. This type of dental therapy, once considered "beauty doctoring," has turned out to be a highly effective cure for both dental and mental ills.

6. When it is necessary to win the confidence of an uneducated patient with a broken down dentition who is totally uninterested in the restoration of function. Although this patient may harbor a latent antagonism to dentists and dentistry, he may not be averse to obtaining an improved smile by a simple, inexpensive, and painless procedure. This usually brightens the patient's outlook toward other dental possibilities.

Other Uses of the Cosmetic Veneer

1. Depending on the nature of the bite, the cosmetic veneer may be used to close or fill in spaces and to hide unsightly lower teeth.

2. An unusual use for a cosmetic veneer has recently come into existence. It is used as a protective measure against certain work-related dental defects. Although the relationship is not always obvious, work-related dental disorders are not uncommon. For example, tailors and dressmakers may develop fissures on the incisors as a result of holding thread and pins between the teeth. Other job-related defects may be observed in the mouths of firemen, bakers, and chefs, and others working near intense heat. These people may exhibit unusual carious involvements of the upper anterior teeth and unusual patterns of *chemical erosion of the enamel.* This may be caused by acid formed by a high concentration of carbon dioxide in the work atmosphere combined with intense heat. In bakers and chefs, enamel surface defects may result from alcoholic solvents produced from flour dust particles. Acids are also produced during the degradation of flour. These processes are enhanced by the moist, hot atmosphere of the kitchen and bakery. Steam and fumes containing volatilized end products of the chemical breakdown of food and enzymes may also contact anterior teeth and contribute to enamel defects. Fortunately, many of these defects may be repaired by remineralization of the enamel if the teeth are protected over a period of time by a cosmetic veneer or by covering the involved surfaces with a composite resin filling material bonded to place by acid etching.

3. Occasionally, the necessity for immediate dental esthetics may extend the use of the cosmetic veneer to an heroic endeavor: the replacement of a congenitally missing upper lateral incisor (Fig. 5–14).

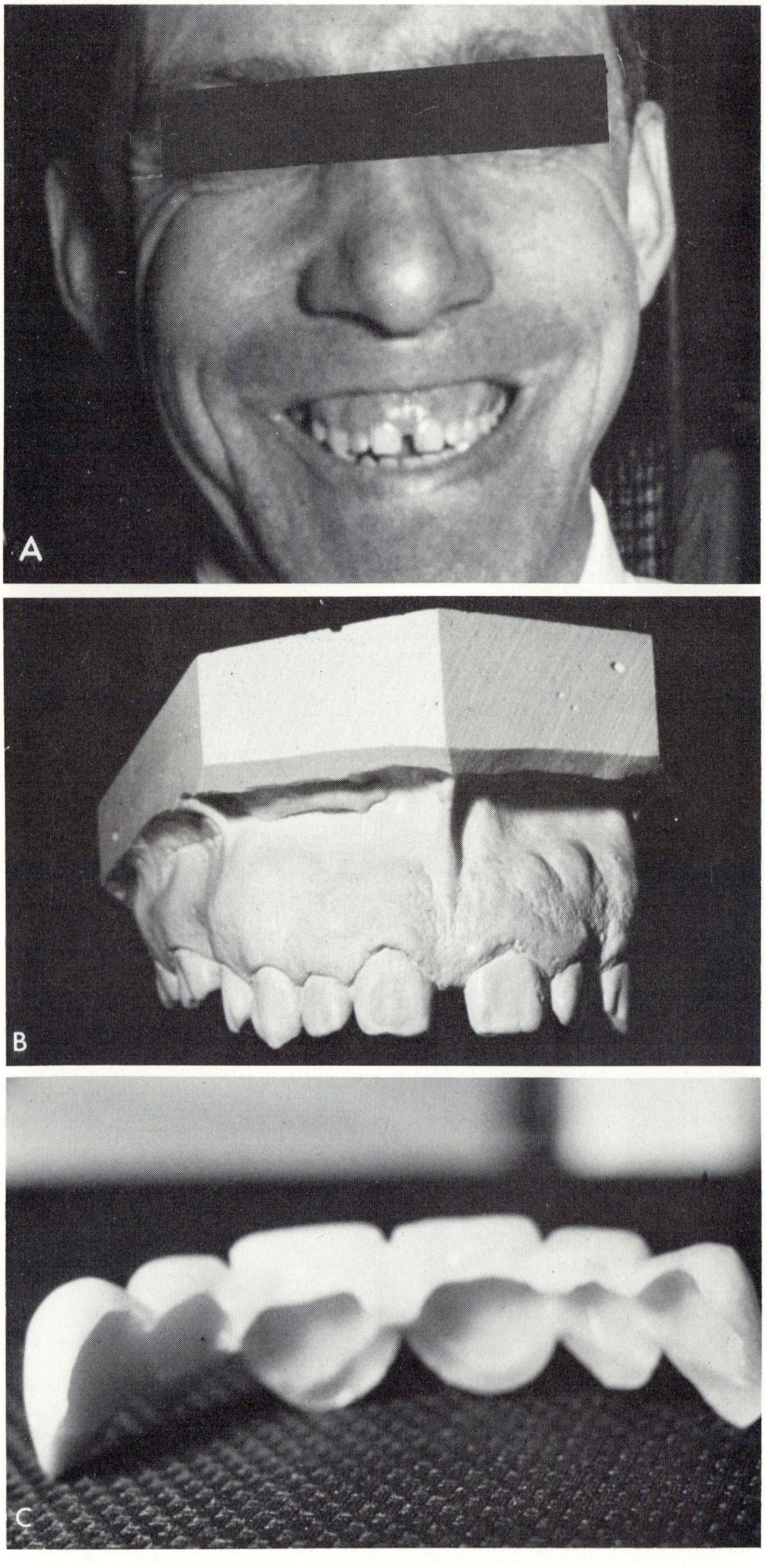

Figure 5–13 *A,* Not every patient is willing or financially able to have electronic or other surgery accomplished to raise the necks of the anterior teeth so that longer jackets may be constructed and the gingival area diminished. *B,* The stone cast of the case involved. Note the large expanse of gingival area. The cosmetic veneer in this case will cover both the tooth and a few millimeters of the gingival area above the tooth. *C,* The cosmetic veneer. This lingual view shows the small area of acrylic resin that overlaps the gingival tissues.

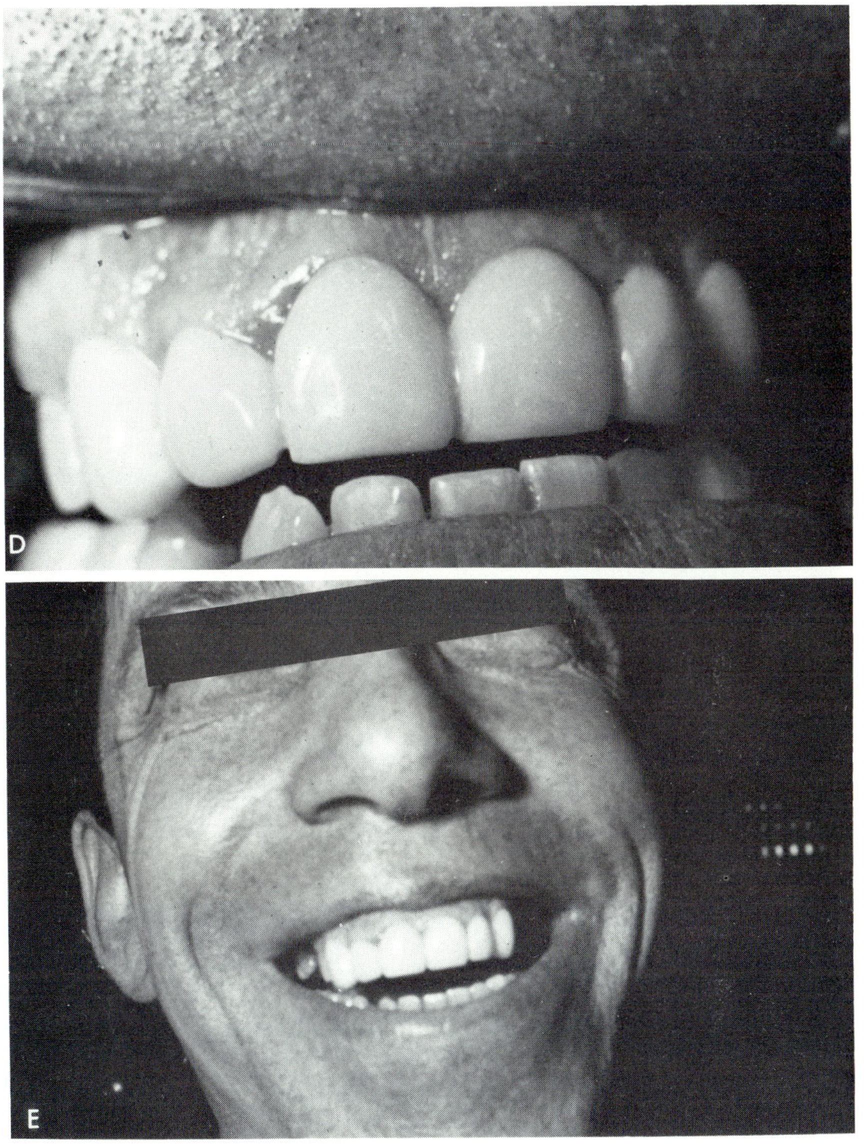

Figure 5–13 *Continued.* *D,* The cosmetic veneer in position, covering both tooth and gingival tissue. The patient is instructed in the limitations of wear when acrylic rests upon the gingiva. *E,* The new look—more tooth, less gum.

Contraindications

1. The cosmetic veneer is contraindicated for the mouth in which there is an edge-to-edge incisal contact.

2. Unless the occlusal relationship allows room (overjet) for acrylic resin to wrap around the incisal edge, a cosmetic veneer should not be made.

3. The cosmetic veneer is not indicated when the upper anterior teeth flare out labially (Fig. 5–15).

4. Upper anterior teeth that have many acrylic resin fillings or cavities should not be covered with a cosmetic veneer.

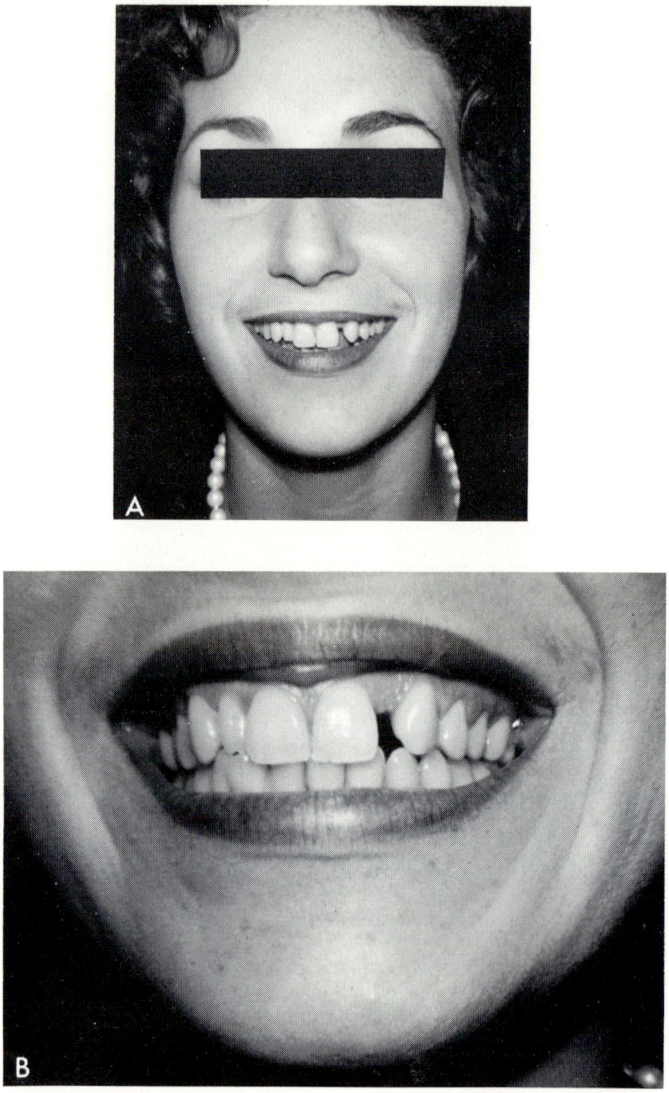

Figure 5–14 *A,* A young adult with attractive upper anterior teeth except for a congenitally missing lateral incisor. *B,* A close look at the smile interrupted by the missing lateral incisor.

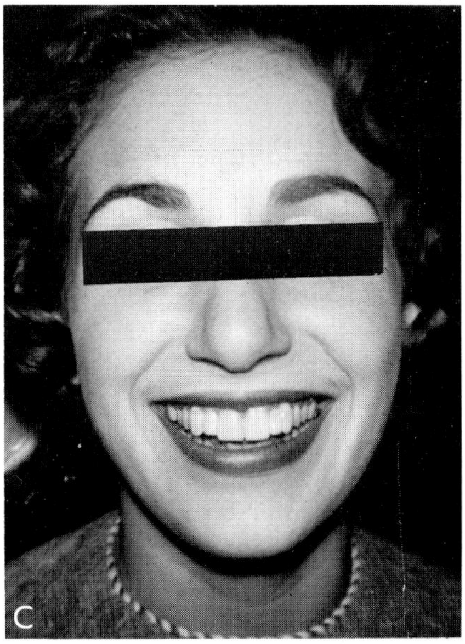

Figure 5–14 *Continued.* *C,* The cosmetic veneer supplies a lateral incisor pontic to close the space.

Maintenance

1. Cosmetic veneers *should not* be cleaned by brushing with a toothbrush and toothpaste. Brushing or scrubbing of any kind will only destroy the surface luster and abrade the resin.[1] Stains may be effectively removed by an overnight soaking in a hypochlorite and water-softener solution (1 teaspoon Clorox, and 2 teaspoons Calgon, in 4 ounces of water).[2] Hot water should be avoided, since it may cause stresses to be released in the acrylic resin resulting in deformation and distortion.[3]

2. When the cosmetic veneer is not being used it should not be allowed to dry out. It should be stored in a small, airtight, glass jar that contains a small amount of moist cotton and a few particles of an antibacterial agent such as methyl- or propylparaben* to prevent bacterial proliferation and odor. All acrylic resins take up and give off water, and in doing so undergo slight dimensional changes. If the cosmetic veneer is allowed to dry out it may be too tight when inserted in the mouth, and breakage may occur.

Practical Considerations

1. Retention may be a concern of the patient prior to treatment. It will not be after the processing of the cosmetic veneer, for it is

---

* Opotow Crown and Bridge Paraben, Teledyne Dental, Elk Grove Village, IL 60007.

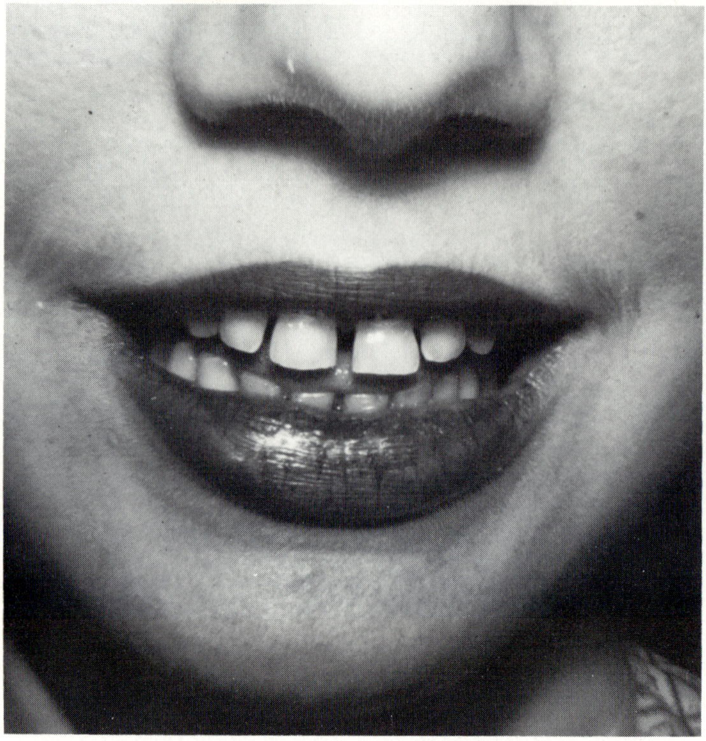

Figure 5–15 Anterior teeth flared out labially, owing to tongue thrust. A cosmetic veneer is contraindicated because of limited space between the teeth and the upper lip and because tongue pressure may evict it or break it. Oral myofunctional therapy is indicated prior to any restorative procedures.

difficult to remove. In fact, some projections and small areas on the contact surface of the resin may have to be ground away to lessen the retention. In this manner, the degree of retention is adjusted until the patient demonstrates the ability to remove the cosmetic veneer. Otherwise, if retention is too positive, breakage may occur when removal is attempted. The excellent retention of a cosmetic veneer is due to the accuracy of fit, the slight dovetailing between the teeth, and the flexibility of the resin, which allows it to spring over small undercuts without breaking.

If retention ever decreases, owing to excessive wear or minor breakage, a denture adhesive powder may be utilized until repair or adjustment is accomplished in the dental office by adding acrylic resin with the brush technique.

2. The patient will experience a stinging sensation when an overflow film of excess acrylic resin contacts the tissues in a confining alginate impression material matrix. This may cause a small amount of discomfort, but only for a very short period of time. It may be prevented, however, by drying the tissues and applying a thin film of mineral oil or dental silicone grease prior to the application of the acrylic resin.

3. All acrylic resin materials contain a slight amount of residual monomer after processing. Although self-curing resins may have slightly more than the heat-curing resins, practically all traces of the residual monomer (extractable by water or saliva) disappear in a few hours after placement in the mouth.

4. Not only are repairs easily accomplished with the resin paint-on brush technique but length, width, thickness, and contour may be modified in the same manner.

5. Modifications of the procedure for the fabrication of the cosmetic veneer presented in this chapter may be utilized. For example, instead of using an alginate impression as a matrix, a silicone putty impression or a vacuum formed plastic sheet may be used to mold the acrylic resin to the teeth.

6. An important precaution in the procedure is the blocking out in the natural teeth of undercuts that may tend to inhibit the initial removal of the hardened resin. Otherwise, efforts to remove the cosmetic veneer may cause it to fracture. After the cosmetic veneer has been removed, grinding adjustments to moderate the retention may be accomplished (Fig. 5–16).

7. Many of the self-curing resins used today have improved color stability, due to the addition of ultraviolet light absorbers. However, there is always a slight change and blending of the color in the first 48 hours after fabrication of the cosmetic veneer. This usually enhances the esthetic effect.

8. Phillips notes that "... the curing of these denture resins at room temperature aids in eliminating many of the processing stresses introduced during heat-curing, with the result that the denture may fit better and be more stable dimensionally."[4] Since polymethyl methacrylate is the resin referred to, and the one used for the cos-

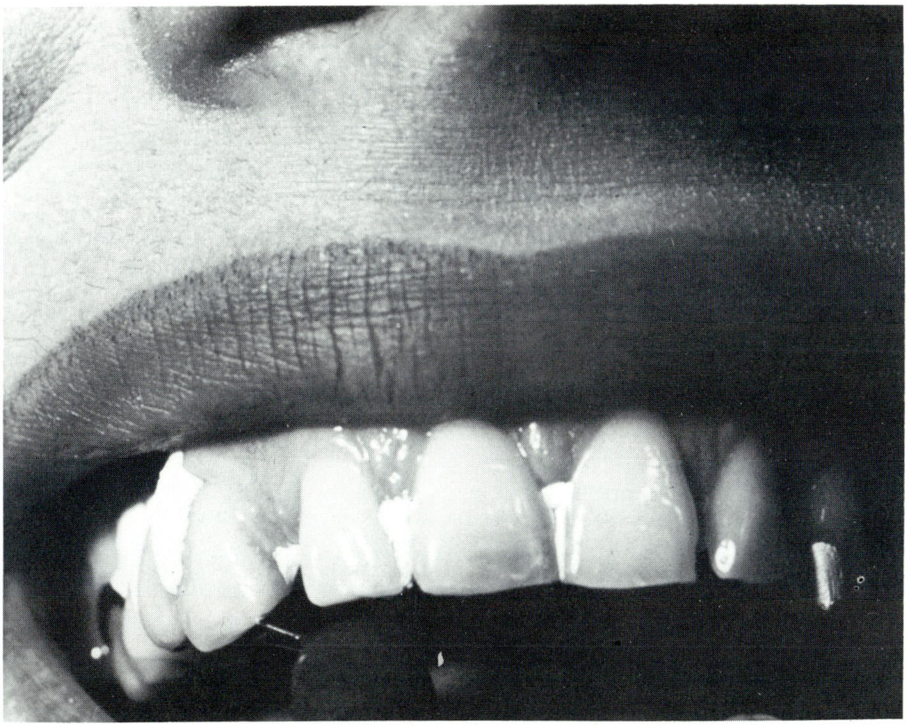

Figure 5–16 An example of a mouth with undercuts blocked out with Cavit in preparation for the fabrication of a cosmetic veneer.

metic veneer, it explains the better fit and dimensional stability of the room temperature-cured cosmetic veneer.

9. As a terminology reminder it should be noted that acrylic resins that are not heat-cured (heat activated) may be designated by the following terms, all of which have the same meaning: self-curing resin, cold-curing resin, room temperature-curing resin, autopolymerizing resin.

10. This method of cosmetic improvement (the cosmetic veneer) should be resorted to more often to help patients in esthetic distress. Especially since it is such an inexpensive and uninvolved procedure.

SUMMARY

Eyelashes, wigs, artificial fingernails, makeup, and many other materials and devices are used to hide unattractive features and to enhance appearance. Cosmetic veneers conceal unattractive teeth and improve the appearance of a smile. This contributes various psychological benefits to a patient, including the restoration of self-confidence. At the same time it enhances the image of dentistry.

Schweitzer, in a book on the treatment and evaluation of problem cases, describes the improvement of esthetics with the use of an "acrylic overlay splint" that is similar to a cosmetic veneer.[5] He points out that esthetics was improved so much that the patient was unwilling to be without the splint. Goldstein, in a recent book on esthetics in dentistry, wisely suggests that an interim procedure such as an "acrylic cosmetic overlay" (similar to the cosmetic veneer) can provide an immediate esthetic result without permanently altering tooth structure.[6] In full accord with these authors, and with respect for their sensitivity to the problems of dental esthetics and the method of treatment, this chapter augments the procedure they suggest with practical considerations and guidelines for improved and less costly therapy through the use of self-curing resin.

REFERENCES

1. Vieira, D. F., and Phillips, R. W.: Influence of certain variables on the abrasion of acrylic resin veneering materials. J. Prosthet. Dent. *12*:720, 1962.
2. Woelfel, J. B.: Newer materials and techniques in prosthetic resin materials. Dent. Clin. North Am. January 1971, p. 71.
3. Craig, R. G., O'Brien, W. J., and Powers, J. M.: Dental Materials. St. Louis, The C. V. Mosby Company, 1975, p. 218.
4. Phillips, R. W.: Science of Dental Materials. 7th ed., Philadelphia, W. B. Saunders Co., 1973, p. 194.
5. Schweitzer, J. M.: Oral Rehabilitation Problem Cases. St. Louis, The C. V. Mosby Company, 1964, p. 263.
6. Goldstein, R. E.: Esthetics in Dentistry, Philadelphia, J. B. Lippincott Company, 1976, p. 248.

six

Materials for Esthetics

If a man will begin with certainties, he will end in doubts, but if he will be content to begin with doubts, he will end in certainties.

Francis Bacon

PORCELAIN AND RESIN

Porcelain and dental resin are the only two materials available that may be used to disguise metal crowns and make them look like natural teeth. Used without metal each of these materials may be fabricated into a translucent tooth-colored crown. Only the porcelain crown has the necessary durability for a final restoration; however, the dental resin crown in its self-cured form makes a most adequate temporary restoration. When used as the veneer component of a gold crown, dental resin makes a durable final restoration; this, in fact, is the restoration of choice over porcelain fused to metal when oral limitations and economic factors dictate the selection. It is important for the dentist to recognize some basic comparisons between these restorative materials, as well as their shortcomings and the factors implicit in their failure.

Comparison

Porcelain is perfectly color stable; dental resin is not. Porcelain resists abrasion; dental resin does not. Unlike porcelain, the sheen and glossy appearance of dental resin are impermanent. Porcelain maintains its luster unless subjected to contact with abrasive materials. The inherent weakness of porcelain, its lack of tensile and shear strength, may be minimized when it is fused (a chemical bond to a large extent) to a cast metal alloy crown that fits the prepared tooth. Dental resin cannot be fused or bonded in any way to metal. It may only be attached by mechanical means. Thermal change, deformation, and other factors contribute to seepage between resin and gold. Seepage is not a problem with the porcelain-metal combination. Porcelain is more likely to break rather than deform under pressure, whereas dental resin will deform readily and resist breaking. Dental resin is more sensitive than porcelain to the expansion and contraction caused by the oral intake of hot and cold foods and beverages. Nevertheless, despite the widely divergent characteristics and the various imperfections of the two materials, both provide esthetic tooth-colored restorations and are used extensively for crowns and fixed partial dentures.

Some Disadvantages of Porcelain Restorations

1. Much of the translucency of porcelain is negated when it is used over metal or opaquing agents.

2. Shrinkage due to the volumetric change that occurs during the firing of porcelain can result in a poor-fitting restoration.

3. Well-defined angles are difficult to produce with porcelain. During firing, sharp angles become rounded. The rounding may destroy the details of an occlusal surface.

4. A minor disadvantage of the porcelain fused to metal restoration is the clicking sounds that may be produced during mastication with opposing porcelain restorations. A more important factor to consider is the impact force transmitted to the periodontium through porcelain to porcelain occlusal contact, which may be detrimental to the biologic health of the underlying hard and soft structures.

5. Porcelain restorations are sensitive to stress concentrations, and brittle fractures may easily occur as a response to overloading. There is also the possibility that the porcelain may separate from the metal to which it is fused.

6. The metal understructure must be thick enough and strong enough to resist flexure. The preparation of an abutment tooth to accept an adequate thickness of metal and porcelain is a threat to the pulpal health of the tooth.

7. Porcelain restorations that contact gold surfaces in occlusion will wear away the gold over a period of time.

Practical Considerations for Porcelain Restorations

1. Since porcelain is fragile, sacrifices must be made for its esthetic benefits. Patients with porcelain restorations should be cautioned to be careful in their eating habits. They must be *constantly alert* to avoid biting cherry, peach, and prune pits, seeds, fish, and chicken bones, and nut shells. They must also be careful at cocktail parties to avoid sliding ice cubes and the sudden contact of elbow, glass, and tooth.

2. Porcelain does not always break at the time of impact. Invisible stresses may lead to subsequent breakage. For this reason, a mallet and an orangewood stick should not be used to refine the seating of a porcelain restoration during cementation. Although seating may be improved slightly, there is no way to know the extent of

stresses inflicted that may ultimately lead to breakage. Adequate seating of porcelain restorations may readily be obtained with strong finger pressure.

3. Porcelain restorations do not have the light absorbing and reflecting qualities of a natural tooth. Brecker[1] noted: "It is impossible to construct porcelain jacket crowns to match every type of tooth without having some difficulty in obtaining color and shade." Actually, all restorations, plastic or porcelain, look different with different lighting or backgrounds. Patients should be advised of these considerations before treatment begins.

4. Two identical porcelain jacket crowns will look different if one is cemented to a tooth that is pulpless or has a metal core or thimble.

5. With the passage of time, a natural tooth next to a porcelain jacket crown will change color. Also, tobacco will stain the natural tooth more readily than it will a porcelain jacket. Eventually the porcelain jacket will stand out as a lighter tooth, although it blended in color with the natural tooth when first inserted.

6. Polycarboxylate cements should not be used with the all-porcelain restoration, since this type of cement does not adhere to porcelain.[2]

7. Zinc phosphate cement is completely opaque and can modify the shade of a porcelain jacket crown because of its light absorption and color. Silicophosphate cement is slightly translucent and less likely to affect the hue.

8. Porcelain fused to metal restorations should be used only when sufficient tooth structure can be reduced to allow for an adequate thickness of metal and porcelain without harming or exposing the pulp.

9. Porcelain fused to metal restorations are contraindicated on very short teeth and on thin, delicate ones.

THE DISCOLORATION OF ACRYLIC RESIN VENEERS

Few things are more distressing to the dentist and his patient than the premature loss of esthetics that results from the discoloration of acrylic resin veneers. The polymer used to disguise a gold cast crown, and for temporary crowns, bridges, and splints, is a material that requires much understanding by the dentist if he is to use it to its best advantage. Acrylic resin can be very perplexing; sometimes it changes color, sometimes it does not. Clinical observations indicate also that the rate of discoloration varies. Sometimes acrylic resin discoloration occurs in a relatively short period of time after insertion, yet at other times adequate color may be maintained over a prolonged period of time. Dentists complain that acrylic resin is an inferior material. "Look how it discolors" is a frequent remark. Nevertheless, there are times when it is indicated, when no other material will suffice. When resin is utilized as a veneer to camouflage metal, there are factors implicit to failure that dentists must recognize. When these factors are understood, conditions can be modified, allowing both a greater degree of success and a comprehensive understanding of the occasional failures.

If the factors leading to the failure of acrylic resins remain unrecognized by the dentist, the resin material may be blamed erroneously for inadequate end-results.

There is a well-accepted philosophy in dentistry: Faulty technique and lack of knowledge concerning the factors involved in success or failure are the true shortcomings of a dental material.

For our purpose, discoloration is defined as a complexity involving internal color modification (yellow, brown, or gray), surface staining, and loss of surface gloss. It can occur during the hardening process as well as during prolonged periods of use.

Shortcomings of Acrylic Resin

Aside from discoloration, each of the general shortcomings of acrylic resin contributes to color modification, as follows:

1. Low Resistance to Wear and Abrasion. The low resistance of acrylic resin to wear and abrasion allows an acrylic resin surface to lose its original polished appearance and to present areas of various degrees of roughness. Stains from food, medicaments, and other sources become deeply engrained and difficult to remove.

2. Inability to Bond to Metal. Because acrylic resin does not bond to metal, thermal changes cause the resin and metal components of a gold veneer crown to expand and contract differently. Separation occurs, and the leakage of saliva, debris, and the end-products of food decomposition imparts a grayish discoloration to the acrylic resin. The inability of the acrylic resin to bond to metal causes it to be very sensitive to separation from the metal when deformation occurs.

3. Deformation under Pressure. Functional occlusal forces not only are capable of deforming the thin walls of a metal casting but also can very readily distort the entire body of acrylic resin adjacent to it. This causes separation, and the leakage that ensues causes the resin to discolor.

4. High Coefficient of Thermal Expansion. The high coefficient of thermal expansion also contributes to discoloration. Hot and cold foods and beverages cause the resin to expand and shrink. This may create spaces between a veneer and casting that allow fluids and debris to enter. Discoloration results from this reduction of the initial adaptation of resin to metal.

5. Polymerization Shrinkage. The shrinkage that occurs during processing is an undesirable feature of acrylic resin. Water sorption may compensate in part for this dimensional change. However, Lamstein and Blechman[3] have shown that the volumetric changes during the curing process cause marginal seepage and a discolored acrylic resin veneer.

CATEGORIES OF DISCOLORATION FACTORS

The factors implicated in the discoloration of acrylic resin veneers may be divided as follows into three categories according to where they originate:

1. During manufacturing and formulation
2. During fabrication and manipulation
   a. In the dental laboratory
   b. In the dental treatment room
3. During utilization
   a. Factors in the mouth
   b. Factors outside the mouth

During Manufacturing and Formulation

Impurities incorporated during manufacture may predispose the resin materials to discoloration, as will certain organic dyes that tend to leach out. Plasticizers should be used sparingly in dental resins. They are used to increase the solubility of the polymer in the monomer and to lessen dough-forming time. However, too much plasticizer may lead to discoloration by leaching out. Cross-linking agents of low purity should not be utilized. Ethylene glycol dimethacrylate, dental grade, is of high purity and is especially effective as a cross-linking agent for dental acrylic.

Other factors that influence discoloration during manufacturing and formulation are as follows:

Poor storage conditions and an extended shelf life

Water-soluble ingredients

The nature and concentration of inhibitor in the monomer and concentration of peroxide used as initiator

The presence of a tertiary aromatic amine.

During Fabrication and Manipulation

a. In the Dental Laboratory

1. DESIGN OF THE BOXING TO HOLD ACRYLIC. Discoloration depends on the following:

Depth of boxing, especially cervical third.

Retention method, undercuts, loops, or beads.

The type of gold utilized. Flash gold-plating avoids a gray look and lessens discoloration due to oxidation on contamination.

2. POLYMERIZATION. Factors involved that may contribute to future discoloration are as follows:

Incorrect amount of monomer, evaporation in the mixing jar, and excessive pressure in the flask.

The use of a red-bulb syringe. When this is placed down in a horizontal position, monomer may flow into the bulb and pick up some of its color and contaminate the resin.

The manipulation of plastic dough with bare hands. Monomer is a good solvent for body oils and will pick up dirt from the hands. Color tests show that it is possible to transfer skin oils to the dough, with measurable changes in the final color.

Porosity leads to absorption of moisture, food, and cleaning materials, and therefore causes staining and odor.

Heat applied too quickly, not enough pressure, packing before dough stage, overly high temperatures, and insufficient mixing of powder and liquid all lead to discoloration.

Rapid cooling leading to the formation of stresses and packing too stiff, causing poor flow and ultimately poor retention must also be avoided.

3. FINISHING AND POLISHING. Heat will depolymerize acrylic resin. Even that amount of heat engendered in routine finishing and polishing may cause depolymerization. A small amount of this on the surface may lead to discoloration. It should be recognized that the speed, heat and dryness involved in polishing gold is transmitted to the resin that is in intimate contact with the metal. To polish acrylic resin a wet polishing wheel should be used at slow speed to avoid excessive local temperatures and the initiation of surface stresses.

The curvature and form of a piece of acrylic resin used to veneer a gold crown is almost identical to the curvature and form of the palate of a complete denture. In fact, an acrylic resin veneer separated from its metal framework looks like a miniature denture palate. The acrylic resin used as a crown and bridge veneer and that used as the denture base material for a complete denture are exactly the same except for a difference in color. The physical properties and handling characteristics of one are similar to those of the other.

A research endeavor has shown that denture bases of heat-curing or self-curing acrylic resins become *warped under routine grinding and polishing.*[4] It is suggested that, whenever possible, no grinding or polishing be done, particularly on the palate sections of these dentures. Tests showed that all these dentures warped when ground under fairly heavy pressure, and that polishing induced still further warping. Distortion was most apparent in the palate sections.

Acrylic resin veneers are subject to the same warpage, and this results in discoloration along the margins that have distorted away from the metal casting. These veneers should be waxed to the proper thickness, foiled, and if possible, finished and polished with *the least possible amount of heat or pressure.*

WETTABILITY WITH SILICON TETRACHLORIDE. A thin film of silica makes resin easy to keep clean and may reduce the potential for staining.[5]

b. In the Dental Treatment Room. The dentist receives the restorations veneered with acrylic resin from his own or a commercial laboratory. At this time adjustments for esthetics, occlusion, contacts and tissue compatibility are made. Final cementation of single crowns follows. For a fixed partial denture or splint, however, biologic evaluation in the form of temporary cementation is called for. *In these manipulations, adjusting and cementing, the dentist has a great opportunity to contribute unknowingly to the future discoloration of the acrylic resin material involved.* This can be minimized when the following are recognized:

1. ADJUSTMENTS. Grinding away occlusal prematurities on the gold crown, and grinding to adjust contact points, to modify contours, and to remove removal buttons *imparts a great deal of heat to the metal and in turn to the acrylic* and to the hand holding it. Sometimes, grinding makes metal so hot it can hardly be held in the hand. This heat is also picked up by the acrylic resin. Not only does it predispose the resin to early discoloration but it also softens it and increases the chances for a "popping out" of the veneer. Grinding the acrylic veneer to modify its thickness or contour will require smoothing, finishing, and polishing. As noted before, these all contribute to warpage and discoloration.
2. TEMPORARY CEMENTATION. Most of the cements used for the temporary cementation of fixed prostheses are formulations of zinc oxide and eugenol. During insertion, an excess of this cement is extruded onto the buccal or labial surface of a restoration. Since a phenolic compound of any type has a deleterious effect on acrylic resin and tends to depolymerize it, the veneers should be protected from contacting the eugenol cement by a previously applied film of silicone grease (Opotow Dental Silicone*). The silicone grease should be smeared over buccal and lingual surfaces and placed into the interproximal surfaces for protection of the acrylic and to facilitate removal of hardened excess cement.
3. FINAL CEMENTATION. "For almost a century zinc phosphate cement has been the most successful dental cementing medium but it is now being replaced by modified zinc oxide–eugenol cements . . ." So reads the first sentence of the chapter on dental cements in the *Guide to Dental Materials,* American Dental Association, Ed. 6, p. 48.

   With the increased utilization of EBA-modified and resin-reinforced zinc oxide and eugenol cement there is a need for the protection of resin surfaces that may be contacted by excess cement. Although silicone grease is recommended for this purpose, clinicians have been known to use petrolatum, carding wax and Albolene oil. These agents should be kept away from the margins. Regardless

---

*Teledyne Dental, Elk Grove, Chicago, IL 60007

of the protective film utilized, the eugenol component may still penetrate and attack the acrylic resin veneer and predispose it to discoloration. Therefore, the excess of zinc oxide and eugenol cement that flows out over an acrylic resin veneer should not be allowed to remain until hardened. It should be wiped away with a cotton roll or gauze immediately after complete seating of the restoration. This will minimize the time of contact of the excess cement and the acrylic resin, and therefore limit the deleterious effect on the resin, since it is related to the length of time they are in contact.

During Utilization

Factors in the Mouth. If all the details and positive considerations of manufacturing, formulation, fabrication, and manipulation of acrylic resin are favorable, the material should not be predisposed to discoloration. However, the true test is now at hand. After installation in the mouth the resin must contend with threats to its color maintenance from within and without the oral environment.

The oral environment is a complex and unique area of dynamic changes that is considered to be as heroic a vicinity as outer space. Although outer space has much larger thermal changes, it does not have the microorganisms, changing pH, and enzyme activity that are found in the mouth. Dental plastics stored in the oral environment are predisposed to the resultant effects of physical, thermal, and chemical attack.

PHYSICAL ATTACK. Acrylic resin is subject to deformation from the great stresses in the oral cavity. Masticatory forces, tongue thrust, and other muscular actions create diverse pressures against fixed restorations. The type of occlusion is a factor of concern. Occlusal and impact forces cause sudden overloads on resins, restorations, and teeth. Also, a premature occlusal contact introduces torque that can deform the metal frame of an acrylic veneer and loosen it, and thus allow leakage and discoloration.

Abrasion caused by gritty particles of food, toothpastes, and toothbrushing may cause a resin surface to become discolored. Thermal changes may cause leakage that leads to discoloration, or they may crack or craze the resin so that stains set in easily.

Teeth and restorations in the mouth are bathed in some degree of moisture most of the time; however, when nasal infections are present, during dental procedures, and in activities such as speechmaking, conditions of excessive dryness occur. Another determinant of the amount of saliva present is emotion, which may be depicted by the wetness of "mouth-watering anticipation" or the dry mouth of fear. The humidity in the mouth may range from zero to 100 per cent. The absorption of water by acrylic resin is of considerable importance, since it is accompanied by dimensional changes.

Bruxism, other oral habits, and periodontal conditions may present a complexity of forces that burden the acrylic resin veneer and contribute to its discoloration.

CHEMICAL ATTACK. Ingested material may play a part in the discoloration of acrylic resin veneers. Food and beverages supply artificial and natural dyes, preservatives, chelating agents, and carbonates. Hot tars from tobacco smoke may discolor resin and natural teeth. However, even more discoloration may be caused by organic solvents in medications, anesthetics, and alcoholic drinks. Alcohol is especially harmful to resin restorations. Its contact with teeth and restorations in the mouth should be minimized. Patients should be cautioned not to savor alcoholic drinks in the mouth for more than a moment. The lingering taste should be replaced by the fast gulp. Alcohol should be swallowed fast to avoid possible harm to resins used for dentures, fillings, or veneers.

Toothpastes also contribute to the chemical attack on acrylic resin. *Accepted Dental Therapeutics*, Ed. 35, American Dental Association, pp. 309–310, lists three popular brands of toothpaste *that contain up to 3 per cent chloroform.* They are Close Up, Macleans and Ultra Brite. Repeated application of a strong solvent like chloroform is deleterious to a resin surface. Acrylic veneers, denture base resin, unfilled resin fillings and composite resin filling materials, resin cements, and pit and fissure sealants are harmed by contact with chloroform. Discoloration and accelerated wear are manifestations of the chemical attack.

With ingested material leading the parade of organic acids, sulfides, ammonia derivatives, and other chemical agents in one direction, another attacking army of chemical agents threatens the acrylic from the opposite direction. From inside the body, *breath, belching, and regurgitation bring new and potent chemicals and gases.* These contribute to the changing chemical nature of the mouth, and to the ever-changing pH. Acetone is a strong solvent that attacks acrylic resin. Because *diabetics may secrete acetone or other ketone bodies during respiration,* porcelain should replace resin in the selection of a restorative material for them. Resin fillings and cements should also be avoided. Silicate fillings and zinc phosphate cement will be more durable in the diabetic mouth.

Under certain conditions, enzymes, acidic products, and other secretions produced by microorganisms digest both the surfaces of teeth *and the restorative materials.*

The modifications to an acrylic resin material caused by contact with various strong chemical agents are not limited exclusively to surface discoloration; tensile strength and resistance to abrasion may also be lowered. This may explain in part why acrylic veneers "pop" out of supposedly retentive crown housings prematurely and why in certain instances they abrade rapidly, exposing the underlying metal.

Factors Outside the Mouth. Not only is acrylic resin material subject to physical and chemical insults from the torture chamber within the mouth, it is also the target for the onslaught of a wide variety of deleterious agents from outside the mouth.

HAIR-SPRAY POLYMERS. In 1958 a relationship between lung disease and hair-spray inhalation was suggested.[6] Since then a large body of *medical* literature has been devoted to this subject.[7-10] The aerosol or pressurized spray can is not as innocent as it looks from its outside packaging. Its function requires the use of gases that may be inhaled, absorbed, or swallowed. If medical science is concerned about spray materials reaching the lungs, dental science should recognize that it can reach the teeth just as easily. Spray-can furniture polish and oven cleaner are only two of a wide variety of sprays used in close proximity to the mouth and teeth. There is no sure method of using sprays to guarantee that they will not enter the mouth. The contents of spray cans are propelled by fluorocarbon, nitrous oxide, and methylene chloride propellants. These materials, plus chemical contents such as aniline dyes, may contribute to the discoloration of acrylic resin veneers.

Other sprays that may gain access to the mouth and have a harmful effect on acrylic resin are perfumes, colognes, after-shave lotions, deodorants, insect repellents, and sun-screen agents. Since substitutes are available for most spray products, patients should be advised to favor them.

LIPSTICK. The application of lipsticks, lip pencils, and lip glosses should be accomplished without contacting teeth restored with acrylic resin. These cosmetics are occasionally smeared over anterior teeth by accident. The chemicals, pigments, and aromatic and coloring agents in some of these products may discolor acrylic resin if allowed to remain for more than a few moments. Patients with acrylic resin restorations should be cautioned to apply lipsticks carefully and to wipe away without delay any of the cosmetic that touches the teeth.

VAPORS. Acrylic resin should not be selected as a restorative material for a patient who might be continuously exposed to gasoline vapors, which will predispose the resin to turn yellow and then brown in a relatively short period of time. In fact, various other vapors have a similar action on acrylic; for example, cleaning fluids, benzene, chloroform, and nail polish remover.

In this age of complex industrial processes, in which new and powerful solvents are being utilized there is always a possibility of exposure which, while apparently harmless to the patient, may have a cumulative effect on the plastic in his dental restorations.

SUMMARY

The widespread use of acrylic resin may be due to its strength, low solubility, ease of fabrication, and excellent initial esthetic qualities. However, all restorative dental materials have a number of shortcomings and imperfections, and acrylic resin is no exception. It has, nevertheless, been a boon to dentistry. For crown and bridge work, acrylic seems to be as satisfactory as any other resin.[11] Where it is indicated to disguise metal, dentists should understand the factors that may cause it to fail its purpose. It is important to know that the discoloration of acrylic resin veneers may be a result of prolonged contact with eugenol cement, the heat of polishing and adjusting, or exposure to fumes, solvents, and various chemical agents. Recognition of these factors and others gives the dentist an opportunity to modify conditions for a greater degree of success.

Assuming that there has been perfection in manufacture and formulation, the acrylic resin veneer will be a successful restorative component if it is well designed with regard to retention, boxing, and occlusal protection; if it is processed and adjusted carefully with concern for contact with heat and chemicals; and if the patient is cautioned to protect against the various internal and external abusive agents.

In conclusion, it should also be noted that many unsuspected factors similar to the ones that contribute to modification of acrylic resin may also be implicated in the failure of other restorative materials in the mouth. For example, although chlorine may not be harmful to acrylic resin, it does attack chromium alloys.[12] A large number of removable partial dentures are constructed from chromium alloys, and these alloys are also being developed for fixed restorations. How does chlorine get in the mouth? It is well known that proprietary cleaning agents or bleaches that contain chlorine should be avoided. One reliable and seldom recognized source of oral contact with chlorine is in the swimming pool. Every mouthful of water the swimmer gets contains chlorine.

REFERENCES

1. Brecker, S. C.: Clinical Procedures in Occlusal Rehabilitation. 2nd ed., Philadelphia, W. B. Saunders Co., 1966, p. 408.
2. Phillips, R. W.: Science of Dental Materials. 7th ed., Philadelphia, W. B. Saunders Co., 1973, p. 546.
3. Lamstein, A., and Blechman, H.: Marginal seepage around acrylic resin veneers in gold crowns. J. Prosthet. Dent. *6*:706, 1956.
4. Mason, H. J.: Extreme warpage of resin dentures in routine grinding and polishing. North-West Dent. *43*:97–99, 1964.
5. O'Brien, W. J., and Ryge, G.: Wettability of poly (methyl methacrylate) treated with silicon tetrachloride. J. Prosthet. Dent. *15*:304–308, March-April 1965.
6. Bergmann, M., et al.: Thesaurosis following inhalation of hair spray. N. Engl. J. Med. *258*:471–476, 1958.
7. Bergmann, M., et al.: Thesaurosis due to inhalation of hair spray. N. Engl. J. Med. *266*:750–755, 1962.
8. Morgan, W. K. C.: Thesaurosis following inhalation of hair spray. Lancet *2*:412, 1959.
9. DeNosaquo, N.: Hair sprays and blood dyscrasias. J.A.M.A., *188*:197, (April 13) 1964.
10. Giovacchini, R. P., et al.: Pulmonary disease and hair-spray polymers. J.A.M.A., *193*:298, (July 26) 1965.
11. Peyton, F. A., and Craig, R. G.: Current evaluation of plastics in crown and bridge resins. J. Prosthet. Dent. *13*:743, 1963.
12. Phillips, R. W., Swartz, M. L., and Norman, R. D.: Materials for the Practicing Dentist. St. Louis, C. V. Mosby Co., 1969, p. 202.

seven

Biophysical Factors Related to Retention

The best laid schemes o' mice an' men
Gang aft a-gley;
An' lea'e us naught but grief and pain
For promised joy.

Robert Burns

Cementation apparently brings a crown and bridge restoration to its conclusion by making it "fixed." Until dental cement is allowed to harden between the walls of the restoration and the prepared teeth, the fixed restoration is still removable. It seems, therefore, that the cement makes it "fixed." And, generally, the connotation is that the cement provides all the retention. Premature loosening of a fixed restoration is referred to as "cement failure." Dentists concerned about retention frequently ask, "What cement shall I use?" or, "What cement do you use?" Unfortunately, they harbor *the erroneous concept that successful retention depends only on a cementing material.* It does not. Retention depends almost completely on certain biophysical factors pertinent to the abutment tooth, the fixed prosthesis, and the oral environment. Actually, no dental cement is adhesive to prepared tooth structure or to the restoration. Nevertheless, cement does contribute to the retention of a fixed restoration, but it is an adjunct to retention and not the sole source. The marginal seal and insulation supplied by a cement may be equally or more important than the aid it gives in retention.

A fixed restoration that is totally dependent on dental cement for retention may eventually loosen.

What, then, determines whether or not a fixed restoration stays fixed? What are the reasons for "cement failures?" And what is the answer to the question, "What cement shall I use?" The answer to these questions is summed up in another question: "What are the biophysical factors involved?" It is certainly true that the effective installation of a fixed retention *is* dependent on the cement employed and the efficacy of the cementation procedure—but there are other very important considerations; namely, *the biophysical characteristics of the structures (restorations and teeth) being joined together.* Various features of the oral environment (the storage place of restoration/cement/teeth) must also be considered significant to the integrity of the cement bond. Indeed, the sealing of an inert foreign body to prepared tooth structure in the moist, heavily stressed human mouth is only partly contingent on cement. It is, however, very dependent on the biophysical factors related to 1) The abutment tooth; 2) the fixed prosthesis, and; 3) the oral environment.

Understanding and recognition of these factors will be helpful not only for successful final cementation but also in *the selection of an appropriate temporary cement* for both temporary and permanent crowns and bridges.

BIOPHYSICAL FACTORS RELATED TO THE ABUTMENT TOOTH

The use of tooth-reduction apparatus to obtain a properly prepared abutment tooth is guided by the need for adequate reduction of the various tooth surfaces to meet biologic, esthetic and preventive requirements. For example, when preparing abutment teeth, the dentist must keep in mind the requirements of space—interproximal space, occlusal space, space for esthetics, gingival space, and the space required to maintain the integrity of the pulp chamber. Each surface is reduced to an adequate depth for a specific reason. Examples follow.

Occlusal Reduction

This is done to allow room for a proper thickness of restorative material. This facilitates the forming of proper occlusal anatomy in the restoration. Proper occlusal anatomy permits the most efficient mastication of food and reduces the load transmitted to the underlying tooth. Adequate occlusal coverage protects against the transmission of impact forces to the cement film that separates it from the tooth structure.

Proximal Reduction

This type of reduction is done to provide parallel walls for retention and enough space for multiple layers of restorative material (cement, metal, porcelain or resin). Most importantly, it provides enough room for the interdental papilla to exist without disturbance. Proximal reduction also allows better tooth to tooth contact areas and marginal ridges.

Buccal and Labial Reduction

Buccal and labial reduction must provide enough room to allow esthetic coverage of the metal crown without causing an excessive buccal bulge. Here also the nature of the gingival margin is of special concern. Its form and placement are influenced by esthetics, cariogenicity, and periodontal conditions.

Lingual Reduction

Although lingual reduction may be of less importance than that of the other surfaces, it is nevertheless of importance as far as resistance to deformation, periodontal health, tongue room, and speech are concerned.

Factors That Influence Retention

The preparation of tooth structure to accommodate a casting is actually *the first step to successful retention.* The tooth must be sculptured to enhance its coupling with the casting. While doing this, the dentist should keep in mind the biophysical factors related to the abutment tooth discussed in this chapter that influence retention and the cement bond. Knowledge of these factors will guide his hand in shaping an abutment tooth for the best possible retention. They are as follows:

Length

Retention increases with an increase in the length of the abutment tooth. In most instances the height or length should be kept to the maximum that allows adequate coverage of the occlusal or incisal surface. However, if the space for occlusal coverage is too thin, the cement may be destroyed by the pounding of the opposing cusps. Thin occlusal coverage allows the transmission of forces. When heavy impact forces are transmitted through the thin occlusal surface of the crown, the cement may fracture. Also, a hole may develop after moderate wear and allow leakage and accelerated disintegration of the underlying cement. Torque may produce loosening of a casting more readily when the cement bond is to a short abutment tooth (Fig. 7–1). A good rule to follow in the preparation of tooth structure is the taller the abutment tooth, the more tapered the walls may be.

Occasionally, when the occlusal surface of a tooth with a short clinical crown is reduced to allow for adequate coverage by a crown, the remaining tooth structure is almost flat and flush with the surrounding gingival tissue. In this instance, it may be helpful to expose more of the crown by cutting away some of the gingival tissue around it, preferably with the wire electrode. For retentive form on a very short tooth all walls should be made as vertical as possible, with little or no taper.

Kaufman, Coelho and Colin[1] have pointed out the importance of abutment length in improving the retention of castings, and this is adequately confirmed by clinical experience. With minimum abutment crown length, increased retention may be provided, not only by more parallel walls, but by multiple pins or by splinting additional abutments.

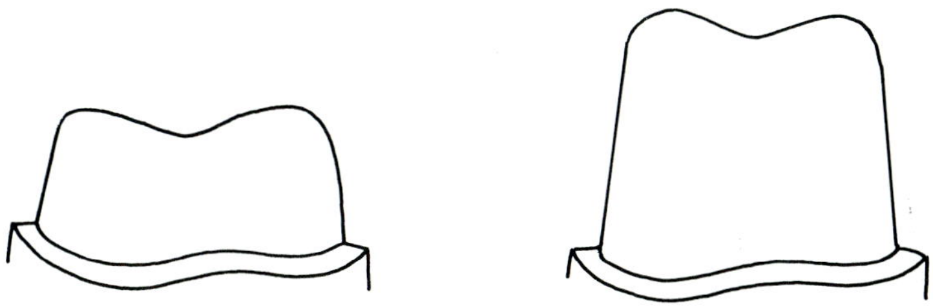

Figure 7–1 Abutment preparations of similar contour, taper, and diameter, but of different length. The short preparation provides less retention.

Taper

The most important factor in the retention of castings is the taper or convergence of the preparation.[1] *Retention increases as the walls of the abutment preparation approach parallelism* (Fig. 7–2). An increase in parallelism is much more important to better retention than an increase in the length of a preparation. An overtapered preparation should be avoided. The "ice cream cone" preparation does not provide for a retentive coupling with a casting. Another good rule to follow in the preparation of tooth structure is the shorter the abutment tooth, the more parallel the walls.

Shape

If cement confined to the occlusal or incisal surface of a prepared abutment tooth must travel around sharp line angles to escape from this area during the seating of a casting, it is sometimes trapped therein and its impeded exit inhibits the complete seating of the casting. Also, stress concentrations in the cement at these sharp line angles on the prepared tooth surface have shown them to be potential sites for failure.[2] Abutment teeth with rounded occlusal or incisal contours allow cement to escape from the occlusal area as the casting is seated (Fig. 7–3). This allows more complete seating of a fixed restoration. The more completely the restoration is seated, the better the retention. Asymmetric shapes resist rotation that could loosen an abutment casting. Intracoronal accessory pits and grooves enhance retention where needed.

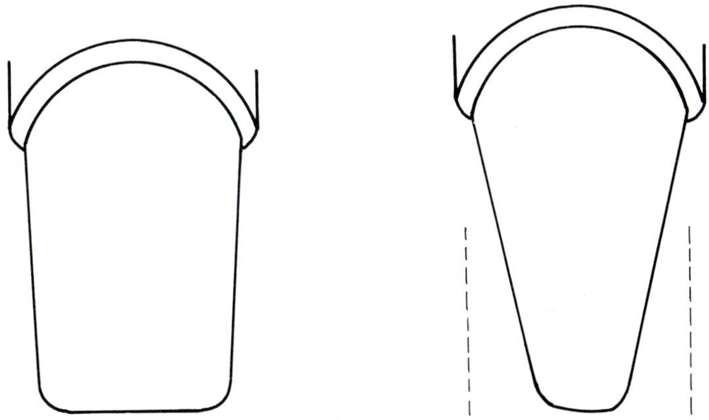

Figure 7–2 An abutment preparation with parallel walls will provide more retention than a similar preparation with tapered walls.

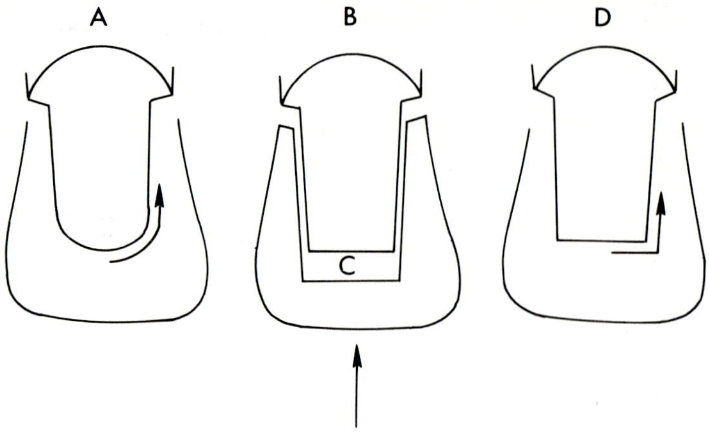

Figure 7–3 A, An abutment tooth with rounded incisal contours allows easier flow and escape of cement as a crown is seated. B, With squared-off or sharp incisal line angles, cement may be trapped in the incisal area (C) during insertion, owing to the slow-down in flow around the sharp corners (D). The ultimate perfection of seating of the crown depends on the extrusion of all the cement at C. Anything that impedes its exit causes a larger ultimate film thickness in this area, faulty seating, and decreased retention.

The shape of a prepared abutment tooth is influenced by the establishment of a full shoulder at the gingival margin. This acts as a guide to the dental laboratory technician, shows the extent of the preparation, allows room for esthetic coverage, and may provide some biologic and periodontal benefits. However, it is not without fault. It has been shown that sharp angles at the gingival shoulders are to be avoided, since these areas are more sensitive to failure than are restorations with rounded line angles.[3] Because of the concentration of forces, a prepared abutment tooth may fracture at the full shoulder area in the mouth of an old patient. A chamfer preparation is more advisable for older and more brittle teeth. Also, caries initiated by the ever-present microleakage may proliferate more rapidly into the acute angle of a full shoulder preparation (Fig. 7–4). Another consideration may be the ease of the flow of escaping excess cement when a crown is seated on a full shoulder preparation as compared to a chamfer preparation. A squared-off full shoulder may impede the

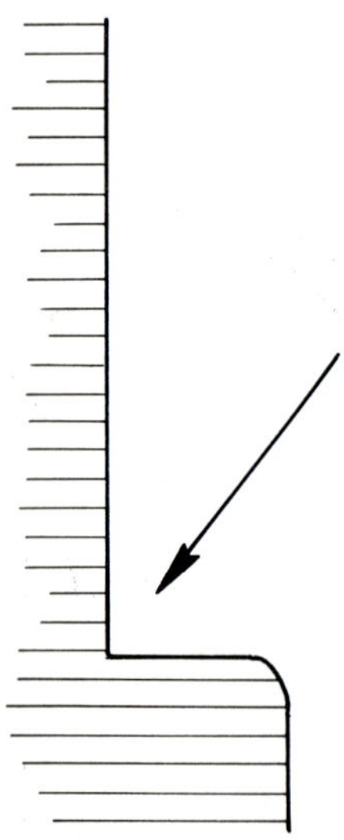

Figure 7–4 The crevice formed by the angle of a full shoulder preparation may be more conducive to the proliferation of recurrent caries than the smooth curved area of a chamfer preparation.

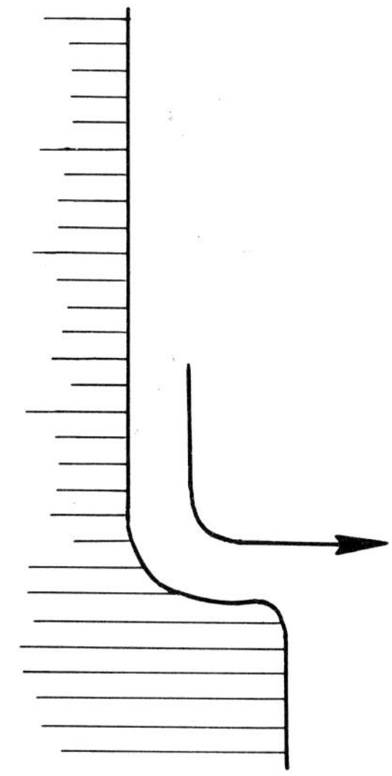

Figure 7–5 Rounded contours anywhere on a prepared abutment tooth facilitate the flow and escape of excess cement and tend to minimize hydrodynamic phenomena.

escape of cement in a manner similar to the aforementioned occlusal and incisal line angle (Fig. 7–5). Occasionally a dentist who is enslaved by the full shoulder concept may cause a pulp exposure in his zealous attempt to create a shoulder where it is not indicated, and sometimes where it is. Another consideration is marginal fit. A discrepancy in the seating of a casting to a full shoulder preparation will cause a poor marginal adaptation at the gingival area. In the same situation, a chamfer margin is better.[4]

The shaping and design of the gingival area of a crown preparation should incorporate the biologic principles of pulp preservation, considerations for the protection of soft tissues, room for esthetics, rounded line angles, and a guideline for finishing, regardless of whether it is designated a full shoulder, a chamfer, or anything else.

In sculpturing an abutment tooth, some surfaces are more important than others for the ultimate retention of a casting. The buccal or lingual surface of an abutment preparation on a posterior tooth may supply resistance to displacement during forceful working occlusion in mastication. Generally, the *lingual wall of the lower preparation* and the *buccal wall of the upper preparation* provide resistance to functional displacement if they have minimal convergence from the long axis of the tooth. If these surfaces are too tapered, resistance to displacement is less, and the upper may be displaced lingually and the lower buccally. Of course, when these surfaces are more vertical, they resist displacement in these directions (Fig. 7–6).

Surface Texture

Although a smooth preparation facilitates impression making, it has been shown that slightly roughened surfaces contribute to a stronger bond. Accordingly, a short preparation or one that lacks the proper parallelism should be roughened slightly before final cementation to enhance retention. Also, a surface notch or indentation on

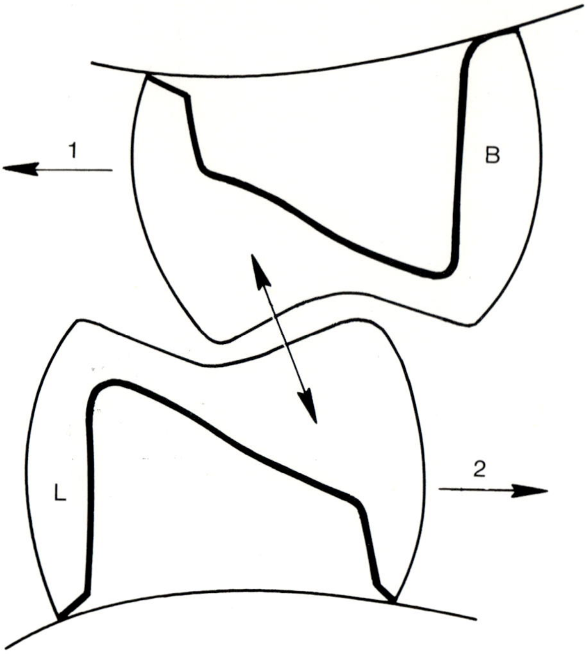

Figure 7–6 After the removal of a large amalgam filling, a gold inlay, or extensive caries, a posterior tooth presents less structure for shaping into a retentive preparation. Regardless of repair of contour with cement, the lingual wall (L) of the lower preparation and the buccal wall (B) of the upper preparation should be tooth structure that is prepared vertically to the long axis of the tooth to resist lingual displacement of the upper (1) and buccal displacement of the lower (2).

opposite walls of the prepared abutment tooth will upgrade retention. These should be made with care to avoid a pulp exposure (Fig. 7–7).

Diameter

Retention increases with an increase in the diameter of an abutment tooth. At constant taper, the abutment tooth with the greatest *unit area* will provide the most effective cement bond. Therefore, whenever a choice must be made for a bridge abutment, the tooth with the greater diameter may be relied upon for more retention.

Mobility

Periodontal conditions that allow movements associated with torque permit an abutment tooth to move out of its cast retainer (Fig. 7–8). Mobile teeth require special consideration in preparation and throughout the course of crown and bridge therapy. Lack of sufficient parallelism and retentive form may result in premature loosen-

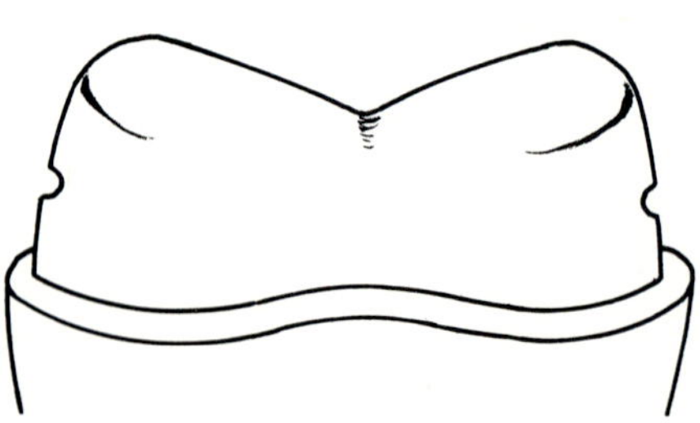

Figure 7–7 Small notches made on the opposite walls of a short abutment preparation just prior to final cementation will greatly improve retention.

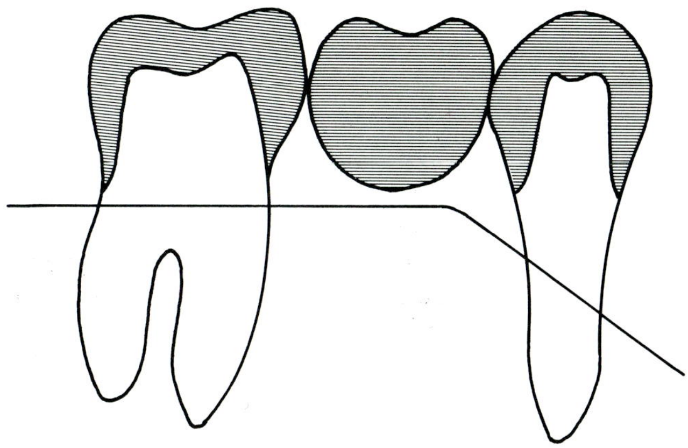

Figure 7–8 Periodontal conditions that allow movements associated with torque may permit an abutment tooth to move out of its cast retainer.

ing after final installation. On the other hand, too much retentive form may be damaging to the periodontium during impression making and other procedures that require repeated removal and insertion of copings or crowns.

The prognosis for a periodontally involved tooth as a fixed bridge abutment may not depend on the crown:root ratio and amount of remaining alveolar bone but on the maintenance of a stable periodontium (absence of periodontal pockets and continuous plaque removal). A stable periodontium is a key factor to a healthy dentition. Nevertheless, a tooth with a poor crown:root ratio is not a good choice for a fixed bridge abutment unless it is attached to more than one other abutment having favorable crown:root ratios. Here again, we must compromise, depending upon the nature, position, and relationship of the other abutments. In many dentitions, compromise is necessary when balanced against an impending totally edentulous state.

It should be recognized that a pier abutment in the middle of an edentulous span requires a very retentive preparation and casting because of the seesaw mobility to which it is subjected.

Nature of Dentin

Depending on age, vitality, and past history, surfaces of cut-tooth structure may differ in texture as much as do fine linen, muslin, and polyester fabrics. These differences occur because the surfaces, or parts of surfaces, of abutment teeth may differ as to the histologic makeup of the dentinal tubules. One surface that presents itself for contact with dental cement may be primary dentin, whereas other surfaces may be secondary dentin, dead tracts, or calcific areas. These variables may account for differences in retention and pulpal reactions. For example, the tubules in secondary dentin are coarser and more irregular than those in primary dentin. A continuous deposition of dentin throughout life tends to reduce the volume of the dental pulp.[5] The new dentin formed throughout the life of the tooth is more amorphous, less tubular, and slightly less regular than primary dentin.[6] This secondary or reparative dentin seems to heal and protect the pulp; also, it transmits less sensation. Dead tracts in primary dentin are due to degeneration and disintegration of the odontoblastic processes that may result from rapidly progressing caries, fractures, operative injuries, and drug application injuries. The tubules in dead tracts are sealed at their pulpal ends and are not as highly calcified as sclerotic dentinal tubules. Primary dentin will respond to injury or exposure of its dentinal tubules by becoming sclerotic. The sclerosis aids in sealing off the dentin by means of tubular calcification. The sclerotic tubule is, therefore, *sealed at both ends.*[7] The dentin under an old and arrested carious lesion presents tubules that are sclerosed and impermeable. This protects the pulp against the penetration of any irritating or acidic restorative material.

Bonding crowns and bridges in young patients is more of a challenge than in older ones. It has been shown that pulpal calcifications, which are a feature of aging, cause a diminution in number of nerves supplying the pulp.[8] This loss of nerves in the pulp may be the reason for the decrease in sensitivity of the teeth of individuals over 40 years of age. It follows, then, that young teeth are more sensitive, have larger pulps, and are wetter than older teeth.[9]

A tooth is a water system.

It should be remembered that air-dried primary dentin becomes moist as tissue fluid ebbs up from the cut tubules. The inherent dryness of non-vital tooth structure contributes a surface predisposed to luting efficiency.

The permeability of the dentin of a tooth is influenced by caries, trauma, age, operative procedures, medicaments, and restorative materials.

BIOPHYSICAL FACTORS RELATED TO THE FIXED PROSTHESIS

The fixed prosthesis should be designed and constructed for effective storage and longevity in the oral environment, so that it may contribute to the *preservation* of the dental structures. This is no less important than function and esthetics. The factors related to the fixed prosthesis that influence retention are as follows:

Accuracy of Fit

An ill-fitting casting is predisposed to premature loosening regardless of the strength of the cement and the adequacy of the preparation. Poor fit permits leakage and allows for both accelerated disintegration of the cement and recurrence of caries. A fixed restoration should fit with a precise and definitive seat, and should resist any movement or rotation. It should also have a small amount of tensofrictional grip. It is not necessary to have a tight-fitting casting for good retention. The tight casting may reduce the thickness of the cement below the optimum in some areas, and thereby reduce the retention value.[10] The tightness of a crown prior to cementation is not predictive of its retentiveness when cemented.[10, 11]

Resistance to Deformation

The ideal restorative material for a fixed restoration should have rigidity. It should resist moving, warping, bending, or changing shape when a force is applied to it. Unfortunately, the ideal material is not available, and lack of sufficient rigidity in a fixed restoration is a frequent cause of failure. All materials are deformed by the application of force. The restorative materials utilized, metal, resin, or porcelain, determine to a great extent the degree of deformation that may be anticipated during function. Occlusal forces tend to open margins. Thin proximal walls should be avoided, for they are easily distorted. The modulus of elasticity of the metal used for casting should be high to avoid bending under torque and torsion. Heat treatment of the metal used for fixed partial dentures is essential for maximum efficiency in function and retention; it increases the yield strength, hardness, and tensile strength of the metal. Deformation of restorative materials under the stress and force of masticatory function may allow leakage and loosening to occur.

Acrylic resin crowns will deform more readily than metal or porcelain crowns. Because deformation causes leakage and loosening of crowns, it is difficult to maintain acrylic resin crowns over an extended period in the mouth without loosening.

Well-fitting crowns of metal or porcelain may be successfully cemented to retentive preparations with a relatively weak cement, such as one of the temporary cements in the low compressive strength range. In the same circumstance, a resin crown would be likely to fail retentively unless a very hard and strong temporary cement was used. In other words, the more deformation, the stronger the cement required. *A final cement for one material may only be a temporary cement for another.* A temporary cement in many instances has turned out to be a "permanent cement" when the biophysical factors caused total resistance to removal. Of course, considerations related to retention must not overshadow those for marginal seal, insolubility, and low film thickness.

Internal Surface Texture

Slightly roughened surfaces on the inside walls of the casting, as well as on the abutment tooth, contribute to the efficiency of the cement bond. Retention may be increased by making an indentation on the inner wall of the casting that precisely overlies a similar concavity on the abutment tooth. When cement fills both facing concavities a plug of cement is thereby created that greatly enhances retention (Fig. 7–9). To upgrade retention, the internal surfaces of crowns should be slightly roughened prior to final cementation.

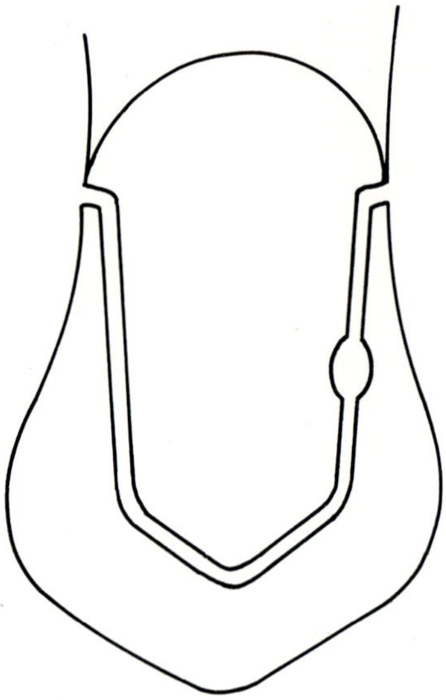

Figure 7–9 When increased retention is required for a long-span bridge or problem situation, make indentations on the abutment preparation and on the inside wall of the casting that faces it. This forms a plug of cement that greatly improves retention.

Length of Bridge Span

Fixed bridges are actually beams supported by abutments. An increased number of consecutive pontics is similar to an increased length of beam. Any beam subjected to a vertical force will deflect at each end. This deflection increases with the length of the beam. Therefore, when occlusal pressure is exerted in the middle of a long-span fixed bridge, the "beam" tends to deflect at each end. The cement bonds at the ends may be strained or broken. However, the short-span bridge with a single pontic exerts very little deflective force on its abutments during function. Where there is no span, of course, there is little or no deflection. This is the case with consecutive teeth that are splinted together with crowns. A series of splinted teeth places the least burden on the cement bond. Schweitzer[12] gives us a clinical documentation of the minimum burden placed on the cementing material when crowns are splinted and no span exists. A four-unit posterior splint of gold crowns veneered with acrylic was secured in a patient's mouth for 12 years by Temrex Cement, a *temporary* zinc oxide and eugenol cement. When the splint was removed by cutting the crowns, the cement was intact and had not dissolved out, even at the margins. We do not suggest the use of a temporary cement such as Temrex Cement for final cementation, but do point out that with splinted crowns and no span even a cement with low strength will suffice for retention. As mentioned above, solubility, marginal seal, and other properties must also be considered in a final cementing material.

For successful retention, the long-span bridge with more than two consecutive pontics should have retentively shaped abutment teeth with emphasis on parallelism, well-fitting castings, cement with high compressive and shear strength, and an overall increase in the occlusal-gingival thickness of the metal (Fig. 7–10).

Design of Fixed Prosthesis

Multiple abutments support one another against flexure and loosening. A series of splinted abutment teeth is subjected to little or no deflective force, and the weakest type of cement provides adequate retention because of the multiplicity of tensofrictional grips. However, when splinted abutment teeth are utilized to maintain a pontic in a cantilever position, a critical engineering problem is involved. A cantilever bridge is a fixed restoration with a free-end pontic. Well-fitting castings on retentively shaped preparations and the strongest cement are prescribed for this type of bridge. In crown and bridge therapy the use of a cantilever bridge is associated with unique engineering and biophysical considerations. The cantilever bridge is used for psychologic and esthetic considerations, to avoid the use of a removable partial denture, to avoid the cutting and preparation of the tooth across the span (the central incisor when the lateral incisor is attached to the cuspid), and occasionally to provide a housing for a precision attachment.

The Mechanics Involved in the Cantilever Bridge

The components of a cantilever bridge make up a seesaw with a rotational center located somewhere near the center of the abutment tooth adjacent to the pontic. Pressure on the pontic causes the seesaw to rotate (Fig. 7–11). When the pontic is depressed, the most remote abutment is raised occlusally. This abutment is under a force of diagonal extrusion. The abutment adjacent to the pontic is the potential fulcrum for torque, torsion and bending. It should always be the thickest and strongest casting. The largest displacing forces are concentrated on the abutment tooth that is most remote from the

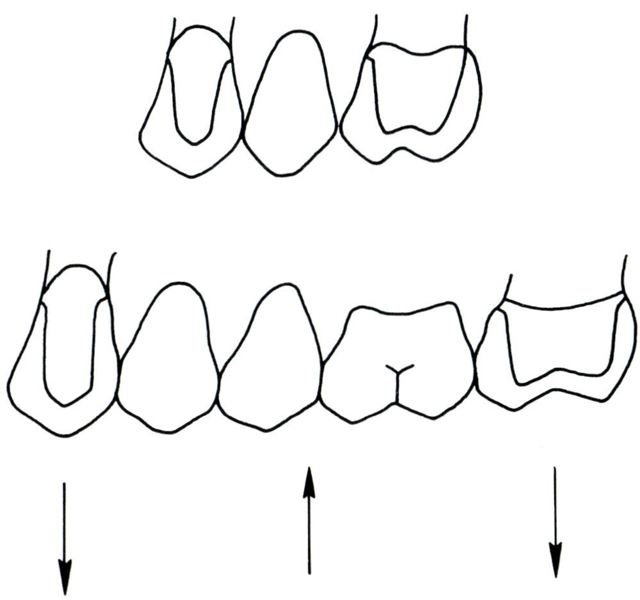

Figure 7–10 The short-span bridge (above) exerts very little deflective force on its abutments during function. However, pressures exerted in the middle of a long-span bridge (below) may cause strain toward deflection at each end. An increased occlusal-gingival thickness of metal will provide a beam more resistant to bending and deflection.

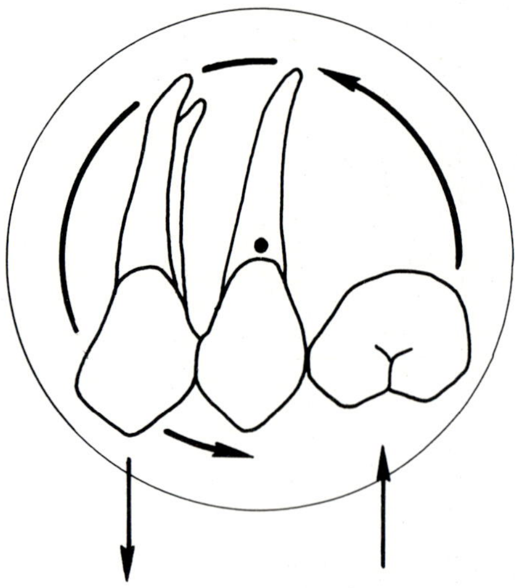

Figure 7–11 Pressure on the pontic of a cantilever bridge causes a rotational effect that is resisted by the bone support of the abutment roots. If the pontic ultimately becomes depressed, the most remote abutment becomes raised occlusally.

cantilever pontic.[13] These forces are directed toward lifting the retainer crown from this abutment tooth. This abutment tooth should therefore have very parallel walls, and the crown should be strong and thick and fit well. It should also extend slightly further into the gingival crevice for the following reasons: the length of the preparation is increased and therefore more retention is obtained, and esthetics will be perpetuated if slight elevation of the tooth and crown occurs after time and function.

BASIC RULES FOR A CANTILEVER BRIDGE

1. A cantilever bridge should have a *single* pontic. No more than one tooth should be replaced.
2. Abutment retainers should be only full crowns.
3. Cantilever bridges should have two or more abutment teeth; however, a lateral incisor may be replaced with one abutment.
4. Good root, bone, crown length, and periodontal conditions should prevail.
5. The pontic should be slightly smaller to present a decreased masticatory surface.

The success of a cantilever bridge will be possible only if the following factors are present.

1. Abutment teeth should have long roots supported by dense bone. Two or more abutment teeth are good—a splint around the arch is better.
2. Retentive abutment preparations should have parallel walls and an asymmetrical component such as a groove or a flattened wall to resist rotation.
3. The abutment preparation farthest from the cantilevered pontic must extend slightly deeper into the gingival crevice.
4. When abutment teeth have a free-end pontic located to the distal, they should be prepared with mesial walls almost vertical to resist rotational loosening. When the pontic is mesial, the distal walls of the preparations should be vertical for the same reason.

5. Full crown castings should be thick, strong, and heat treated for maximum metallurgical properties.

6. The retainer crown adjacent to the pontic should be the thickest and strongest.

7. Soldered joints should be thick and strong or be eliminated by an abutment-pontic casting.

8. The buccal-lingual width of the cantilevered pontic should be narrowed and the mesial-distal extension reduced, so that a smaller masticatory surface is obtained.

9. There must be good occlusal contact on the retainer crown most remote from the pontic to maintain its position and counteract elongation.

10. The nature of the opposing arch is important. Pressure on the pontic is less when it occludes with a complete denture than with (in declining order) a multiple-unit fixed bridge, natural teeth, or a removable partial denture.

11. Strong cement must be applied effectively to obtain the most complete and accurate seating.

12. The gingival base of the cantilevered pontic should face the edentulous tissue area with slightly less positive contact than the usual bridge pontic, and with a highly polished metal or glazed porcelain surface. Acrylic resin is not recommended in this area.

13. Good occlusal balance and proper occlusal morphology plus adequate sluiceways will facilitate chewing and cause less stress on the abutment teeth during mastication.[14]

Escapeways

The presence or absence of escapeways for cement influences the extent of seating of well-fitting abutment castings. Retention depends on the degree of seating. The more completely a casting seats, the more retentive it is.

The viscosity of the cement and related hydrodynamic phenomena create a resistance to the complete seating of a casting.[15] The resistance to seating is greater when abutment walls are more nearly parallel. Since castings do not seat completely, occlusal and marginal relationships are rendered less precise. All efforts should be made to minimize this unavoidable loss of accuracy. The presence of escapeways in full crown castings, such as grooves or planned occlusal vents, makes possible ease of seating, more complete seating, and increased retention.

When the fluid in an automotive brake line escapes through a break in the system, hydraulic pressure is lost, and the brake foot pedal is easily pressed to the floorboard. Similarly, full crowns are pressed down into place easily and completely when the usual hydraulic kickback is eliminated by a vent (a planned opening). The *viscosity* of zinc phosphate cement is a prime contributor to the hydraulic problem, and most of the research and writing on venting deals exclusively with this cement. In contrast, alumina EBA cement has minimal viscosity and very low surface tension, and crowns secured with this cement go into place easier and more completely.

Venting is not necessary. To repeat—venting is specific to zinc phosphate cement because of its viscosity. Venting is not clinically significant with alumina EBA cement.

BIOPHYSICAL FACTORS RELATED TO THE ORAL ENVIRONMENT

The oral environment is a complex and unique area of dynamic changes. It is referred to both as a disaster area, and as a torture chamber for materials. It is an unusual theater of activity because everything in it is continuously changing: its shape, temperature, pH, chemical content, moisture content, enzyme activity, and bacterial proliferation. As a result of the hostile and changing conditions present in the mouth, restorative materials and cements are threatened with rapid destruction. They are predisposed to the resultant effects of thermal, chemical, galvanic, and physical attack in this oral arena.

Some mouths present more hostile conditions than others. A fixed restoration that may be successfully retained in one mouth may fail prematurely in another. The survival of a fixed prosthesis in the mouth depends not only on the chemistry, stresses, habits, occlusion, and individual characteristics of the oral environment to which it is exposed but also on the following biophysical factors that influence retention.

Thermal Changes

When hot and cold foods such as ice cream and coffee are introduced into the mouth, sudden temperature changes occur that may range from near freezing to near boiling. As a result, all structures in the mouth—tooth, casting and cement—expand and contract differently according to the thermal coefficients involved, allowing separation to occur and leakage to ensue.

Chemical Changes

Various dilute organic acids, sulfides, ammonia derivatives, and other chemical agents in the form of liquid or solid foods or medicaments parade through the oral cavity. In the opposite direction, emanating from the stomach or lungs, are other chemicals in solid, liquid, or gaseous form emerging from the mouth as a result of breathing, belching, and various degrees of regurgitation. The solubility of dental cements is increased when certain chemical solutions predominate. Washout of cement and marginal leakage is influenced by the changing chemistry of the mouth, and possibly by potentially destructive enzymes. Changes in pH occur that are related to ingested foods and their breakdown by-products which lie adjacent to the cement line. Since the rate of salivation varies, the moisture content of the oral cavity may readily change and influence not only chemical activity but also the dryness required for cementation.

Oral Galvanism

When two dissimilar metals are bathed in an electrolyte solution, a difference in electrical potential is created. This may happen in a mouth containing different metallic restorative materials such as gold, silver, steel, and vitallium. The saliva acts as the electrolyte and the dissimilar metals as the anode and cathode, from and to which electrical current flows.

The clinical side effects of this situation include a metallic taste, hypersalivation, and irritation of the mucosa. Pulpal pathosis may be caused by the galvanic current.[16] It has been shown that exfoliative glossitis and other lesions may also result from the galvanic phenomenon. The pH of the saliva and the electrolyte content of the mouth are important factors in the production of the untoward reactions. Symptoms disappear when the metallic materials are removed.

Stress

There are great stresses in the oral cavity. Average biting stresses on a single tooth may range as high as 30,000 pounds per square inch. Masticatory forces, tongue thrust, and other muscular actions create diverse pressures against fixed restorations. The nature of the occlusion is a factor that influences retention. Occlusal forces can fracture cement. A premature occlusal contact can introduce torque that will shatter the cement bond. Habits such as bruxism, dietary abnormalities, and periodontal conditions may present a complexity of forces that burden the cement bond.

Mechanical Forces

Other dental prostheses may bring pressure to bear upon the cemented crown or bridge, and influence the success or failure of retention. The multiple-unit fixed bridge or full-arch splint that occludes with a cemented restoration may be considered a powerhouse of opposing force. Its weighty influence may contribute to loosening. In contradistinction, a complete denture exerts a minimal amount of opposing force to a cemented prosthesis. Pressures and resultant deformation may also be the result of a sharp cusp on an opposing tooth or an opposing restoration of harder metal or unglazed porcelain. There are forces and torque associated with the insertion, removal, and function of removable partial dentures that depend on cemented castings for internal or external retention. Occasionally, the cemented cast retainers succumb to these forces, and loosening occurs.

PRACTICAL CONSIDERATIONS FOR BETTER RETENTION BASED ON BIOPHYSICAL FACTORS

1. On the short tooth that may pose a problem for retention parallelism should be increased.
2. Castings will fit better and cementation will be easier if long preparations are tapered.

3. An asymmetric preparation resists rotation. To avoid symmetry, flatten or groove one wall of the preparation.

4. Round off all occlusal, incisal, and shoulder line angles.

5. To enhance retention, roughen the abutment preparation prior to final cementation.

6. Reduce tooth surfaces enough to fabricate a crown with walls thick enough to resist deformation.

7. To upgrade retention, roughen the inside walls of a casting.

8. The long-span bridge should have less convergent walls than the short-span bridge.

9. The cantilever bridge requires abutments with very parallel walls.

10. Preparations may be more tapered for a splint of consecutive abutments when no span is included.

11. The abutment preparations for a bridge that opposes a large porcelain bridge or full arch splint should be very retentive.

12. The abutment preparations for crowns that will provide external or internal retention for a removable partial denture should be very retentive.

13. A fixed bridge occluding with a complete denture has diminished retentive requirements.

14. Remember that young teeth are more sensitive, wetter, and more difficult to bond to than older, dry teeth.

SUMMARY

Crowns and bridges depend not only on dental cements and the technique of cementation for lasting retention but also on the biophysical factors related to the abutment tooth, the fixed prosthesis, and the oral environment. These biophysical factors contribute to, or work against, successful retention. The dentist who recognizes them is forearmed. He may modify some of these factors to overcome unfavorable conditions. Besides their influence on retention, the factors referred to in this chapter must also be considered when removing a cemented restoration and when selecting a temporary or final cement.

REFERENCES

1. Kaufman, E. G., Coelho, D. H., and Colin, L.: Factors influencing the retention of cemented gold castings. J. Prosthet. Dent. *11*:487–502, 1961.
2. Nicholls, J. I.: Crown retention. Part 1. Stress analysis of symmetric restorations, J. Prosthet. Dent. *31*:179, February 1974.
3. Colin, L., Kaufman, E. G., and Papirno, R.: Stress concentrations in full crown restorations. N.Y. State Dent. J. *29*:370, 1963.
4. Douglass, G. D.: Principles of preparation design in fixed prosthodontics. J. Acad. Gen. Dent., April 1973, p. 25.
5. Seltzer, S., and Bender, I. B.: The Dental Pulp. Philadelphia, J. B. Lippincott Co. 1965, p. 213.
6. Seltzer, S., and Bender, I. B.: The Dental Pulp. Philadelphia, J. B. Lippincott Co. 1965, p. 214.
7. Gardner, A. F.: Pathology of the dental pulp with clinical correlations. *In*

Practical Dental Monographs, Chicago, Year Book Medical Publishers, Inc., May 1963, p. 29.
8. Bernick, S.: Effect of aging on the nerve supply to human teeth. J. Dent. Res. *46*:694, 1967.
9. Toto, P. D., et al.: Effect of age on water content in human teeth. J. Dent. Res. *50*:1284, 1971.
10. Lorey, R. E., and Myers, G. E.: The retentive qualities of bridge retainers. J.A.D.A., *76*:568, March 1968.
11. Kaufman, E. G.: The retention of crowns before and after cementation. N.Y.U. J. Dent. *25*:6, 1967.
12. Schweitzer, J. M.: Oral Rehabilitation Problem Cases. St. Louis, C. V. Mosby Co., 1964, p. 251.
13. Schweitzer, J. M., Schweitzer, R. D., and Schweitzer, J.: Free-end pontics used on fixed partial dentures. J. Prosthet. Dent. *20*:120, August 1968, p. 132.
14. Antonoff, S. J.: The status of cantilever bridges. N.Y. State Dent. J. *38*:275, May, 1972.
15. Jorgensen, K. D.: Factors affecting the film thickness of zinc phosphate cements. Acta Odont. Scand. *18*:479, 1960.
16. Gardner, A. F.: Pathology of the dental pulp. Dent. Clin. North Am., November 1961, p. 632.

eight

Crown and Bridge Cementing Materials

Research in its highest expression is open-minded inquiry for truth, to be found and revealed unreservedly for the information, instruction, advantage, and welfare of all.

William J. Gies

Dental cement is the most used adjunctive material in crown and bridge therapy. It is a constant link that not only retains, but protects, seals, insulates, and repairs tooth structure. It may also soothe pain and allow for a trial evaluation of a fixed partial denture. A few years ago the universal dental cement was zinc phosphate cement. Today in dentistry there is no single cement considered suitable for all usages, but various dental cements are available and are selected for use according to physical, esthetic, or biologic requirements.

LUTING AGENTS FOR FIXED RESTORATIONS

These agents include:

1. Phosphoric acid cements—
   a. Zinc phosphate cements
   b. Silicophosphate cements
   c. Water-settable cements

2. Zinc oxide and eugenol cements
   a. Simple zinc oxide and eugenol cements
   b. Resin-fortified zinc oxide and eugenol cements
   c. Ethoxybenzoic acid (EBA) cements

3. Resin cements
   a. Acrylic resin cements
   b. Composite resin cements
   c. Polycarboxylate cements

All cements used in the final cementation of fixed restorations are based on zinc oxide, except for the acrylic resin and composite resin cements. Zinc oxide, in various forms, reacts with phosphoric acid, eugenol, and polyacrylic acid. By themselves, hardened dental cements are not durable and are weak and brittle. They resemble the shell of an egg or a very thin film of glass with a surface that is hard and difficult to scratch, and yet breaks up very easily. When cements are covered by stronger restorative materials, however, they are protected to a large extent from breakage and dissolution.

Since barnacle cement, glass-ionomer cement, and cyanoacrylate cement have not as yet been shown to be applicable to the luting of crowns and bridges, they are not included in this discussion. With the exception of the simple zinc oxide and eugenol cements and the resin-fortified zinc oxide and eugenol cements, which are mainly used as temporary cements and bases, the agents considered in this chapter have all been proposed for the final cementation of crowns and bridges. However, there are reservations and limitations with regard to the utilization of some of them.

PHOSPHORIC ACID CEMENTS

Zinc Phosphate Cements

Zinc phosphate cement, the universal cementing medium, has functioned adequately over the years because its compressive strength was enough to withstand mechanical forces. In recent years, however, with the trend toward re-evaluation of methods and materials, and with the increasing emphasis on the biological responses to dental materials, the shortcomings of zinc phosphate cement have been brought into sharper focus. Research reports have indicated that these cements may be injurious to the pulp, have poor sealing qualities, and are relatively soluble in dilute organic acids.

Skinner[1] noted that zinc phosphate cements are inadequate for luting fixed restorations, and that there is no method to prevent their solution in mouth fluids. Phillips[2] states that the use of zinc phosphate cement as a base under permanent restorations is decreasing in popularity. Without a doubt, zinc phosphate cement has many inherent disadvantages. It causes pulpal irritation and sensitivity. It does not adhere to tooth structure, and has poor sealing ability. Because of its high viscosity, well-fitting castings are difficult to seat without prepared escapeways. It increases enamel solubility, generates heat, and tends to shrink on setting. It must be kept dry before setting and wet afterward. Its low pH persists for many hours after setting has occurred. Tissue tolerance is poor, and it exhibits no appreciable antibacterial properties.

Despite these shortcomings, zinc phosphate cement has been widely used because of its ideal handling characteristics, and because *no other cementing material was available.* Zinc phosphate cement sets hard and strong. The setting time is readily controlled. Excess cement is easily removed and does not adhere chemically to acrylic resin veneers as do zinc oxide and eugenol and acrylic resin cements. It also provides adequate thermal insulation. Its use in conjunction with cavity liners decreases some of its shortcomings. However, the addition of a few drops of eugenol to zinc phosphate cement sabotages its prime virtue, for the eugenol lowers the strength, hardness, and abrasion resistance of the cement and, since eugenol is incapable of neutralizing the acid, the pH remains below 2. Although pain and sensitivity may be obtunded by the eugenol, the potential for pulpal damage still exists. Antibiotics, antiseptics, fluorides, and other agents have been added to zinc phosphate cements to impart bacteriostatic properties and to reduce the acid solubility of adjoining enamel, but these measures have been relatively unsuccessful over any extended period of time.

Filtration

Zinc phosphate cement exhibits an unusual but typical phenomenon called filtration.[3] On occasion, during the seating of well-fitting crowns with this cement, a filtration process causes the mixed cement to separate into a powder and a liquid. As a result, isolated areas of cement liquid and other areas of powder alone exist between the restoration and the tooth structure. Each separated component is undesirable; the liquid alone is highly acid and the powder alone is subject to easy and fast dissolution. As a result, crowns work loose, owing to the resultant poor retention. At the same time, concentrated areas of liquid acid may cause pulpal injury, and a washout of liquid areas that extend to crown borders may allow recurrent decay. The degree of this filtration is influenced by the pressure of cementation, the viscosity of the cement, and the taper of the preparation. Rounding of the occlusal line angles and venting of the crowns will minimize the problems of filtration.

Soluble, Sooner Than Later

According to recent research,[4] the solubility of phosphoric acid-type cements (zinc phosphate, hydrophosphate, and silicophosphate) is appreciably greater when exposed to water *early* rather than late: the longer the time lapse before contact with water, the lower the solubility of the cement. It seems that these cements should be protected from oral fluids more carefully than is commonly done. Therefore, immediately after crowns, bridges or inlays are installed in the mouth with this type of cement, a cavity varnish should be applied to all of the margins to protect against early dissolution.

The Nature of the Bond

Neither zinc phosphate cement nor any other cement (including polycarboxylate cement) is "truly adhesive" to prepared dentinal structures. Any apparent "adhesion" or retention is obtained by the mechanical interlocking of the cement between the tooth structure and the restoration. The cement film provided is reasonably strong but is very brittle, and a slight shearing movement is capable of initiating a fracture of the bond. A cement that would provide a more resilient film, such as a resin material or a zinc oxide and eugenol cement, would have a distinct advantage if other properties were also adequate.

Certified Dental Zinc Phosphate Cements

Today in dentistry only four dental zinc phosphate cements are certified as Type 1, fine grain. What does this mean? It means that of all the many zinc phosphate cements manufactured today for the dental profession, only four meet the American Dental Association Specification No. 8 for use in the cementation of crowns, bridges, and inlays.[5] All the others probably cannot pass the relatively new requirement for film thickness (under 25 microns). The four Type 1, fine grain, zinc phosphate cements recommended for the cementation of precision castings are as follows:

1. Elite Cement, IDT Corp.
2. Fleck's Extraordinary, Mizzy, Inc.
3. Modern Tenacin, L.D. Caulk Co.
4. S. S. White Zinc Improved, S. S. White Co.

Zinc Phosphate Cement—Good Characteristics

Sets hard and strong.
Setting time is easily controlled.
Excess cement is easy to remove.
Does not adhere to acrylic resin.
Provides thermal insulation.
Has a low film thickness.

Zinc Phosphate Cement—Bad Characteristics

Irritating to dental pulp.
Poor sealing ability.
Soluble in dilute organic acids.
High viscosity and surface tension.
Increases enamel solubility.
Generates heat on setting, and shrinks.
Its low pH persists for hours.
Tissue tolerance is poor.
No antibacterial properties.
Causes a filtration phenomenon.

Practical Considerations

1. Vital abutment teeth should be protected from contact with a zinc phosphate cement by a thin film of a copal type cavity varnish. Young teeth need more careful protection than old teeth, and primary dentin needs more protection than sclerotic dentin.

2. A mix of zinc phosphate cement made on a cool glass slab is stronger, less soluble, and shrinks less than a mix made on a warm glass slab.

3. The more powder mixed into the liquid, the greater the strength and the less the solubility of the cement will be.

4. The cement liquid should be dispensed only at the moment of spatulation. The bottle should be capped tightly immediately. If the cement liquid is carelessly exposed to air the water content will be altered and the setting time changed, and its physical properties will be reduced.[6]

5. The timing of the spatulation is important. Slow, smooth, and careful additions of powder into the liquid, spread out over a large area of the cool glass slab will dissipate much of the heat of the chemical reaction, slow the reaction down, and allow the incorporation of more powder. A stronger, more insoluble cement will result.

6. Saliva will weaken unset zinc phosphate cement; therefore, moisture should be carefully removed from the gingival crevice prior to cementation or the most critical portion of the cement, that providing the marginal seal, will be compromised.

7. The cement should be applied first to the fixed prosthesis, before any cement is placed on the prepared tooth in the mouth. Otherwise, the body temperature may accelerate the set of the cement and cause crystallization that could interfere with complete seating.

8. Occlusal adjustments to newly cemented restorations should be delayed. The heat, pressure, and vibration of grinding may disrupt the integrity of the cement film at the stage of initial setting and encourage washout and premature loosening.

9. Immediately after cementation of a restoration a cavity varnish should be applied to all margins, before the saliva-removal apparatus is removed. In this manner, the cement will be somewhat protected against early dissolution.

10. The selection of a zinc phosphate cement for the effective cementation of a fixed restoration should be made only from those cements that meet the requirements of American Dental Association Specification No. 8, listed therein under Type 1.

11. Zinc phosphate cement is readily softened by hydrogen sulfide, and is attacked by various corroding agents in the mouth, depending on the diet and the bacteria that predominate. The cement is more soluble also when the pH of the mouth is decreased. The patient with a mouthful of cemented restorations

should be specifically cautioned against acidic soft drinks, and also be instructed in other aspects of proper nutrition.

Silicophosphate Cements

As the name implies, these are combinations of silicate cement and zinc phosphate cement. They are stronger than the zinc phosphate cements and appear to be slightly less soluble. Silicophosphate cements are the only luting materials utilized in the cementation of fixed prostheses that possess a degree of translucency. They are indicated primarily for the cementation of porcelain jackets.

The recently introduced composite resin cement, Epoxylite CBA 9080,* is also a translucent cementing material. In selected instances (loose-fitting porcelain jackets) and with proper pulp protection, this luting agent will supply a strong, insoluble bond without loss of translucency.

Zinc phosphate, polycarboxylate, and EBA cements are opaque materials, and the final cementation of porcelain jackets (especially thin ones) with these cements may result in less than the total translucency required for proper esthetics. However, an opaque cement will not detract too much from the final esthetic value of a thick porcelain jacket crown. The thick porcelain jacket will more than likely cover a non-vital tooth with a post preparation or an overly prepared vital abutment tooth with a great deal of sensitivity. In the latter instance, if the retentive form of the preparation is adequate and of sufficient length, a well-fitting thick-walled porcelain jacket is ideally cemented with an alumina EBA cement.

Commercial products such as Lucent** and Fluoro-Thin† are examples of silicophosphate cement. All exhibit high strength, are translucent, and possess anticariogenic properties by virtue of the fluoride they contain. The greater the silicate component, the more the fluoride uptake in enamel and the greater the reduction in acid solubility.[7] Silicophosphate cements usually do not extrude into a thin enough film to allow complete seating of a well-fitting casting. Fluoro-Thin (Fig. 8–1), however, seems to have less film thickness than the usual silicophosphate cement. Both Fluoro-Thin and Lucent meet the cementing media film thickness requirement of the American Dental Association Specification No. 21, Type 1. In fact, they are the only silicophosphate cements that do.

Silicophosphate cements generally take a long time to set and are as irritating to the pulp as other phosphoric acid-containing materials. Cavity liners should be employed when these cements are utilized. Despite the higher strength of this cement it does not seem to retain castings any better than zinc phosphate cement.

Silicophosphate cements are mixed like zinc phosphate cement or like silicate cement, depending upon their formulation and the manufacturer's directions.

---

*Lee Pharmaceuticals, South El Monte, CA 91733
**L. D. Caulk Co., Milford, DE 19963
†S. S. White Dental Products, Phila., PA 19102

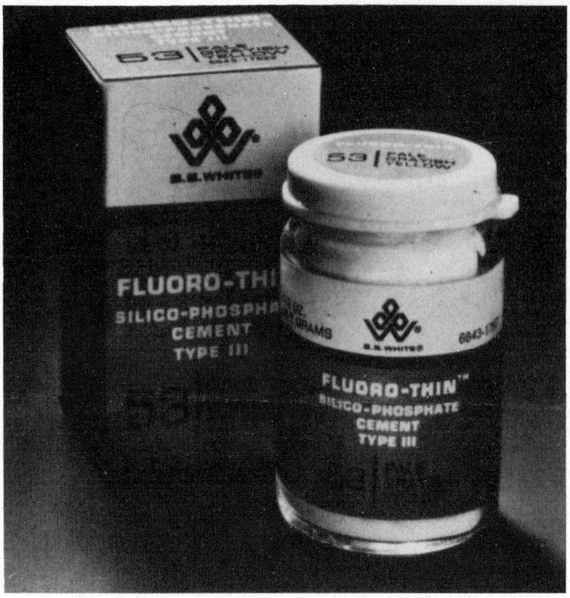

Figure 8–1 An example of a silicophosphate cement.

Practical Considerations

1. Silicophosphate cements require the same cool glass mixing slab and the same care of the liquid as the zinc phosphate cements.

2. Vital abutment teeth should be coated with a thin layer of a copal type cavity varnish prior to contact with this cement. In fact, very careful pulp protection is necessary because of the low initial pH of these cements.

3. Since the sensitivity to moisture is similar to that of the zinc phosphate cements, the same dryness requirements and protection after setting are necessary.

Water-Settable Cements

Water-settable zinc phosphate cements were developed in Japan in 1959. They are also called hydrophosphate cements and zinc hydrophosphate cements. Instead of mixing this cement powder with a phosphoric acid liquid, water is used as the liquid component. At first, this would seem to have an attractive potential: no phosphoric acid liquid and possibly improved shelf life and storage over zinc phosphate cement. Since the acid nature of zinc phosphate cement is a drawback, mixing with water seemed more benign than mixing with acid. However, none of the promise came true. Water-settable cement powder is like instant frozen orange juice concentrate, add water to make orange juice or add water to make "instant" zinc phosphate cement.

Tests have shown these cements to be even more acidic than zinc phosphate cement,[8, 9] and they may therefore have a more detrimental biologic effect on the pulp. They also do not meet the accepted values for various physical properties. They are inferior to the conventional zinc phosphate cement in compressive strength, have higher film thickness and solubility, and, since they are very hygroscopic, have poor keeping qualities.[10] Water-settable cements are not suitable for crown and bridge therapy.

ZINC OXIDE AND EUGENOL CEMENTS

Simple Zinc Oxide and Eugenol Cements

Ferdinand Magellan died in 1521 while searching for a route around the world and a cargo of cloves. The same cloves he was seeking are used today in the kitchen for roasting hams, stewing fruits, and baking apples. They also supply the oil of cloves from which eugenol is derived. Oil of cloves is made up of about 85 per cent eugenol, the other 15 per cent being terpenes and other components. Its medicinal value is derived from the eugenol content. Oil of cloves has had a long and popular history in dentistry as an anesthetic and antiseptic. The United States Pharmacopoeia states that oil of cloves is "traditionally" used for application to the gums and teeth. Dentistry, therefore, is responsible for recognizing the unique contribution of eugenol. Eugenol combined with zinc oxide was introduced into dentistry as a replacement for creosote just before the turn of the century. Over the years, eugenol mixtures have been used as periodontal dressings and under restorations with or without a pulp exposure. For pulp capping, however, calcium hydroxide has replaced zinc oxide and eugenol mixtures. Nevertheless, many dentists overlay the calcium hydroxide dressing with a zinc oxide and eugenol cement. A great deal of impressive evidence favorable to the use of zinc oxide and eugenol pastes has been gathered. There is no doubt of the palliative effect of this compound as an obtundent. The discomfort caused by an aching tooth can often be relieved when the zinc oxide and eugenol paste contacts the exposed pulp or dentin. It is generally recognized that zinc oxide and eugenol cements possess much better compatibility than most dental materials with both the hard and soft tissues of the mouth, relieve pain, and provide a good seal to tooth structure. Therefore, they have found a wide range of applications in dentistry: as temporary fillings, sedative bases, cementing media, soft tissue packs, and, with modifying agents, as impression pastes.

In crown and bridge therapy zinc oxide and eugenol cements are widely used as therapeutic bases and for the temporary and final cementation of fixed restorations. These cements are recognized for their unique sedative effect upon pulpal tissue. A simple mixture of zinc oxide and eugenol is weak and sets slowly, but it relieves pain. How many other agents are available for the treatment of a painful tooth? Zinc oxide and eugenol is *the only cement in dentistry* that will soothe and sedate the dentin and pulp. Indeed, zinc oxide and eugenol is a unique and magical material.

Zinc oxide and eugenol cements are mildly antiseptic and are less irritating to prepared tooth structure than any other. Since a simple mixture is weak and sets slowly, it must be modified to be stronger and set faster. Many different agents may be added to zinc oxide and eugenol mixtures, not only to improve strength and decrease setting time but also to improve solubility, modify surface tension, and increase antibacterial activity. Zinc oxide and eugenol cements vary greatly, and many formulations have been juggled and manipulated to achieve a desired end-product. Some of the many substances used in zinc oxide and eugenol formulations and the reasons for their use are given in Table 8–1.

Corn oil, menthol, oleic acid, oil of rose, Canada balsam and Peruvian balsam may be added to the formulations for various reasons.

A simple zinc oxide and eugenol formulation may be zinc oxide, USP, and eugenol, USP, with a small percentage of zinc acetate to speed up the set (Fig. 8–2). Various commercial products contain zinc oxide and eugenol with zinc acetate, resin or rosin, and corn oil or cottonseed oil. Although generally the zinc oxide and eugenol cements are in powder and liquid form, some have fillers, plasticizers, and other ingredients so that they may be dispensed in collapsible tubes. Examples of both types of zinc oxide and eugenol cements are as follows:

Powder and liquid—

Temrex Cement, Interstate Dental Company
After Prep, Teledyne Dental Products
ZOE 2200, L.D. Caulk Company
Pulprotex, L.D. Caulk Company
Moyco ZRE, J. Bird Moyer Company
Anodyne Temporary Cement, L.D. Caulk Company
Tempak, Westward Dental Products
S.S. White Z.O.E., S.S. White Company

Collapsible tubes—

Opotow Temporary Cement, Teledyne Dental Products
Cavitec, Kerr Manufacturing Company
Interstate Temporary Cement, Interstate Dental Company
Temp-Bond, Kerr Manufacturing Company

TABLE 8–1 ADDITIVES USED TO MODIFY ZINC OXIDE AND EUGENOL CEMENTS

Substance	Reasons for Use
Hydrogenated resin	Strength, smoother working characteristics
Parabens	Lower surface tension, strength, antibacterial activity, delay set
Ethoxybenzoic acid	Strength, antibacterial activity, lower surface tension
Alumina (aluminum oxide)	Strength
Fused quartz	Strength
Polystyrene	Strength
Poly (methyl methacrylate)	Strength
Zinc acetate	Decrease setting time
Glacial acetic acid	Decrease setting time
Mineral oil	Increase surface tension, viscosity
Thymol iodide	Antibacterial agent

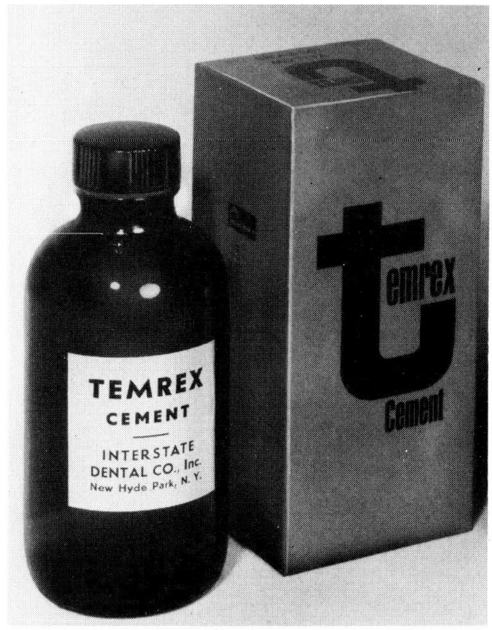

Figure 8–2 A simple zinc oxide and eugenol cement. This cement has no resin or rosin in the powder, but has a small percentage of zinc acetate to accelerate the set. The liquid is pure eugenol except for about 1 per cent of oil of rose.

Eugenol vs Zinc Oxide and Eugenol

Eugenol mixed with zinc oxide produces a far different reaction in the mouth from that produced by eugenol alone. Eugenol is an irritating material and should not be used alone in the mouth. However, the small amount (optimum) of eugenol that diffuses from a hardened mass of zinc oxide and eugenol is beneficial. It soothes, sedates, obtunds pain, and is antibacterial.

Many substances that are beneficial when used in proper amounts are harmful when used otherwise. For example, fluorides in large amounts are harmful to the human body, and yet small amounts are beneficial because of their anticariogenic value. A small amount of chlorine may be used to purify the water in a swimming pool; yet it would be dangerous to swim in a pool full of chlorine. Vitamins A and D are valuable in small amounts and harmful in large amounts. Dentists use dangerous materials in the mouth. Amalgam, polysulfide rubber impression materials, and silicate cement are involved with toxic components such as mercury, lead peroxide, and phosphoric acid. Obviously, many potentially harmful materials may be beneficial if they are used correctly in the optimum percentage and formulation. This is true with eugenol. The key to understanding is recognition of the fact that *eugenol alone and zinc oxide mixed with eugenol* have entirely different irritative characteristics.

Langeland[11] states that eugenol may cause irritation to the pulp and "that is the reason why excess eugenol should be squeezed out of the zinc oxide and eugenol mix." Granger[12] says that "eugenol should not be used repeatedly on fully dried teeth, as it is a pulp irritant and repeated applications on dry teeth can cause pulp involvement in deep preparations." Roydhouse[13] states that "eugenol is irritating to soft tissues." Frigoletto[14] warns, "I do not suggest the use of eugenol on a deep lesion or near an exposure because it may kill the pulp." Rotberg and deShazer[15] showed that eugenol removes calcium from dentin. Schilder and Amsterdam have demonstrated the inflammatory characteristics of free eugenol.[16] Various other investigators have reported on the untoward effects of eugenol.[17-19] *Hardened mixtures of zinc oxide and eugenol, however, appear to be well tolerated by the hard and soft tissues.*[20]

Even though eugenol may obtund pain, when used alone on prepared tooth structure it is a pulpal irritant.

The irritating effect of eugenol may be minimized if the tooth to which it is applied is old or sclerotic. Nevertheless, it is a mummifying agent. Yet, mixed with zinc oxide, it forms a cementitious mass that hardens and is beneficial to tooth structure. Just the right amount of eugenol effuses from the hardened mass of cement. *This small amount given off is the optimum amount of eugenol for effective therapy.* The point is this: just the right amount, the optimum amount, of a substance is necessary for the desired effect.

Full strength eugenol should never be applied directly to prepared tooth structure. Only traces of eugenol that emanate from a hardened mixture are beneficial to the tooth. The smaller the amount the better. Compared to other zinc oxide and eugenol cements, EBA cements have approximately two thirds less eugenol in their makeup, and therefore give off a minimum amount of eugenol. A zinc oxide and eugenol cement containing a lesser amount of eugenol is less likely to have an effect on the polymerization of a composite resin material. Although a number of these resins will set regardless of the presence of zinc oxide and eugenol, when less eugenol is present, the potential for altered physical properties is less. As to how much eugenol should be used in a zinc oxide and eugenol product, Molnar[21] states that "... only the least amount of eugenol should be added to obtain a reaction product of optimum physical properties."

Not All Zinc Oxide and Eugenol Cements Are the Same

A rose is a rose is a rose may be a poetic truism, but not all zinc oxide and eugenol is zinc oxide and eugenol. The zinc oxide and eugenol mixtures referred to in various research reports and dental literature both here and abroad are not always the basic or characteristic mixtures that are generally used. The term "zinc oxide and eugenol" covers a large family of very diverse formulations, just as the term "animal" covers many differing forms. A mouse cannot substitute for a mule, nor can a cancer investigator merely report that he used animals. Yet the dental literature abounds with references to zinc oxide and eugenol. Which zinc oxide and eugenol? Are chemical additives involved; are there modifications of any of the components? Is resin or rosin in the powder, the liquid, or both? Indeed, the term "zinc oxide and eugenol" does not tell the whole story. Not all zinc oxide and eugenol cements are the same. In some, *both powder and liquid contain a large amount of resin.* Compared to formulations with just an accelerator in the powder and just eugenol as the liquid, the resin-fortified materials have a number of different physical properties and characteristics. For example, they are usually much stronger, set faster, have a larger film thickness, react differently with paraben additives, and diffuse a larger amount of free eugenol after hardening. It is misleading to apply conclusions derived from testing one zinc oxide and eugenol cement to all other zinc oxide and eugenol cements. There are at least three different categories of this material in the unfortified state.

1. Zinc oxide, USP, and eugenol, USP (nothing else)
2. Zinc oxide, USP, and eugenol, USP, with the usual additives, such as resins, rosins, and chemical agents.
3. Zinc oxide, USP, and eugenol, USP, with unknown ingredients, antibacterials, or antibiotics.

As far as zinc oxide powder is concerned, there are different grades, particle sizes, and methods of manufacture. There are also different types of eugenol of different reactive ability. Packaging, storage, and shelf life also influence product variation.

In routine clinical use, many zinc oxide and eugenol cements with various types of components are known to provide the usual biologic benefits and physical characteristics, and there is no need to further identify the formulation. However, in the testing, research and evaluation of these materials there should be more specificity, for, despite the main differences, dental literature and research reports continue to refer to that nebulous material "zinc oxide and eugenol." Which zinc oxide and eugenol? The answer is seldom designated. *This is a large flaw in contemporary dental materials research.* If a zinc oxide and eugenol mixture is referred to in testing procedures it should be identified with the details of its formulation. Otherwise, research reports involving biologic compatibility and physical properties lose validity. This may explain some of the controversy and conflicting conclusions and opinions that exist regarding the pulpal effect, pulp-capping ability, sealing ability, and solubility of zinc oxide and eugenol mixtures.

Resin-Fortified Zinc Oxide and Eugenol Cements

Zinc oxide and eugenol cements may be fortified with various resins. Polystyrene may be present in the liquid or polymethyl methacrylate in the powder, or perhaps a resin or a rosin in both the powder and the liquid. Nevertheless, zinc oxide and eugenol cements may only be strengthened to a limited degree with resins, and therefore they are indicated for temporary cementation rather than final cementation.

ZOE, B&T* and Fynal* are examples of resin-fortified zinc oxide and eugenol cements. Polymethyl methacrylate is probably the reinforcing agent in both products.[22] These cements are significantly stronger than simple zinc oxide and eugenol cements. The degree of reinforcement seems to depend largely on particle size and on the uniformity of distribution of the resinous and inorganic phases of the powder components.[22] Fynal (Fig. 8–3) is not as strong and insoluble as EBA cements such as Zebacem* and Opotow Alumina EBA Cement,** and may be better used as a strong temporary cement. It is very adequate for use with acrylic resin temporary coverage on short preparations or long-span bridges, or in other situations requiring strong retention for temporary coverage.

Both the simple zinc oxide and eugenol cements and the resin-fortified ones are used as temporary cements. They are of great value to the dentist in crown and bridge procedures. He reaches for this type of material 1) to sedate deep painful areas in prepared teeth, 2) to seal and protect abutments with temporary coverage after preparations are accomplished, 3) to re-cement temporary coverage after impression making or other procedures are accomplished, 4) to temporarily cement the finished fixed bridge or splint for a period of biologic evaluation.

A great deal of success in crown and bridge therapy is related to the understanding and effective utilization of zinc oxide and eugenol. Its pain-relieving effect may be due to its anodyne action

*L.D. Caulk Company, Milford, DE 19963
**Teledyne Dental, Elk Grove Village, IL 60007

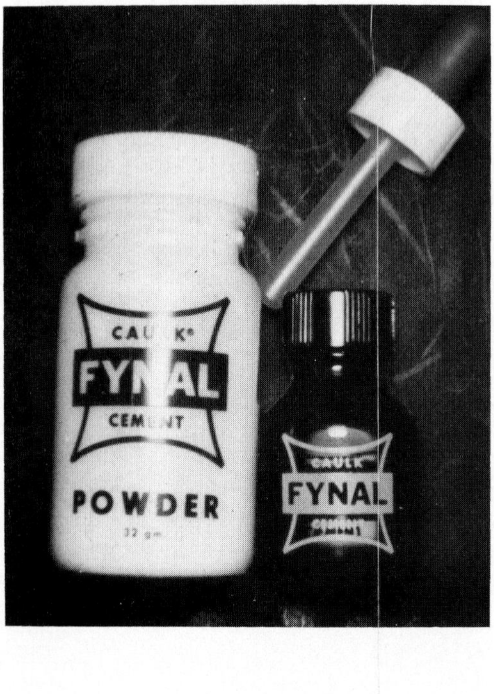

Figure 8–3 An example of resin-fortified zinc oxide and eugenol cement.

and to its ability to seal tooth structure because of good initial adaptation. When the initial adaptation to tooth structure or the marginal seal is broken by loosening, deformation, or passage of time, or a combination of these factors, leakage of irritating oral fluids may cause pain and hypersensitivity. It is erroneous to blame the zinc oxide and eugenol material instead of the leakage for the sensitivity or pain. Temporary coverage or final restorations cemented temporarily with zinc oxide and eugenol cement usually yield comfortable, pain-free abutment teeth if they do not function over a period of time in the mouth while loose and leaking. Therefore, every effort should be made to provide retentive preparations, well-fitting restorations, and temporary cementation with a cement selected according to the biophysical factors involved so that premature loosening will be avoided.

ANTIBACTERIAL ACTIVITY

According to Peyton and co-workers,[23] an antibacterial agent in a dental cement would be effective to the extent that the set cement is soluble. Otherwise, the antibacterial agent would be locked in. This may readily apply to a zinc phosphate or a resin cement. However, the reaction of zinc oxide and eugenol seems to be both a chemical and a physical process, and solubility may or may not be necessary for an antibacterial agent to function in this type of cement.

The following hypothesis should be considered: In the set mix of a zinc oxide and eugenol cement, some of the eugenol may be absorbed by the zinc eugenolate produced by the reaction, and also by the unreacted zinc oxide powder.[24, 25] The presence of free eugenol in the set mix can be demonstrated even after several months, and this eugenol not in total chemical combination with the other ingredients can be extracted to some degree from the set mix.[26] This ability to be extracted, or *freedom potential,* of the eugenol may explain in part its efficacious action of continuous therapy to the dental pulp. It may also be reasoned that *a drug with antibacterial action that is soluble to a degree in eugenol will continue to have this value, since its activity will not be totally restricted within the set cement.*

Crown and bridge parabens* are antibacterial agents that are soluble in eugenol. The above conjecture may explain their beneficial effect as additives to various zinc oxide and eugenol formulations.

A study showing the absence of bacteria under a temporary zinc oxide and eugenol material suggests that bacteria under this type of material may not survive and increase in number to an extent that is histologically detectable.[27]

Bartels[28] notes: "The ideal sterilizing agent should show microbial specificity and be innocuous to pulpal tissues. Of the classic substances used for this purpose, only one appears to possess these qualifications. Zinc oxide-eugenol cements have in addition the valuable

---

*Teledyne Dental, Elk Grove Village, IL 60007

characteristic of effecting sedation. Their continued use is highly recommended."

Ethoxybenzoic Acid (EBA) Cements

The old saying, "A chain is only as strong as its weakest link" is particularly applicable to crown and bridge prosthesis, where success or failure is so dependent upon the cementation procedure and the cementing materials. For almost a hundred years zinc phosphate cement has been widely used as a cementing medium for crowns and bridges. In recent years various studies have pointed out the shortcomings of this cement.

One of the most important considerations in placing prosthetic restorations on vital teeth is to preserve the normal condition of the pulp, yet abutment teeth that have survived the abuses of preparation and impression making are subjected, ironically, to an irritating acid cement that has the potential to destroy them. Although cavity varnishes and calcium hydroxide liners are often used to offset the injurious effect of acid cementing media, these measures are only partially effective. Studies have revealed various degrees of penetration to the pulp despite their use.

An investigation by Bender, Seltzer, and Kaufman,[29] which revealed the entrance of microorganisms into the tubules during full crown preparation, suggested another function of the cementation procedure: *therapy to the injured pulp* in both temporary and permanent cementation. Since zinc oxide and eugenol cement mixtures are so effective in their therapeutic action on the dental pulp, a great deal of research in the past two decades has been involved with the improvement of this material for use in the permanent as well as the temporary cementation of fixed prostheses. There has always been a need for a final cement that does not require the associated protection of the abutment teeth that zinc phosphate cement does.

As mentioned before, zinc oxide and eugenol cements are the least irritating of the dental cements and provide an effective seal against marginal leakage. Their pH, or hydrogen ion concentration, is between 6 and 8, even at the time of contact with the prepared tooth. In comparison, the pH of zinc phosphate cement at this time is below 2, and free acid may be present at a pH lower than 4.7 for periods up to six hours after the phosphate cement has set. The solubility of zinc oxide and eugenol mixtures in dilute organic acids, in distilled water, and in the oral fluids is quite similar to that of zinc phosphate cements. Although this cement has low abrasion resistance, the shortcoming may decrease in significance when the cement is covered with a well-fitting full cast crown. One characteristic of a good dental cement that a zinc oxide and eugenol mixture lacks is compressive strength. Progress has been made toward improving this physical property, and its use has been extended to the *final* as well as the temporary cementation of fixed prostheses. In either case, it should be used with full cast crown retainers that are well fitted to retentively prepared teeth.

Laboratory tests and clinical observations have shown zinc oxide and eugenol cements to offer certain advantages other than that of sedation:

1. Consistency, slab temperature and mixing technique are not critical to the ultimate physical properties.
2. Crowns seat easier and *more completely*, and with less pressure than when zinc phosphate is utilized.
3. After insertion, dryness need not be maintained until setting occurs.
4. Initial adaptation to tooth structure is superior to other cements.
5. They are bacteriostatic and bactericidal on several organisms likely to be present in caries.

The use of zinc oxide and eugenol cements for final cementation has increased in popularity. The commercial products initially available were used with caution because of their low strength and poor resistance to abrasion. Even the stronger zinc oxide and eugenol cements available today should be limited to 1) full cast crowns rather than inlays and three-quarter crowns, 2) abutment teeth of adequate length and retentive form, and 3) situations presenting other favorable biophysical factors.

Various additives have been utilized in attempts to improve the strength properties of zinc oxide and eugenol, but the best agent for this purpose is *o*-ethoxybenzoic acid (EBA). The initial report by Brauer and co-workers[30] in 1958 showed a considerable increase in solubility associated with the increase in compressive strength. It was suggested then that the EBA cements be utilized as dental impression pastes or temporary fillings. In 1961 Phillips and Love[31] in the course of biologic testing reported that EBA formulations had superior tissue tolerance compared with zinc phosphate cement. In 1962 Brauer and co-workers[32] announced EBA formulations that exhibited *reduced solubility* as well as improved compressive strength. A few years later another report by Civjan and Brauer[33] compared the physical properties of EBA formulations with ordinary zinc oxide and eugenol and zinc phosphate cements. The EBA cements had much better physical properties than zinc oxide and eugenol cements, and showed compressive, tensile, and shear strengths that approached those of zinc phosphate cements. The material now seemed promising for use as improved sedative bases and pulp-capping and cementing media. This work was part of the dental research program conducted at the National Bureau of Standards. Utilization as cementing media for crowns and bridges was now indicated, pending clinical evaluation.

In 1965 Horn[34] reported a clinical study of the EBA cement. He stated that "... observations of greater duration are required for a more complete appraisal of this cement. However, indications that reflect its merit and the criteria for its usage are rapidly accumulating. EBA cements may be effectively utilized for the final cementation of individual full cast crowns and short-span bridges according to the dictates of the biophysical factors involved."

The "triad of evaluation" (see Chapter I) encompassing physical, biologic, and clinical research was now complete. Nevertheless, research and development in this area continued and the original EBA cement evolved into alumina EBA cement.[35] In this cement, alumina is used instead of quartz as a strengthening agent. The alumina EBA cement proved to be a substantial improvement. It provided not only greater strength but also lower film thickness, lower solubility, and easier manipulation. The uses of this cement were now extended beyond the situations suggested above.

Evaluation of a New Cement

How is a new cementing material appraised? Is it sufficient merely to test its physical properties in the laboratory? If it compares favorably with the physical values outlined in the American Dental Association Specification No. 8 for zinc phosphate cement, will it qualify for use in the mouth? How is sealing, insulating and therapeutic ability assessed? What about pulpal reactions and tissue tolerance? Are viscosity and surface tension low enough to allow for adequate seating and wetting? Do antibacterial properties enhance its ability to offset the deleterious effects of marginal leakage? Is it easy to manipulate?

The answers to these questions may be derived to some degree from laboratory testing and clinical research. However, clinical research of this sort presents many difficulties. What justifies its inception and when does it end? Only time will tell. In the meantime, it is essential to accept the guidelines of the available specifications (A.D.A.) for certain physical and chemical properties, to augment this with biologic testing and clinical investigations, and to allow clinical experience to accrue for subsequent appraisal.

The Formulation of an Alumina EBA Cement

An alumina EBA cement consists of a powder composed of zinc oxide (64 per cent), aluminum oxide (30 per cent) and hydrogenated rosin (6 per cent), and a liquid that is mostly *o*-ethoxybenzoic acid (62.5 per cent) and approximately one-third eugenol (37.5 per cent) See Table 8–2.

TABLE 8–2 THE FORMULATION OF AN ALUMINA EBA CEMENT

An alumina EBA cement should be compounded according to the formulation developed, tested and documented by the National Bureau of Standards.*

POWDER	
Zinc oxide	64%
Aluminum oxide	30%
Hydrogenated rosin	6%
LIQUID	
o-Ethoxybenzoic acid	62.5%
Eugenol	37.5%

*Brauer, G. M. et al. Aluminum oxide as a reinforcing agent for ZNOE-EBA cements. J. Dent. Res. *47*:622, 1968.

It has long been known that zinc oxide and eugenol mixtures are sensitive to modification by benzoic acid derivatives.[36] The *o*-ethoxybenzoic acid modifies the consistency and surface tension of a zinc oxide and eugenol mixture, allowing for an increased take-up of the powder component. In this type of mixture, it "opens the door" for an abundance of the strengthening agent, aluminum oxide, as well as for the zinc oxide and the hydrogenated rosin. The hydrogenated rosin contributes to improved insolubility, and the alumina contributes to the improvement of compressive and shear strength. The alumina also lowers the film thickness and improves the handling characteristics. An alumina EBA cement may attain a compressive strength of approximately 12,000 psi, and have a 24-hour solubility of 0.05 per cent[37] and a film thickness of 20 microns.

Examples of Alumina EBA Cement (Fig. 8–4)

Opotow Alumina EBA Crown & Bridge Cement, Teledyne Dental (Fig. 8–5)
Zebacem C & B Cement, L. D. Caulk Company
ProCem with Alumina, Professional Products Company
Buffalo Alumina EBA Crown & Bridge Cement, Buffalo Dental Manufacturing

Clinical Observations with an Alumina EBA Cement

1. During mixing, the EBA cement shows an unusual surface tension pattern, in that it flows readily and yet exhibits a viscosity resistance to manipulation. After the 60 seconds allotted to the mix, however, a uniformly smooth and readily flowable slurry of low viscosity is obtained.
2. There is a minimum of resistance to complete seating during the insertion of fixed restorations.
3. No pain or sensitivity after cementation is acknowledged.
4. In selected cases, tests with ice-cold water seemed to indicate excellent insulation. Although this effect could be due to the ability of the cement to obtund pain, the aluminum oxide is known to have good insulating ability.
5. The EBA cement sets in the mouth in two or three minutes but remains plastic on the mixing slab for 10 minutes, allowing more than ample working time.
6. Excess cement is difficult to remove from the restoration at first, but has a "self-removing" quality with further hardening and the passage of time.
7. No restorations have loosened prematurely.

Clinical experience with alumina EBA cement has now accrued for more than a decade. Paffenbarger[38] states: "After a century of dominance, the zinc phosphate cements are being replaced by zinc oxide and eugenol cements, modified by orthoethoxybenzoic acid (EBA), and the polycarboxylate cements, which have high retention to a number of dental materials including enamel." The development of alumina EBA cement represents substantial progress toward improving the biologic installation of crowns and bridges. It is a direct result of the ever-increasing emphasis on biologic considerations in restorative dentistry. Nevertheless, it is important to recognize the shortcomings as well as the advantages of any restorative material.

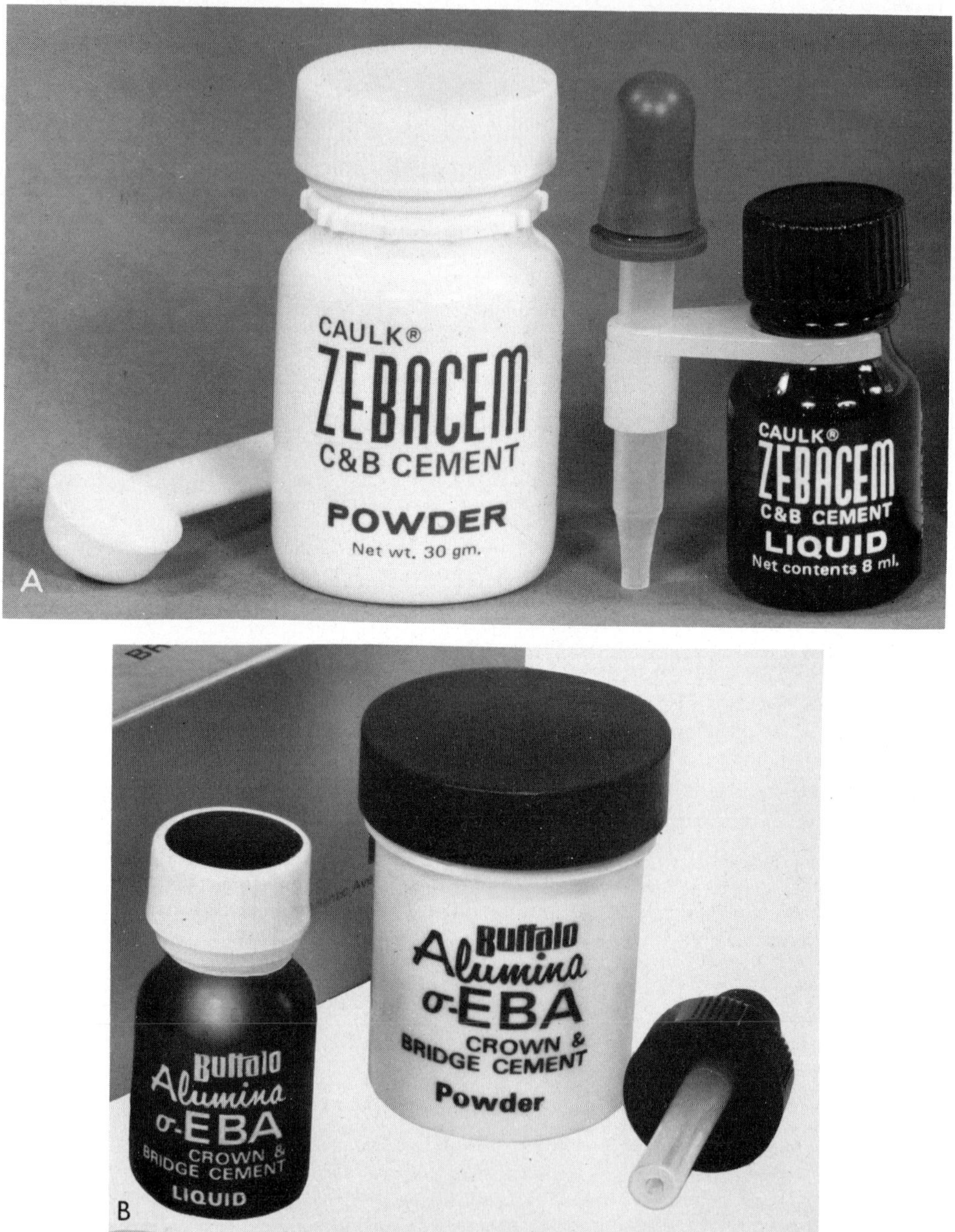

Figure 8–4 Examples of alumina EBA cement.

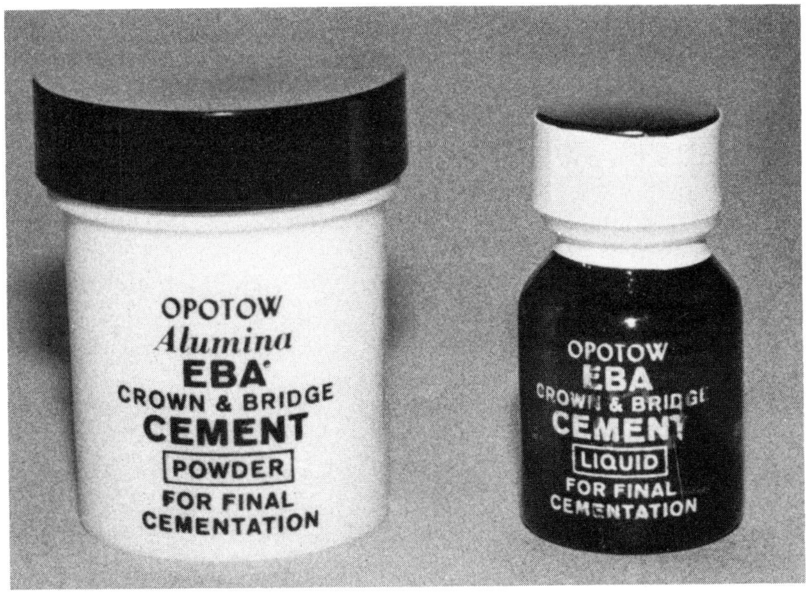

Figure 8–5 The original EBA cement, modified with alumina. This cement is compounded according to the formulation shown in Table 8–2.

Alumina EBA Cement—Good Characteristics

Painless cementation and sedative effect on sensitive abutments.

Extended working time, probably the longest of any cement.

Fast setting in the oral environment.

Good compressive and tensile strength.

Low film thickness and low solubility.

Biologic compatibility with hard and soft tissues.

Good insulation values, both thermal and galvanic.

Mixing technique is simple and non-critical.

Low viscosity and surface tension.

Moisture control is not critical prior to cementation. Abutments should be dry.

Dryness need not be maintained after insertion.

Antibacterial activity (enhanced by the benzoic acid derivative).

Restorations seat easier and with less hydraulic kickback.

Venting is not necessary for precise seating.

Clean-up is easy. Slab and spatula are simply wiped with tissue.

Alumina EBA Cement—Bad Characteristics

Resistance to abrasion is poor.

Excess cement may be difficult to remove.

Acrylic resin veneers require protection from excess cement.

Too opaque for translucent porcelain restorations.

Hasty seating is required due to fast set in mouth.

Slow ultimate hardening requires that function be delayed six to eight hours.

Setting is very sensitive to moisture and humidity.

Practical Considerations

1. Prior to final cementation, crowns or bridges should be seated on the abutment teeth in the mouth a few times to familiarize the operator with the path of insertion. This is important to minimize any delay in obtaining a complete seat, since the cement starts to set very soon after it passes the lips and enters the warm, moist oral atmosphere.

2. Lubricate interproximal spaces and acrylic resin veneers with a thin film of silicone grease to facilitate the removal of excess cement and to protect the resin from the deleterious action of the eugenol component of the cement. Do not lubricate the complete restoration, however, as it then will become too slippery to hold and may be dropped. This would further complicate the inherent nervous tension involved in every final cementation procedure. Final cementation is indeed an exciting, heart-palpitating moment of truth.

3. Be sure to shake the *powder* bottle. As a result of storage, the settling of components, and electrostatic surface interaction attraction, there may be clustering of the ingredients in the powder bottle. Turn the powder bottle upside down and shake a few times. Then turn upright and tap once or twice to settle the powder prior to opening.

4. Turn away, and do not breathe heavily on the mixing slab during spatulation. Condensation of warm breath on the glass slab will accelerate the set of the cement.

5. Do not fill up the entire crown with cement or it and the abutment tooth will be lost from sight under a sea of cement. It is necessary to line only the inside walls of the crown with a small amount of cement, depending of course on the tolerance of fit. The cement will flow out over the entire internal interface.

6. If the liquid component turns dark yellow or brown, there is no need to be concerned, for it will still function effectively regardless of its color. In fact, the same is true for the eugenol component of any other zinc oxide and eugenol cement. Exposure to air and light causes certain chemical and physical changes in eugenol that seemingly allow it to *improve with age*.[39]

7. Contact with chloroform or acetone will remove nearly all the eugenol from a hardened mix of zinc oxide and eugenol cement, resulting in complete disintegration of the cement.[40] For this reason, a zinc oxide and eugenol cement should not be selected as a final cement for diabetic patients. Also, patients should be cautioned not to use a chloroform-containing toothpaste such as Ultra Brite, Macleans or Close up.[41]

8. Immediately after completion of a mix of zinc phosphate or polycarboxylate cement, the cement must be applied without delay. Speed is important at this time; otherwise, the zinc phosphate cement may thicken, and the polycarboxylate cement may lose its gloss. In fact, all cements should be applied *immediately* after completion of the mix, with the exception of alumina EBA, which *has more working time than any other cement.* After the mix is completed with this cement, there is no race against changing consistency, loss of gloss, or premature hardening. There is ample time to apply the cement to a dozen castings, assuming, of course, that tropical heat or humidity does not prevail. Alumina EBA cement is also thixotropic (becoming thinner and more fluid on beating, whipping, or fast spatulation), so that if the cement applied to the first few crowns of a full arch splint start to thicken slightly by the time cement is applied to many others, further spatulation within the confines of a crown will restore the original fluidity.

Effect of Zinc Oxide and Eugenol on Dental Resins

Zinc oxide and eugenol cements may come in contact with dental resin as excess overflow or as a luting film on the inner walls of a crown. These cements, by virtue of the phenolic radical of the eugenol, are known to inhibit polymerization of certain resins. They are, therefore, contraindicated for use on any tooth on which self-polymerizing resin is to be utilized. Even after the polymerization of an acrylic material has occurred, contact with zinc oxide and eugenol elicits certain unstudied phenomena that may be observed clinically. The resin may change color or the hardness of the contacted surface may be modified. Eugenol attacks most dental resins and may cause them to soften and craze.[42] Other changes in physical properties may also occur. Although eugenol tends to depolymerize dental resin, its action seems to be limited as far as depth of penetration is concerned. For example, the inner surfaces of an acrylic resin jacket crown cemented with zinc oxide and eugenol are attacked by the action of the cement. Depolymerization and a chemical reaction ensue, and, as a result, the inside resin surface is modified. The cement adheres to the surface because of the chemical reaction. Subsequently, if the temporary cement film is removed, the resin interface is softer than the outside surface of the jacket crown, which is still hard and polished. The reaction may at times proceed completely through a very thin crown, causing surface discoloration, but this is seldom seen in a resin crown of average thickness.

Thousands of temporary acrylic resin jackets and bridges are cemented successfully every day with zinc oxide and eugenol cement. This cement has excellent initial adaptation to tooth structure, and also adhesion based on chemical reaction with the inside walls of the resin. However, this ideal association may be marred by poor operative technique. If the dentist allows the excess cement to slobber over the external surfaces (especially the labial) of the acrylic resin restoration and harden thereon, the resin will be attacked on the external surface, and be predisposed to discoloration, crazing and softening. This will be prevented if the excess cement is kept to a minimum, and is removed *as soon as it is extruded.* Excess cement should always be wiped away immediately with gauze or cotton to limit the time it is in contact with the resin. The measure of the harmful action of the eugenol on the resin is related to the extent of time they are in contact. As a precautionary measure, resin surfaces may be protected prior to cementation by the application of a thin film of silicone grease.

The excess of both temporary and final zinc oxide and eugenol cement should be wiped away immediately if the restoration being cemented is all resin or has a resin veneer component so that the untoward effect of the eugenol will be minimized.

The Story of the Bumblebee

Research chemists and materials science experts map out the intricacies of the unusual chemophysical interaction of zinc oxide and eugenol and show by documented laboratory tests that the hydrolytic instability of this mixture casts doubt on its durability and effectiveness as a dental cement.[43] This parallels the story of the bumblebee. In the past decade this humorous story has been applied to many seemingly impossible situations and it applies here also. Scientists weighed the bumblebee and measured his body and his wingspread. After measuring the force he exerted with his musculature, they went into a conference with slide rules, made some computations, and came up with the final conclusion that according to all principles of aerodynamics it was totally impossible for the bumblebee to fly. Nevertheless, the bumblebee does fly.

Similarly, zinc oxide and eugenol cement, despite the many pseudo-scientific doubts cast on its functional efficacy, serves with remarkable *clinical satisfaction* in crown and bridge therapy. Even a *temporary* zinc oxide and eugenol cement,* shown to have high solubility[44] and poor sealing ability[44] retained a fixed splint (gold and acrylic resin) in the mouth for over 12 years with adequate seal and retention.[45] Various dental books[46–48] by top clinicians suggest the use of this hard-setting temporary zinc oxide and eugenol cement (which would not qualify today as a final cement) for the permanent cementation of crowns and bridges.

It is difficult to devise significant laboratory tests that will correlate with clinical results. It has been shown that laboratory testing is not always reliable in predicting the durability of a material in clinical service. Despite laboratory indications of mechanical shortcomings, many dentists have had biologic benefits and clinical success with EBA cements for more than a decade.

---

*Temrex Cement

RESIN CEMENTS

Acrylic Resin Cements

About 25 years ago dental resin cements were introduced as outright substitutes for zinc phosphate cements, and occasionally were advertised as being definitely superior cementing materials. It was claimed that they adhered to tooth structure. They did, but only when dry. The initial bond was soon lost in the presence of moisture. Today, although acrylic resin cements are available commercially, they are recognized to be of limited value in crown and bridge prosthodontics.

Acrylic resin cement is unfilled polymethyl methacrylate (PMMA) cement. It is similar to the unfilled direct filling resin, but its powder may have some mineral fillers. The liquid appears to be largely methyl methacrylate monomer.

Three commercial PMMA cements were tested for bonding characteristics:[49] Grip,* Justi Resin Cement,** and Smith's Resin Cement.† None of these cements showed superiority in bonding with enamel or dentin, and claims that these cements would adhere to wet surfaces were found to be untrue.

The acrylic resin cements available today are not suitable for the cementation of crowns and bridges because of their poor handling characteristics. They have a short manipulation time. They shrink on hardening, expand on sorption of water and have a high thermal expansion; therefore, dimensional stability is less than adequate. Microleakage, which may be related to these factors, poses a threat to the health of the tooth. It is almost impossible to remove the excess hardened cement from interproximal spaces and gingival margins so that a smooth coalescence of tooth and casting will prevail around the circumference of the tooth. In the cementation procedure, excess resin cement will adhere to adjacent surfaces of plastic veneers and acrylic resin fillings unless adequate provision is made for the protection of these surfaces. Eugenol and other phenolic compounds inhibit polymerization and may prolong the time of setting indefinitely. Resin cements will not set properly on tooth structure that was previously in contact with zinc oxide and eugenol temporary cement. For biologic and therapeutic benefits, it would be preferable to utilize the zinc oxide and eugenol, and forsake the resin cement. Another biologic consideration: Acrylic resins are highly irritating to the pulp, regardless of whether they are used as filling materials or cements. Despite claims to the contrary, resin cements exhibit no greater adhesion to tooth structure under mouth conditions than do zinc phosphate cements. They are useful, however, in reattaching resin veneer facings to metal,[50] possibly because they demonstrate a thinner film thickness than zinc phosphate cement.

---

*L. D. Caulk Company, Milford, DE 19963
**H. D. Justi Co., Philadelphia, PA 19104
†Lee Smith Co., Teledyne Dental, Elk Grove Village, IL 60007

Composite Resin Cements

Modern composite resin restorative materials may be modified to serve as crown and bridge cements. A composite resin cement is based on the adduct of diglycidyl ether of bisphenol A and methacrylic acid and contains various ultrafine mineral fillers. The resin is diluted to a viscosity suitable for crown and bridge cementation with a low viscosity dimethacrylate monomer.

Research[51] related to a new filled resin cementing material, CBA No. 9080* (Fig. 8–6), indicates that this cement offers insolubility, improved adhesion to gold, porcelain, and acrylic resin, and high compressive and tensile strength characteristics. Unfortunately, this cement requires acid etching of tooth structure and sandblasting of gold alloys to obtain good mechanical adhesion. It is also irritating to the pulp.

All factors considered, composite resin cement is probably the strongest, *most insoluble,* and most durable cement available. However, the dentist should keep in mind a biologic consideration, pulp protection, and a physical shortcoming of the cement, large film thickness. Also, composite resin cement sets very slowly if the mix is too thin. The removal of excess cement does not seem to be a problem, as it is with the unfilled resin cement. However, a prompt removal of excess cement prior to setting is suggested to avoid the necessity of grinding it away after hardening.

Various other composite resin filling materials based on the same chemical system may be modified to a viscosity suitable for crown and bridge cementation by diluting a mix of the material with ethanol or a mixture of isopropyl alcohol and phenyl carbinol (Ease**). The same physical and biologic considerations are involved.

*Lee Pharmaceuticals, South El Monte, CA 91733

**Transon Corporation, Fenton, MO 63026

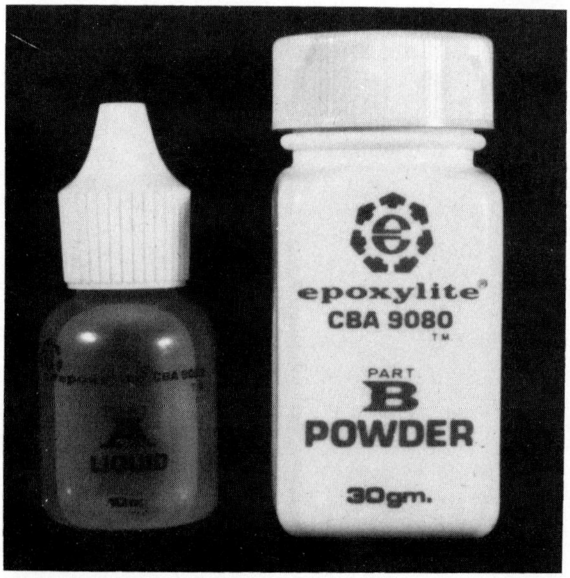

Figure 8–6 An example of a composite resin cement.

The composite resin cement is especially indicated for difficult retention problems involving endodontically treated teeth, for the cementation of posts and cores, and for the re-cementation of old fixed prostheses that must be salvaged for economic reasons. Composite resin cements, despite advertising claims, are not adhesive. It has also been shown that the cavity cleanser, a concentrated citric acid solution recommended to enhance the adhesive ability of the composite resin cement, will increase the undesired pulpal response.[52]

Composite Resin Cement—Good Characteristics

Virtually insoluble in water
High compressive and tensile stength
Good adhesion to gold alloy
Translucent

Composite Resin Cement—Bad Characteristics

Irritating to dental pulp
Timing of excess removal is critical
Large film thickness

Practical Considerations

1. The mixed composite resin cement should look glossy and be flowable, and yet not be too thin or the end product will be unsatisfactory. A mix that is too thin will also have a very substantial delay in setting. On the other hand, if too much powder is used, and the mix is thicker, there will be a reduction of working time and an increase in film thickness.

2. Pressure should be maintained on restorations seated with this cement for three to four minutes. Within the first 15 seconds after seating, and while pressure is being maintained, excess cement should be wiped away with cotton rolls or gauze squares. Then, dental floss should be pulled through contact points and interproximal spaces to remove excess cement (before 30 seconds has elapsed). While seating pressure is still maintained, the accessible margins may be cleaned of excess cement with a little alcohol on a small cotton pellet.

3. Dryness need not be maintained after complete seating.

Polycarboxylate Cements

A relatively new type of resin cement that utilizes an aqueous solution of polyacrylic acid (made from acrylic acid) is called polycarboxylate cement. It has also been called zinc polyacrylate cement, zinc polycarboxylate cement, and polyacrylic acid cement. The powder is mostly zinc oxide with a small amount of magnesium oxide. In fact, the powder is quite similar to that of zinc phosphate cement.

When the zinc oxide powder is mixed with the polyacrylic acid liquid a plastic paste is formed which passes through various elastomeric stages before setting to a hard opaque mass. Similar to other resins, glossy, stringy and rubbery stages are included. Its prime virtues are as follows:

1. It has better adhesion to tooth structure than any other dental cement; more to enamel, less to dentin.
2. It is as bland and non-irritating to the pulp as zinc oxide and eugenol cement.
3. It is almost as strong as zinc phosphate cement in compressive strength and possibly stronger in tensile strength.

Actually, polycarboxylate cement is not new. This cement is proof again of the age-old saying, "There is nothing new under the sun." Twenty-five years ago Bauer[53] patented a dental cement consisting of a powder of zinc oxide and magnesium oxide, and a polymeric acrylic acid liquid. He noted that "the phosphoric acid of other dental cements can be replaced entirely or partially with monomeric or polymeric acrylic acid."[53] The new cement, however, had low compressive strength, less than that required by the American Dental Association Specification No. 8 for dental zinc phosphate cement. It was probably for this reason that the new cement was not pursued farther at that time.[54] In 1966, Smith[55] developed the modern zinc polycarboxylate cement, indicating that other properties, such as adhesion and pulpal compatibility, were just as important as high compressive strength. He reported the results of clinical and histological studies, and suggested that the setting cement chelates with the calcium ions in the mineral phase of enamel and dentin to provide adhesion.[56]

The polyacrylic acid liquid is more viscous than other cement liquids. Therefore, the incorporation of a small amount of powder results in a slurry that looks and feels thick. However, a too thin mix is a frequent problem in the manipulation of this cement. This results in a hardened cement of low strength and high solubility.[57] If the liquid is exposed to air for more than a few minutes it will lose water by evaporation,[57, 58] and the mix will become even more viscous. It has been shown that the longer the exposure time of the cement liquid to the atmosphere, the thicker the resultant film thickness.[58] For this reason, a liquid should be dispensed only at the moment it is to be spatulated. A calibrated syringe dispenser is effective for controlling the proper powder–liquid ratio (Fig. 8–7).

Although various investigators have reported that polycarboxylate cements have low compressive strength compared with zinc phosphate cement, they are still strong enough for effective clinical utilization. Also, despite lack of unanimity among tensile strength studies, the polycarboxylate cement is comparable or superior to zinc phosphate cement in this strength property. A shortcoming of the

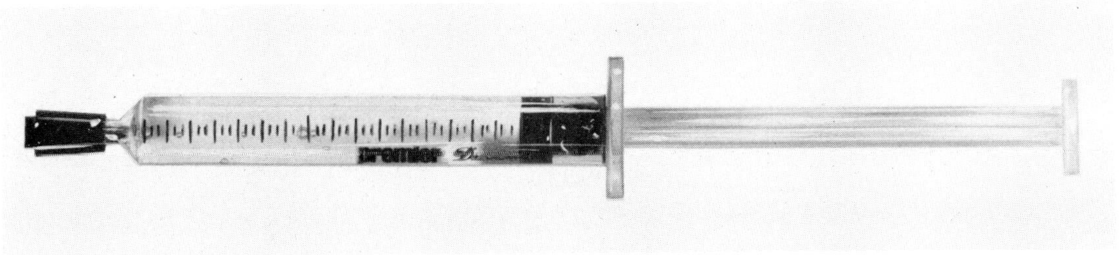

Figure 8–7 A calibrated syringe used for dispensing the liquid component of the polycarboxylate cement Durelon.

polycarboxylate cement is its *early solubility*. Immediately after placement, and while going through the early stages of setting (polymerization), *it is very sensitive to contact with water*. The dentist must protect it from moisture, or the material will dissolve away and present a weakened and irregular surface. Setting time will also be prolonged. After placement to restore contour, any contact with lip, cheek or tongue will result in distortion and stringing out of the cement, and should be avoided. The cement may be placed and shaped with a plastic instrument dipped in alcohol.

The solubility value of the polycarboxylate cement after hardening seems adequate.[59] Values for long-term solubility have not been definitively established.

The properties of polycarboxylate cements depend on the composition of the powder and liquid, and on the molecular weight of the polyacrylic acid. These properties may vary widely if the powder and liquid components are modified. It has also been shown that certain manipulative variables influence the characteristics of a polycarboxylate cement.[58] It would therefore be impractical to present the multiplicity of numerical values attributed to the physical properties of the many variations of this cement. Instead, note the following general description of a polycarboxylate cement.

Polycarboxylate Cement in a Nutshell

Good compressive strength (slightly less than zinc phosphate).
Good tensile strength.
Adequate film thickness and setting time.
Early solubility is critical.
Regular solubility seems adequate.
Long-term solubility is suspected of being poor.[60–62]
High viscosity.
Good adhesion to enamel.
Sticks to dentin better than any other cement.
Excellent pulpal compatibility.
Reacts with stainless steel, forming a chemical bond.
Does not adhere to gold, porcelain or acrylic.

The Stages of Polymerization of Polycarboxylate Cements

Polycarboxylate cements are resin materials and as such go through similar stages of polymerization. The first stage is glossy, the second stringy, the third rubbery, the fourth hardening. Each stage of setting is of practical clinical significance. For example, excess cement should be removed only during the initial soft or glossy stage, or after the material has hardened completely.

1. Glossy stage. This is the initial stage after mixing. Polycarboxylate cement should be applied to tooth structure only during this initial "glossy" stage of the mix. In fact, it should be used only, at all times and for all purposes, in the glossy stage. It is *in this stage only* that the cement manifests its adhesive ability. Once past this stage of polymerization it should be discarded.

2. Stringy stage. For some time after the glossy stage has passed, the cement should not be touched with finger or instrument or it will string out into a sticky, stringy cobweb.

3. Rubbery stage. Excess cement should not be removed during the "rubbery" stage of setting. Otherwise, there is a chance that some cement will be pulled out from under a margin of a crown and produce a void that could ultimately harbor food and bacterial debris.

Polycarboxylate Cement—Good Characteristics

Adheres to enamel.
Sticks to dentin effectively.
Non-irritating to the pulp.
Good compressive and tensile strength.
Adequate film thickness.

Polycarboxylate Cement—Bad Characteristics

High viscosity and surface tension.
Difficult to judge consistency of mix.
Dimensionally unstable.
Poor long-term solubility.
No sedative effect on pulp.
No antibacterial value.
Short working time.

Three commercial cements, Durelon,* (Fig. 8–8) Poly-C,** and Zopac,† were among the first polycarboxylate cements available after development. Some others that appeared thereafter are PCA‡, Chemit,§ and 3M Brand|| (Fig. 8–9).

The Problem of Dimensional Stability

Polycarboxylate cement is problematic as far as dimensional stability is concerned,[60] and may expand minutely or modify its shape in the time that elapses between impression making and the final in-

*Premier Dental Products Company, Norristown, PA 19401
**Amalgamated Dental, London, England
†The Lorvic Corporation, St. Louis, MO 63134
‡S. S. White Dental Products, Philadelphia, PA 19102
§H. J. Bosworth Co., Chicago, IL 60605
||3M Dental Products, St. Paul, MN 55101

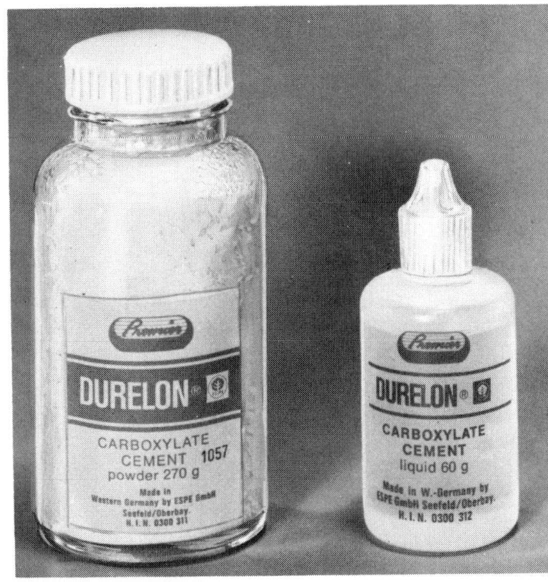

Figure 8–8 Durelon was the first cement of this type available as a commercial product.

sertion of a crown. This characteristic of the cement is readily apparent to the dentist who observes the hardened mix on the pad or glass slab. It will curl up and peel away from a glass mixing surface if allowed to set and harden thereon for many hours (Fig. 8–10). Also, the top sheets of a paper mixing pad will curl up in the various forms of distortion of the remaining film of hardened cement (Fig. 8–11). The cement will also separate easily and peel away from plastic spatulas and instruments, although it adheres tenaciously to stainless steel instruments. Therefore, it is important to consider any dimensional change of a polycarboxylate cement used as a core material or

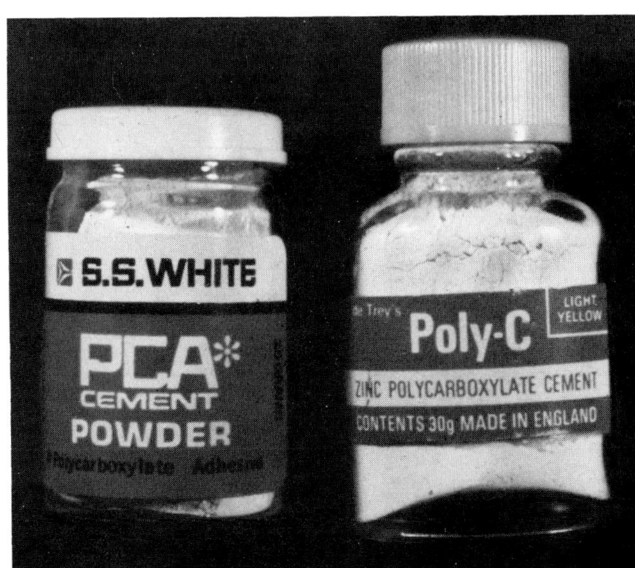

Figure 8–9 Examples of polycarboxylate cements.

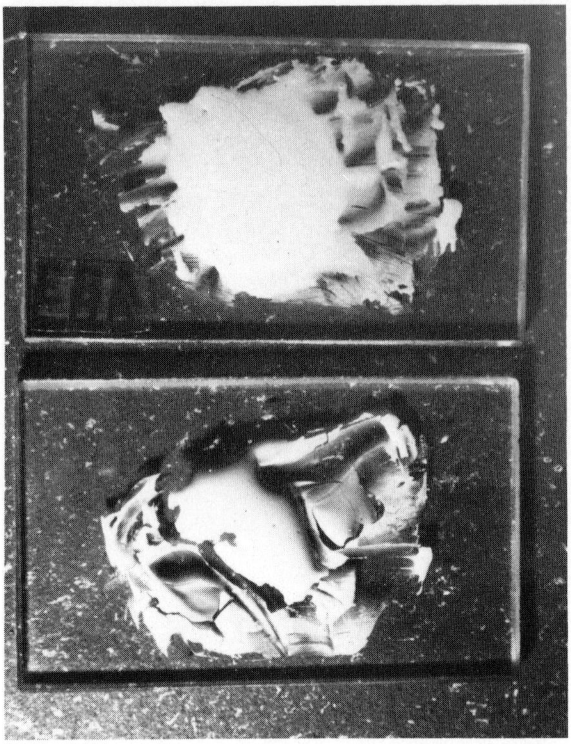

A

B

Figure 8–10 A comparison of cement mixes on glass slabs. After hardening, the EBA cement remains flat and unchanged, and the polycarboxylate cement curls away from the glass slab.

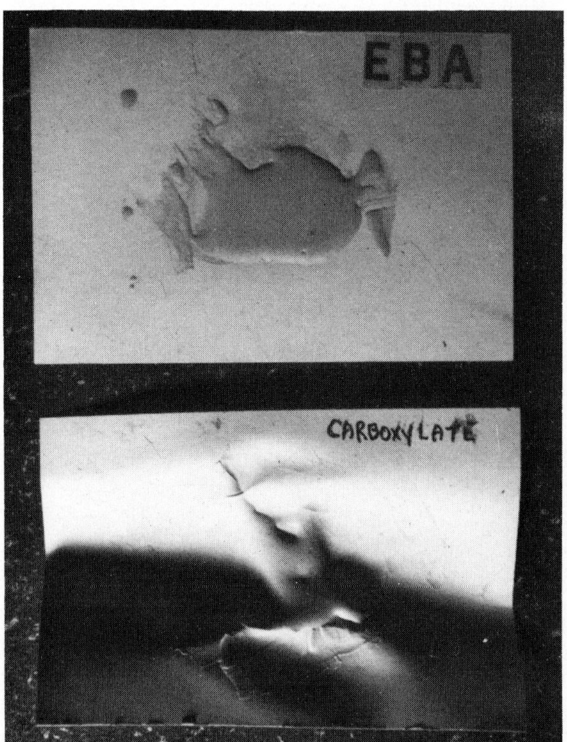

Figure 8–11 A comparison of cement mixes on paper pads. After hardening the top paper sheets were removed. After a few hours the polycarboxylate cement and paper sheet were distorted.

to repair a large area of a prepared tooth. For when the surface of the cement is exposed to the oral environment a change in surface topography may result. The impression made prior to fabrication may include the original surface area of the cement. When the restoration is completed, the fit may be too tight or may bind, owing to the dimensional change of the cement. However, a sandpaper disk applied to the cement surface will improve the fit and allow for a more passive insertion.

A Problem of Retention

Polycarboxylate cement is recognized as being very adhesive to dental enamel and, to a lesser degree, to dentin. Although it has not been shown to be truly adhesive to dentin in vivo, *it does adhere to dentin better than any other available cement.* It also adheres very strongly to steel. Just try to clean it off a stainless steel spatula after it has set. The manufacturer's direction sheet cautions the dentist to be sure to clean it from the steel mixing spatula immediately. In fact, according to Rupp[63] the polycarboxylate cements were formulated especially for the purpose of cementing stainless steel to enamel. Polycarboxylate cement has *no adhesion to gold.*

Polycarboxylate cement has the best adhesion to dentin of all available cements.

These considerations illuminate a method for solving certain problems of retention for porcelain-over-metal crowns or fixed bridges. When abutment teeth are very short, or of less than desirable retentive form, or when the span involved is very long, or when other challenging biophysical factors are involved, the selection of a steel alloy restorative metal such as Howmedica Microbond NP* is more appropriate than gold. Use of this non-precious metal bonded to porcelain and a polycarboxylate cement that adheres to both it and the abutment teeth will help solve the problem of retention.

Practical Considerations

1. The most unique property of the polycarboxylate cement is its adhesive ability. However, polycarboxylate cements do not bond chemically to gold, porcelain, or resin. Zinc phosphate cement seems to stick to alumina or porcelain surfaces better than polycarboxylate cement because these materials are more easily etched by the stronger phosphoric acid liquid.[64]

2. Strict adherence to the proportioning, mixing, and timing of application appears to be essential to routinely produce a cement of optimum physical properties.

---

*Howmedica Incorporated, Dental Division, Chicago, IL 60632

3. Polycarboxylate cement is the only cement that is normally mixed with a spatula made of a material (stainless steel) with which it is chemically reactive. It would be interesting to compare the properties of a carboxylate cement mixed with a stainless steel spatula with those mixed with a plastic spatula to determine if the reactivity of the cement with the spatula causes modification of any physical properties.

4. Acid etching does not enhance the bond strength of a polycarboxylate cement; instead, it appears to decrease the bond strength.

5. Like zinc oxide and eugenol cement, polycarboxylate cement has poor resistance to abrasion.

6. When fitting crowns to abutment teeth that have been repaired with a polycarboxylate cement, reduce the surface area of the cement portion of the preparation with a sandpaper disk to allow for a better, less binding fit.

7. Some commercial polycarboxylate cement liquids will gel after storing for a few months at ambient temperatures, and become unsuitable for cementation.[65]

8. An increased powder-liquid ratio plus a delay in applying the cement may result in a reduction of adhesive ability.[58] Also, an increased powder-liquid ratio may increase strength properties and film thickness.[58]

9. Polycarboxylate cement is not recommended for direct pulp capping, because it does not stimulate reparative dentinogenesis, and it is not bactericidal.[66]

10. Because of high solubility during the first five minutes after placement in the mouth, polycarboxylate cement should be protected from contact with moisture, or marked washout and weakening of the cement will occur.

11. Polyacrylic acid is highly acidic, with a pH of about 1.5. The cement mix which may be as low as pH 4, shows the same pattern of acidity and modification after set as does zinc phosphate cement.[67] The polymeric organic acid, however, does not seem to have the same irritant effect as the mineral acid found in zinc phosphate cement. This may be because polyacrylic acid is both weaker and less mobile than phosphoric acid. Its ability to travel into dentinal tubules is restricted by its high molecular weight and its tendency to become bound to tissue proteins.[68]

12. Polycarboxylate cement is a resin system, and as such takes up and gives off water in dissolution under various conditions. Also, if excess cement is removed during the rubbery phase of

setting, some material may be pulled out from under the margins of the casting, leaving a void.

13. A mixture of polycarboxylate cement is more viscous than a comparable mixture of zinc phosphate cement. A cement with high viscosity makes the seating of full crowns difficult. An important point to remember is that cements with high viscosity are more effective when venting (a planned opening) is utilized. Venting is of lesser significance when using cements of low viscosity.

14. A polycarboxylate cement will provide *a longer working time* if the mixing is accomplished on a cool glass slab and the powder is refrigerated. Do not keep the liquid (polyacrylic acid) in the refrigerator, however, for its shelf life may be shortened.

15. Finally, and of utmost significance, polycarboxylate cement provides no antibacterial activity and no sedative or anodyne action. Therefore, *claims that this cement has the same biologic effect on the dental pulp as zinc oxide and eugenol are misleading.* In biologic evaluations[59, 66, 69, 70] polycarboxylate cements have been shown to be mild and nonirritating to the dental pulp. In this respect it is similar to zinc oxide and eugenol cement. But it must be emphasized that it does not obtund pain, and it does not provide antibacterial activity.

A Comparison of Alumina EBA and Polycarboxylate Cements

Although the EBA and the polycarboxylate cements have been available for almost a decade, they are still considered relatively new cements. When dentistry comes to grips with new materials there is always a certain amount of clarification required to balance overenthusiastic advertising claims and misdirected personal opinions regarding the selection and proper utilization of these materials. It seems cogent, therefore, to compare these cements in order to clarify some of the issues. The practical comparison in Table 8–3 does not delve into chemical composition and the numerical values of physical properties. Instead, the basic physical properties pertinent to crown and bridge cementation, the handling characteristics, and the biologic considerations involved will be the categories of comparison.

The physical, mechanical, and handling characteristics of restorative materials have always been important in dentistry. In recent years, however, there has been increased emphasis on the biologic values of these materials. Today, new materials must be evaluated according to biologic considerations. Two relatively new dental cements have been compared. These cementing materials have many similar properties as well as many widely divergent characteristics. Only polycarboxylate cement shows *adhesion to tooth structure.* Only alumina EBA shows *anodyne action.* They are both

TABLE 8–3 COMPARISON OF ALUMINA EBA AND POLYCARBOXYLATE CEMENTS

	Alumina EBA	Polycarboxylate
Physical Properties		
Strength	Slightly higher in compressive strength	Slightly higher in tensile strength
Film thickness	Similar	Similar
Setting time	Similar	Similar
Solubility	Similar	Similar
Early solubility	Good	Poor
Long-term solubility	Questionable	Questionable
Viscosity	Low	High
Adhesion	None	Excellent
Dimensional stability	Good	Poor
Handling Characteristics		
Mixing technique	Easy, non-critical	Concern for consistency and glossy stage
Working time	Abundant	Limited
Dryness	Not critical	Critical, must be maintained
Removal of excess	Difficult at first, easy later	Rubbery stage must be avoided
Cleanup	Easy, wipe with tissue	Difficult. Wash with water at once
Shelf life	Excellent	Limited
Biologic Considerations		
Pulpal compatibility	Excellent	Excellent
Tissue compatibility	Good	Excellent
Anodyne action	Unexcelled for relief of pain	None
Antibacterial activity	Good	None
Minute pulp exposure repair	Good	Does not stimulate calcific bridging

moderately strong and extrude into thin films. Although they both set in the mouth in a reasonable length of time, alumina EBA has better viscosity, early solubility, dimensional stability, working time, and shelf life. Biologically, they both are nonirritating and compatible with the dental pulp and the soft tissue, but only alumina EBA is antibacterial, and can soothe abused tooth structure and obtund pain.

SUMMARY

Dental cements play an increasingly vital role in the successful accomplishment of a fixed restoration. Initially, crown and bridge therapy involves the use of cementitious materials for protection, repair, and sedation of prepared abutment teeth; later, for biologic evaluation of the fixed restoration; and, ultimately, for retention, marginal seal, insulation, and abutment therapy. The dentist reaches for a dental cement therefore for 1) the bases of deep cavities in abutment teeth, 2) the contouring of abutments, 3) the temporary cementation of acrylic resin temporary coverage,

4) the temporary cementation of the final restoration, and lastly 5) the final cementation of the fixed prosthesis.

Of all the cementing materials available for crown and bridge therapy, the only material that can actually contribute a measure of therapy is zinc oxide and eugenol cement. In this era of increasing concern for biologic considerations, the unique value of zinc oxide and eugenol is often overlooked. It is time for dentistry to look at this material in a more appreciative manner. Every dentist and researcher (and perhaps patients too) should recognize that *no other material* that exists in this world can relieve the pain of an aching vital tooth like zinc oxide and eugenol. This cementitious material is the best reliever of pain in a vital tooth; no ifs, ands, or buts. Any material that obtunds pain, kills germs and seals tooth structure is a very valuable and unique asset in restorative dental therapy.

Fortunately, fortified cements such as the EBA cements have evolved from research designed to upgrade the strength of zinc oxide and eugenol mixtures. Aided by recognition of the biophysical factors involved in the retention of fixed restorations, dentists may utilize zinc oxide and eugenol cements in final cementation to meet biologic requirements such as pulpal compatibility, tissue tolerance, formation of reparative dentin, and antibacterial activity. Aside from the stronger pain-relieving cement, today's cements offer the dentist certain other advantages: for *better adhesion*—the polycarboxylate cement; for *extra strength and insolubility*—the composite resin cement; and for *esthetics (translucency) and anticariogenic activity*—the silicophosphate cement.

Unfortunately, today no specification exists for zinc oxide and eugenol or polycarboxylate cements, although committees are preparing them currently. When the forthcoming specifications are available only cements that fulfill their requirements should be selected. Without a specification to set standards for appropriate physical properties, manufacturers may easily cut corners and economize on ingredients and formulation procedures, and subsequently provide substandard dental materials. Since these products may be dispensed in the original package and with the same name as a cement tested for adequacy at some prior date, the dentist may utilize these materials with a false sense of security.

REFERENCES

1. Skinner, E. W.: Some recent technical advances in dental materials. J. Am. Dent. Assoc. *66*:176, 1963.
2. Phillips, R. W.: Report of the Committee on Scientific Investigation of the American Academy of Restorative Dentistry. J. Prosthet. Dent. *14*:554, 1964.
3. Jorgensen, K. D.: Factors affecting the film thickness of zinc phosphate cements. Acta Odont. Scand. *18*:479, 1960.
4. Swartz, M. L., Sears, C., and Phillips, R. W.: Solubility of cement as related to time of exposure in water. J. Prosthet. Dent. *26*:501, November 1971.
5. Council on Dental Materials and Devices: Certification program for dental materials: List of Certified Dental Materials and Devices revised to Jan. 1, 1976, J. Am. Dent. Assoc. *92*:163, 1976.
6. Norman, R. D., et al: Properties of cements mixed from liquids with altered water content. J. Prosthet. Dent. *24*:410, 1970.

7. Phillips, R. W., et al: Zinc silicophosphate cement: Influence of composition on the acid solubility and fluoride content of enamel. J. Prosthet. Dent. *29*:628, June 1973.
8. Simmons, F. F., D'Anton, E. W., and Hudson, D. C.: Property studies of a hydrophosphate cement. J. Am. Dent. Assoc. *76*:337, February 1968.
9. Laswell, H. R., et al: Evaluation of water activated zinc phosphate dental cements. J. Tenn. Dent. Assoc. *51*:14, 1971.
10. Paffenbarger, G. C.: Dental cements, direct filling resins, composite and adhesive restorative materials: A resumé. J. Biomed. Mater. Res. (Symposium), p. 363, 1972.
11. Langeland, K.: Biologic considerations in operative dentistry. Dent. Clin. North Am., March 1967, p. 131.
12. Granger, E. R.: Practical Procedures in Oral Rehabilitation. Philadelphia, J. B. Lippincott Company, 1962, p. 264.
13. Roydhouse, R. H.: Better Clinical Use of Materials in Dentistry. Chicago, Year Book Medical Publishers, 1962, p. 21.
14. Frigoletto, R. L.: Pulp therapy in pedodontics. J. Am. Dent. Assoc. *86*: 1345, June 1973.
15. Rotberg, S. J., and deShazer, D. O.: The complexing action of eugenol on sound dentin. J. Dent. Res. *45*:307, 1966.
16. Schilder, H., and Amsterdam, M.: Inflammatory potential of root canal medicaments. Oral Surg. *12*:211, 1959.
17. Torneck, C. D.: Reaction of hamster tissue to drugs used in sterilization of the root canal. Oral Surg. *14*:730, 1961.
18. Coolidge, E. D.: Reaction of dog tissue to drugs used in root canal treatment. J. Am. Dent. Assoc. *19*:747, 1932.
19. Pohto, M., and Scheinin, A.: Microscopic observation on living dental pulp. The effect of oil of cloves and eugenol on the circulation of the pulp in the lower rat incisor. Suom. Hammalaak. Toim. *55*:185, 1959.
20. Brauer, G. M.: A review of zinc oxide-eugenol type filling materials and cements. Rev. Belg. Med. Dent. *20*:323, 1965.
21. Molnar, E. J.: Residual eugenol from zinc oxide-eugenol compounds. J. Dent. Res. *46*:645, 1967.
22. Civjan, S., et al.: Characterization of zinc oxide-eugenol cements reinforced with acrylic resin. J. Dent. Res. *51*:107, 1972.
23. Peyton, F. A., et al: Restorative Dental Materials, St. Louis, C. V. Mosby Co., 1960, p. 471.
24. Copeland, H. I., et al.: Setting reaction of zinc oxide and eugenol. J. Res. Natl. Bur. Stand. *55*:133, 1955.
25. Smith, D. C.: Setting of zinc oxide-eugenol mixtures. Brit. Dent. J. *105*:313, November, 1958.
26. Molnar, E. J.: Residual eugenol from zinc oxide-eugenol compounds, J. Dent. Res. *46*:645, 1967.
27. Brannstrom, M., and Nyborg, H.: Pulp reaction to a temporary zinc oxide/eugenol cement, J. Prosthet. Dent. *35*:185, 1976.
28. Bartels, H. A.: Cavity sterilization. A recommended procedure. Dent. Clin. North Am., November 1960, p. 659.
29. Bender, I. B., Seltzer, S., and Kaufman, I. J.: Infectability of dental pulp by way of dental tubules. J. Am. Dent. Assoc. *59*:466, 1959.
30. Brauer, G. M., White, E. E., and Moshonas, M. G.: The reaction of metal oxides with *o*-ethoxybenzoic acid and other chelating agents, J. Dent. Res. *37*:547, 1958.
31. Phillips, R. W., and Love, D. R.: The effect of certain additive agents on the physical properties of zinc oxide-eugenol mixtures. J. Dent. Res. *40*:294, 1961.
32. Brauer, G. M., Simon, L., and Sangermano, L.: Improved zinc oxide-eugenol type cements. J. Dent. Res. *41*:1096, 1962.

33. Civjan, S., and Brauer, G. M.: Physical properties of cements, based on zinc oxide, hydrogenated rosin, *o*-ethoxybenzoic acid, and eugenol. J. Dent. Res. *43*:281, 1964.
34. Horn, H. R.: The cementation of crowns and fixed partial dentures. Dent. Clin. North Am., March 1965, p. 65.
35. Brauer, G. M., McLaughlin, R., and Huget, E. F.: Aluminum oxide as a reinforcing agent for zinc oxide-eugenol-*o*-ethoxybenzoic acid cements, J. Dent. Res. *47*:622, 1968.
36. U.S. Patent 2,936,242. Brauer, G. M. Cements from metal oxides and chelating agents, May, 1960.
37. Craig, R. G., O'Brien, W. J., and Powers, J. M.: Dental Materials. St. Louis, C. V. Mosby Company, 1975, p. 104.
38. Paffenbarger, G. C.: Guide to dental materials and devices: A historical review. J. Am. Dent. Assoc. *84*:1333, June 1972.
39. Nahas, M. S., et al.: Eugenol improvement due to aging. A laboratory appraisal, Austral. Dent. J. *20*:283, October 1975.
40. Brauer, G. M.: A review of zinc oxide-eugenol type filling materials and cements. Rev. Belg. Med. Dent. *20*:323, 1965.
41. American Dental Association: Accepted Dental Therapeutics. 35th ed., 1973/74, p. 309.
42. Phillips, R. W., Swartz, M. L., and Norman, R. D.: Materials for the Practicing Dentist. St. Louis, C. V. Mosby Co., 1969, p. 51.
43. Wilson, A. D., and Batchelor, R. F.: Zinc oxide-eugenol cements: II. Study of erosion and disintegration. J. Dent. Res. *49*:593, 1970.
44. Norman, R. D., Swartz, M. L., and Phillips, R. W.: Studies on film thickness, solubility, and marginal leakage of dental cements. J. Dent. Res. *42*:950, 1963.
45. Schweitzer, J. M.: Oral Rehabilitation Problem Cases. St. Louis, The C. V. Mosby Co., 1964, Vol. 1, p. 251.
46. Brecker, S. C.: Crowns. Philadelphia, W. B. Saunders Co., 1961, p. 485.
47. Granger, E. R.: Practical Procedures in Oral Rehabilitation. Philadelphia, J. B. Lippincott Co., 1962, p. 281.
48. Brecker, S. C.: Clinical Procedures in Occlusal Rehabilitation. Philadelphia, W. B. Saunders Co., 1958, p. 42.
49. Swartz, M. L., et al.: A laboratory and clinical investigation of certain resin restorative and cementing materials. Part 1. In vitro tests on adhesive characteristics. J. Prosthet. Dent. *5*:698, 1955.
50. Schweitzer, J. M.: Oral Rehabilitation Problem Cases. St. Louis, C. V. Mosby Co., 1964, Vol 1, p. 263.
51. Lee, H., and Swartz, M. L.: Evaluation of a composite resin crown and bridge luting agent. J. Dent. Res. *51*:756, 1972.
52. Eriksen, H. M.: Pulpal response of monkeys to a composite resin cement. J. Dent. Res. *53*:565, 1974.
53. Bauer, W.: Verfahren zur Herstellung von selbsthartenden Massen, insbesondere fur zahntechnische Zwecke, D.B.P. Nr. 966,278 vom 18. 12. 1951.
54. Hoffmann, D.: Physical and chemical properties of certain dental cements. Quintessence Internat. *2*:109, February, 1970.
55. Smith, D. C.: Improvements relating to surgical cements. Brit. Pat. No. 1.139.430, 30.12.1966.
56. Smith, D. C.: A new dental cement. Brit. Dent. J. *125*:381, 1968.
57. Smith, D. C.: Dental cements. Dent. Clin. North Am., *15*:3, 1971.
58. Kafalias, M. C., Swartz, M. L., and Phillips, R. W.: Effect of manipulative variables on the properties of a polycarboxylate cement. Austral. Dent. J. *20*:73, 1975.
59. Jendresen, M. D., and Trowbridge, H. O.: Biologic and physical properties of a zinc polycarboxylate cement. J. Prosthet. Dent. *28*:264, September, 1972.
60. Mortimer, K. V., and Tranter, T. C.: A preliminary laboratory evaluation of polycarboxylate cements. Brit. Dent. J. *127*:365, 1969.

61. Moser, J. B., Brown, D. B., and Greener, E. H.: Short-term bond strengths between adhesive cements and dental alloys. J. Dent. Res. *53*:1377, 1974.
62. Moser, J. B., et al.: Solubility and water absorption of orthodontic cements. J. Dent. Res. *54*:280, 1975.
63. Rupp, N. W.: Intermediary base and cementation. *In* Baum, L.: Advanced Restorative Dentistry. Philadelphia, W. B. Saunders Co., 1973, p. 59.
64. McLean, J. W.: Polycarboxylate cements—five years experience in general practice. Brit. Dent. J. *132*:9, 1972.
65. Crisp, S., Lewis, B. G., and Wilson, A. D.: Gelation of polyacrylic acid aqueous solutions and the measurement of viscosity. J. Dent. Res. *54*:1173, 1975.
66. El-Kafrawy, A. H., et al.: Pulp reaction to a polycarboxylate cement in monkeys. J. Dent. Res. *53*:15, 1974.
67. Phillips, R. W., Swartz, M. L., and Rhodes, B.: An evaluation of a carboxylate adhesive cement. J.A.D.A. *81*:1353, December, 1970.
68. Wilson, A. D.: Zinc oxide dental cements. *In* Von Fraunhofer, J. A.: Scientific Aspects of Dental Materials. London, Butterworths, 1975, p. 185.
69. Truelove, E. L., Mitchell, D. F., and Phillips, R. W.: Biologic evaluation of a carboxylate cement. J. Dent. Res. *50*:166, 1971.
70. Barnes, D. S., and Turner, E. P.: Initial response of human pulp to zinc polycarboxylate cement. J. Can. Dent. Assoc. *37*:265, 1971.

nine

Some Pertinent Considerations Related to Dental Cements

If you want a dream to come true, you must first have the dream.

Carl. O. Boucher

A PRACTICAL COMPARISON OF DENTAL CEMENTS

A large amount of information related to the testing of crown and bridge cement has been made available both in lectures and in the literature. Laboratory measurements of compressive strength, tensile strength, setting time, film thickness, solubility, flexural strength, adhesive strength, linear shrinkage, thermal conductivity, and other physical characteristics have all been published. Unlike the results of biologic testing, which speak for themselves, the values for physical testing are more likely to require translation into bread-and-butter practicality. An understanding of the biologic considerations involved in the use of the cement and in its clinical and handling characteristics is also necessary. A practical comparison of dental cements (assuming adequate values for strength, film-thickness, and solubility, and other physical properties) should include the criteria shown in Table 9–1.

PRACTICAL QUESTIONS RELATED TO PHYSICAL PROPERTIES

In considering various cementing materials, dentists may be puzzled by the following questions:

1. How much compressive strength is necessary for the successful retention of a metal casting?
2. Does the laboratory measurement of film thickness indicate the extent of the final seating of a crown or bridge?
3. How important is the setting time of the cement?

TABLE 9–1 A PRACTICAL COMPARISON OF DENTAL CEMENTS

Type of Cement	Adequate Set Under Water	Protection with Silicone Grease**	Removal of Excess Cement	Adhesion	Viscosity and Surface Tension	Pulp Protection Required	Working Time
Zinc phosphate and silicophosphate	No	No	Easy	None	High	Yes	Limited
Alumina EBA	Yes	Yes	Difficult at first, easy later	None	Low	No	No limit
Polycarboxylate	No	No	Problematic*	Excellent	Very high	No	Limited
Composite resin	Yes	Yes	Problematic*, difficult	None, except by acid etching to enamel	Very high	Yes	Limited

*Gel or rubbery state may allow pulling out of material from under crown margins.
**For acrylic resin and nonbonding surfaces.

4. What factors influence the marginal seal of a crown?
5. What factors influence the oral solubility of a cement?

The answers to these questions and to many others about dental cements are usually obscured by a large amount of numerical values and statistics that, unfortunately, vary according to the source (i.e., where they are obtained, by whom, and how). Research measurements of the physical properties of the same cement may differ in testing laboratories located in different geographic areas (see Chapter 1). Nevertheless, the aforementioned questions may be answered without numerical values as follows:

1. The amount of compressive strength required in a cement to retain a casting has not been determined. Indeed, the minimal retentive requirement for cementing materials has not been defined, probably because of the many variables and biophysical factors that are involved.

2. No. The final seating of a crown or bridge is governed by the ultimate film thickness, and this is influenced by the factors shown in Table 9–2.

3. The importance of the setting time of the cement is related to the timing and ease of excess removal, the working time, the control

TABLE 9–2 FACTORS INFLUENCING THE ULTIMATE FILM THICKNESS AND MARGINAL AND OCCLUSAL ACCURACY

Taper and contour of preparation
Cement escapeways in restoration
Force used in seating restoration
Length of time force is maintained
Hydrodynamics
Timing and technique of cement application
Viscosity of cement
Surface tension of cement
Temperature of cement
Amount of cement powder in liquid
Particle size of cement powder
Flow resistance of surfaces involved

of early solubility, and the need for immediate occlusal adjustments by grinding. It is more important with some dental cements than it is with others.

4. The marginal seal may be transient at best. The factors that influence the marginal seal are as follows:
    a. Thermal changes
    b. Deformation
    c. The oral chemistry
    d. The solubility of the cement
    e. The fit of the restoration
    f. Recurrent caries
    g. Capillary action

5. The oral solubility of a cement is influenced by the following:
    a. The accuracy of the fit. This governs the access of the dissolving media to the cement.
    b. The nature of the media; that is, the type and amount of liquids such as carbonated beverages, vinegar, drugs, medicaments, and lemon juice.
    c. The turbulence of the media, such as salivary flow, fluid pressure, rinsing forces, muscular actions, and oral habits.
    d. The deformation of castings under functional pressure.
    e. Temperature variations causing expansion and contraction of crowns.
    f. Enzymes, microbiologic action, and pH changes.
    g. General health. Belching, regurgitation, and respiration bring powerful dissolving agents into the mouth.
    h. The powder to liquid ratio of the cement, and its manipulation.

The answers to the questions have been brief, but they are further embellished later in this chapter in the discussions on retention, film thickness, setting time, marginal seal, and solubility.

A SHARP FOCUS ON THE ACTUAL FUNCTIONS OF DENTAL CEMENT

Retention

No dental cement is truly adhesive to prepared tooth structure. Cement is an adjunct in the retention of a fixed restoration and not the sole source. In fact, a fixed restoration that is totally dependent on dental cement for retention may eventually loosen. The retention of crowns and bridges is based primarily on the biophysical factors involved in the coupling of a well-fitting casting to a retentively shaped abutment tooth. The cement merely fills in the space between the walls of the casting and the walls of the tooth. A mechanical bond is formed when the cement hardens in the minute irregularities of the facing surfaces. The *effectiveness of the bond* depends upon the following:

(1) the compressive, shear and tensile strength of the cement;
(2) the ultimate film thickness (the thinner the film the better the

bond and the greater the degree of seating. The ultimate film thickness depends on pressure, time, temperature, and other factors [see Table 9–2]);

(3) the accuracy of the fit of the casting (tensofrictional grip);

(4) the retentive form of the abutment tooth—taper, length, contour;

(5) the surface texture of the tooth and the inside of the casting;

(6) the metallurgical makeup of the casting (resistance to deformation);

(7) the differences in the coefficients of thermal expansion of casting, cement, and tooth;

(8) the nature of the coupling (i.e., inlay, three-quarter crown, or full crown); and

(9) the extent of the area subjected to the mechanical bond (the diameter of the abutment tooth).

It should be emphasized that all dental cements used to retain crowns and bridges do so by mechanical interlocking and not by virtue of any adhesive ability.

There is a large amount of criss-crossing of information and confusion concerning the ability of some cements to be "adhesive" to certain surfaces under certain conditions. This issue is clouded further by clinicians and manufacturers who stress the importance of materials that are adjunctive aids for true adhesion but are of little significance to mechanical bonding, such as surface conditioners, cleansers, primers, and surface energy activators. Just as it is impossible for a woman to be a "little bit pregnant," so too it is impossible for the luting of a crown to be "a little adhesive." Any retentive coupling of tooth and crown that is not bonded by a truly adhesive luting system must depend totally on mechanical bonding. Therefore, as long as retention is mechanical it will simply depend on a cement hardening between the imperfections of the facing surfaces of a retentive preparation that is coupled with a well-fitting casting.

Although a dental cement is usually assessed by its compressive strength, it is recognized that tensile strength and shear strength are also pertinent considerations in the functioning of a dental cementing material. High compressive strength is usually associated with the ability of a cement to provide retention. Although the FDI and the ADA specifications set a minimum value for tests of the compressive strength of a zinc phosphate cement, the minimum compressive strength required for its clinical use, or for that of any cement, has not been determined. The ADA specification No. 8 for dental zinc phosphate cement requires a minimum compressive strength at 24 hours of 9956 psi (700 kg per sq cm). A dental cement with a compressive strength of 8000 psi (562 kg per sq cm) has nevertheless been considered adequate for final cementation.[1,2] Actually, depending on the biophysical factors involved, a cement with a compressive strength of 7000 psi may even be adequate.

A more realistic approach for determining the retentive strength of a cement is the diametral test, in which tensile strength is determined by use of a compression test across the diameter of a cylindrical specimen. Cementing crowns to preparations and pulling them off in a vertical direction is an unrealistic way to evaluate the retentive ability of a dental cement. This force is the complete opposite of that which results from normal oral function. Forces of vertical removal are rarely engendered by the typical functional forces exerted on a cemented restoration in the mouth.

As mentioned above, the retention of crowns and bridges is based primarily on the coupling of a well-fitting casting to a retentively shaped abutment tooth and upon the biophysical factors involved. However, two other factors strongly influence retention. They are the crushing strength of the cement,[3] and the extent of seating of the crown on the preparation. A crown that is incompletely seated with a strong cement may not be retained as well as a crown that is fully seated with a weaker cement. It should be noted that retention increases when the following are increased:

1. Parallelism
2. Length of preparation
3. Surface area of preparation (diameter)
4. Roughening of facing surfaces.

Marginal Seal

The cement should preserve the integrity and health of the prepared tooth structure by providing a seal against saliva, bacteria, and the irritating end-products of food stagnation. This function is partially dependent on the solubility of the cement utilized. Unfortunately, the most insoluble cement falls victim to the ravages of thermal change, deformation, and other phenomena. Since there is always a potential for leakage, a cement with antibacterial properties may function as a secondary line of defense against bacterial invasion.

The margins of restorative materials that are in contact with tooth structure do not seal the area. Therefore, leakage occurs and may allow the ingress of oral fluids, bacteria toxins, soluble ions, and debris. *This is referred to as microleakage.* It may lead to pulpal sensitivity, caries, staining of margins, and pulp pathology. To prevent microleakage, a restorative material should combine chemically with the tooth surfaces and should also expand and contract to the same degree as the tooth during temperature changes. *No dental restorative material has this ability.* There is no filling material, cement, or other type of restorative material available in modern dentistry that will effectively seal the interface between a tooth and a restoration in the oral environment. Because of the lack of a chemical bond between restorative material and tooth structure, microleakage is a constant factor for failure. The degree of microleakage is a measure of the acceptability of a restorative material.

In fixed restorative dentistry the solubility of the cement is just one of many factors that influence the marginal seal. Other factors to be considered are as follows:

1. Accuracy of the fit of the restoration.
2. Temperature fluctuations.
3. Thermal conductivity of restorative material.
4. Cementation technique.
5. Strength of the tooth-cement-restoration "mechanical" bond.
6. Cavity varnish.
7. Deformation.
8. Film thickness.
9. Capillary action.
10. Recurrent caries.
11. Changing oral chemistry.
12. Penetrability of chemical agents in food and certain types of partial regurgitation.

Although many of the above factors have been discussed at length in dental literature, few observers have recognized the influence of capillary action. Capillary penetration exists between restorative materials and tooth structures.[4] Just as alcohol runs up the wick of an alcohol lamp, and ink goes into a blotter, and coffee climbs into a lump of sugar, so too does fluid in the mouth run into the crevices between tooth, cement, and restoration. The degree of penetration is influenced by the narrowness of the crevice, the surface tension of the liquid (oral fluid), and the extent to which the liquid wets the solid surfaces. Decreasing the size of the crevice by improving the adaptation of the restorative material will increase capillary pressure and penetration. Paradoxically, this poses a more significant threat to the marginal seal of well-fitting restorations than does the lesser capillary intake of ill-fitting restorations with poor adaptation.

The phenomenon of *capillarity,* or *capillary penetration,* which was originally identified by Leonardo da Vinci, is an interesting result of the surface tension of liquid. A simple demonstration of capillarity may be given by placing a clean glass tube with a very fine bore in a glass of water; the water will rise up the tube against the effect of gravity. The smaller the inside diameter of the tube, the higher the water will rise. A rise similar to that in the glass tube will take place between two photographic plates or glass slabs placed together and stood upright in a shallow ink solution; the rise of the ink between the plates will be seen through the glass. Further, if a thin wedge is introduced between the plates at one side the result will be as shown in Figure 9–1, the rise at the wedge side being *much lower* than at the other. It is probable, therefore, that microleakage due to capillary action between the facing surfaces of tooth and restoration will be less in areas of poor fit than in areas of extended intimate contact.

Since marginal leakage is an inherent shortcoming of dental restorative materials, the clinician must appreciate the importance of protecting the pulp under all restorations. The best way to do this is with proper cavity lining materials. Varnishes of copal resin and liners of calcium hydroxide and zinc oxide and eugenol cements

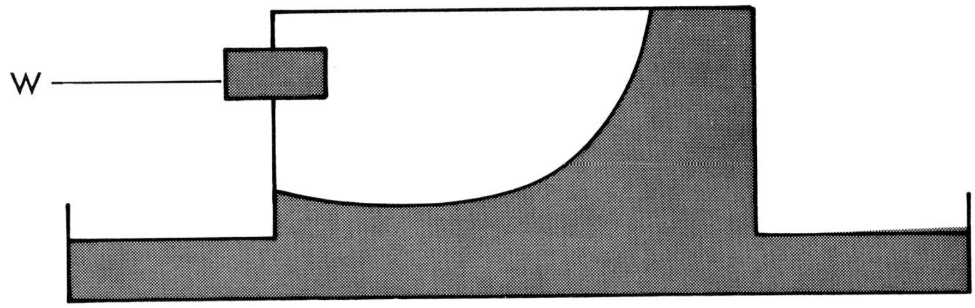

Figure 9–1 Two flat glass plates placed together and standing upright in ink. The rise of the ink between them will be obvious. If a thin wedge (W) is introduced between the plates at one side, the rise at the wedge side is much lower than at the other.

decrease leakage when applied to the walls of dentin adjacent to the pulp. Zinc phosphate cements, however, were not found to have this effect.[5, 6] Since zinc phosphate is a porous, permeable liner and has an acidic effect on the pulp, its use is contraindicated for pulp protection.[5]

Microleakage is based on a series of phenomena and is a serious threat to preventive dentistry. The clinical skills of the dentist and his knowledge of the physical and chemical nature of restorative materials plays an important role in minimizing this problem.

Insulation

The cementing medium should insulate the prepared tooth structure from galvanic activity as well as thermal change.

Therapy

In the light of the increasing emphasis on the biological compatibility of restorative dental materials, an ideal cement should not only be non-irritating, it should also provide therapy to abused dentinal and pulpal tissues.

THE FALLACY OF FILM THICKNESS

The intimate contact relationship of any two facing surfaces is modified and rendered less precise when another material, no matter how thin, is interposed between them. Likewise, a crown that contacts tooth structure along a closely adapted margin immediately after fabrication will no longer be closely adapted to that margin when a thin film of cement is introduced between them in the cementation procedure. This is one of the most challenging of the problems involved in the cementation of a fixed prosthesis and probably one of the least understood.

Naturally, the thickness of the particle size of the cement is of substantial significance. A granular cement of large particle size will not allow the most intimate seating of a crown; nor will it press out into a very thin film between two plates of glass weighted by 15 kg as required by the American Dental Association Specification No. 8 for dental zinc phosphate cement. This specification limits the thickness of a cement for the luting of fixed restorations to 25 microns. However, *the ultimate clinical film thickness* after the final cementation of the casting is only partially related to the film thickness of the cement as measured in the laboratory test. In dental cementation procedures the film thickness of the cement is modified and reduced by the dissolution of the cement particles in the liquid, by chemical reaction, and by the pressure of spatulation and the force of seating.

The preciseness of the clinical seating of the casting, the ultimate film thickness, and marginal and occlusal accuracy are influenced by the factors shown in Table 9–2.

At constant taper, height, and fit a cement of low viscosity and low surface tension will allow more effective seating than a cement of high viscosity and surface tension, regardless of the particle size of the cement powder.

Since dental cement is required for the installation of crowns and bridges, an error of approximately the thickness of a thin film of the cement is always introduced when final cementation is accomplished. As a result, previously established margins and occlusal relationships are disturbed. This problem cannot be solved; it can only be minimized. Dentist and patient must live with this necessary shortcoming. A film will always exist even if a crown is vented; there is no way to avoid it. Venting will not solve the problem; however, it may help decrease the ultimate film thickness when a cement of high viscosity is used. For all practical purposes the dentist may cope with this problem by endeavoring to keep the ultimate film of cement to a minimum. To accomplish this he must be aware of the factors that influence the ultimate film thickness (Table 9–2). These factors explain why the evaluation of clinical film thickness by laboratory testing cannot be effective. As a result of these laboratory tests, some dental cements are advertised to have such low film thickness that the dentist can be sure that restorations will seat completely. Obviously, it takes more than a thin cementing material to insure the complete seating of crowns and bridges.

An often overlooked consideration that influences the ultimate film thickness is the nature of the surfaces that will be covered with the cement. The size, shape, texture, and contour of these surfaces influence *flow resistance.* Just as cement may flow differently over metal or glass surfaces, and form different film thicknesses thereon, it may also flow differently (with different flow resistance) on dentin or enamel, or on different types of dentin, or on metal posts and cores.

If the dentist recognizes the factors that influence the ultimate film thickness of cemented restorations, he may modify some of them to obtain the most favorable marginal adaptation and occlusal accuracy. A cement that meets the ADA specification for film thickness should be used. It should be mixed to a thin consistency on a cool slab in a cool atmosphere. It should be applied without delay at the beginning of its practical working time. It should be seated with substantial but controlled force, and maintained under this seating pressure until initial setting has occurred.

THE DILEMMA OF SETTING TIME

The time that elapses from the beginning of mixing the components of a cement until the mixture hardens is referred to as the *setting time.* This time may be influenced by ingredients, accelerators, particle size, temperature and moisture, depending on the type of cement. When a cement sets too fast, appropriate manipulation and placement are hindered. When a cement takes too long to set in the mouth, the removal of excess cement is delayed and time is wasted, and a threat to the integrity of the cement may occur if function ensues before strength to accommodate it has developed. However, a long setting time on the mixing surface is of little significance.

The dentist mixing zinc phosphate cement for crown and bridge cementation may suddenly find himself between "the devil and the deep blue sea." As he incorporates powder into the liquid, slowly building up to an appropriate consistency, his dilemma becomes increasingly apparent: If too much powder is taken into the liquid, the consistency may be too thick for the complete seating of the abutment castings. If too little powder is incorporated, a weaker and more soluble cement will be produced and it will set very slowly; also, the cement will be more acidic and pose a threat to pulpal health. The low pH of a thin mix may have a harmful effect on a vital pulp even if a cavity varnish has been applied. The real dilemma, however, starts the moment the proper consistency is attained. Now the race is on. There must be no delay. The race is between the dentist's application and insertion of the cement in the mouth and the advancing chemical reaction that thickens the cement and causes it to set. Timing and coordination at this time is very important. One false move, or poor timing, and the hard-earned occlusion is faulted and the crown margins will no longer coincide with the margins of the preparation. Another detriment to the effort is the inadvertent incorporation of moisture in the form of condensation from the surface of a glass slab that is too cold. Conversely, a glass slab that is too warm will accelerate the set of the cement.

A somewhat similar situation may be encountered when a polycarboxylate cement is utilized. These resin cements proceed rapidly into the usual stages of chemical reaction. Any undue delay may result in crusting and the loss of the initial glossy sheen of the first stage. The ability of these cements to adhere to tooth structure depends on application before the sheen fades away. If multiple abutment crowns are involved, the cement placed in crowns 1, 2, and 3 may be thickening by the time cement is placed in crowns 4, 5, and 6.

The only crown and bridge cement that resolves this setting-time problem to some degree is the alumina EBA cement. With this material, the dentist may make a mix, relax, and go out for a "quick lunch." There is no race; anyway, not at this time. The slurry of mixed cement remains thin on the slab for an extended period of time depending on temperature and humidity. In fact, after a few minutes' delay, it may even be thinner. If for some reason, such as high humidity or temperature, the mixture thickens slightly, it will become thinner if it is spatulated again. It is a thixotropic material and as such becomes more fluid when stirred. Therefore, the dentist may place this cement in the many abutment crowns of a full arch splint and then go back to the first few placed and stir them with a small instrument to regain fluidity if necessary.

EBA cements are sensitive to the moisture and warmth of the mouth, where they react quickly and set fast. With this cement, the race begins *after the cement has passed the threshold of the lips* and entered the mouth. Speed is now essential, for the restoration must be seated in the shortest possible time. Any undue delay may detract from seating efficiency. It is strongly suggested that before cementation the dentist rehearse the path of insertion with a few trial insertions.

The setting time of a cement in the mouth is significant with regard to the following:

1. Removal of excess
2. Initiation of function
3. Refinement of seating of crowns
4. Early solubility of the cement
5. Marginal seal
6. Grinding to adjust occlusion

THE PHENOMENON OF SOLUBILITY

The solubility and disintegration of a cement is obviously of great clinical significance. It is difficult to draw practical conclusions regarding the solubility of a cement, however, if the solubility is to be determined by immersion in distilled water (American Dental Association Specification No. 8), since in the oral cavity this value depends somewhat on the changing chemistry of the oral fluids to which the cement is exposed. Nevertheless, the laboratory test used for a relative comparison of one cement to another, and for screening dental cements for clinical use, utilizes tests of solubility and disintegration in distilled water. Cements have also been tested and compared in dilute organic acids common to the mouth. Since the mouth is not a simple container of distilled water, or for that matter of dilute organic acids, and since there are large differences in the dynamic chemistry of every oral environment, plus the concomitant activity of many complex and unknown factors, *in vitro* solubility tests do not have much clinical meaning. Various *in vivo* tests have endeavored to evaluate the durability of dental cements,[7, 8, 9] but they too only scratch the surface of our understanding of the complex phenomena involved in solubility, and merely substantiate what is clinically obvious.

Both abrasion resistance and solubility have been designated as factors in the intraoral disintegration of dental cements.[7] Low resistance to abrasion is easy to understand, but solubility per se is a nebulous consideration. It is not a simple matter of one substance dissolving in another, but a series of interrelated phenomena. As far as the washing away of dental cements is concerned, what we have been calling "solubility" is in actuality a complexity that may be termed "breakdown disintegration," only a small part of which is caused by simple solubility (one substance dissolving in another). The factors that may be implicit in the breakdown disintegration of a dental cement are as follows:

1. Changing oral chemistry
2. Enzyme activity
3. Microbiologic action
4. pH changes
5. Bruxism and clenching
6. Turbulence of oral fluids
7. Thermal changes (hot and cold food habits)
8. Deformation of restoration and tooth structure
9. Dietary habits
10. Plaque and caries index
11. Capillary action
12. Medication
13. Diseases (diabetes, etc.)
14. Intercrevicular fluid
15. Oral electric currents may liberate metallic ions from a restoration.

Early Solubility

According to recent research,[10] the solubility of phosphoric acid-type cements (zinc phosphate, hydrophosphate, silicophosphate) is appreciably greater when exposed to water *early* rather than *late*. The longer the time lapse before contact with water, the lower the solubility of the cement. It seems that these cements should be protected from oral fluids more carefully than is commonly done. Therefore, immediately after crowns, bridges, or inlays are installed in the mouth with this type of cement, a cavity varnish should be applied to all margins. "Early" solubility deserves more clinical consideration than solubility measured at 24 hours or 7 days, as suggested in new and old specification tests. For that matter "long-term" solubility is also very meaningful to durable and successful crown and bridge therapy.

TO VENT OR NOT TO VENT

In the process of cementing full cast crowns, the fluid cement is confined between the internal walls of the casting and the facing tooth structure. The seating force causes the cement to escape through progressively smaller openings at the margins. When the crown is almost seated the force exerted on the confined fluid cement inaugurates an hydraulic pressure that is antagonistic to the complete seating of the crown. The resistance to seating is greater when the walls of the preparation are almost parallel. If castings do not seat completely, both occlusal and marginal relationships are rendered less than precise. Every possible effort should be made to minimize this unavoidable loss of accuracy. One method is to make a vent, or planned opening, in the occlusal surface of a crown so that the cement trapped under pressure can escape. The purpose of venting is to put a hole in the hydraulic system so that it cannot engender resistance to seating as long as the cement under pressure has a way to escape. It must be recognized, however, that *the escape of cement depends on factors other than the presence of a vent.* Escape depends on (1) the location of the vent; (2) the fit of the casting; (3) the taper and contour of the preparation; (4) the viscosity and surface tension of the cement; (5) the force applied to seating and the time this force is maintained; and (6) the space established inside the casting to allow for a cement film.

The hole in the crown may be closed after cementation with amalgam, gold foil, or a plug of gold.

Successful venting is not a total panacea. It does not provide perfection of seating; it only minimizes the error caused by interposing the cement between the preparation and the casting. This error can also be minimized by using a cement with low surface tension and low viscosity at the correct consistency, with proper timing of application, abundant force at seating, and the maintenance of this force.

Hydraulics is a branch of engineering science that deals with the practical application of the laws of hydrodynamics. The chief physical properties of a fluid that affect its motion are its density, viscosity, and compressibility. Viscosity varies with temperature. It should be noted that a liquid in motion possesses energy by virtue of its velocity and its pressure. Hydraulic pressures vary with cements of different viscosities and surface tensions. Venting is of less significance when a cement of low viscosity and low surface tension is used. A minimum of hydrodynamic phenomena are involved when an alumina EBA cement is used.

Research projects on the effects of venting full cast crowns are quite popular. In this monotonous parade of data, each experimental procedure shows the same thing—that a vent in a well-fitting crown allows the least discrepancy when the crown is cemented. All this splitting of hairs is specifically related to the utilization of a cement with appreciable viscosity, such as a phosphoric acid or a polyacrylic acid cement. Too many dentists are being misled into believing that all they have to do to insure complete seating is to make a vent in each crown. This is not true. The error initiated by introducing cement between the tooth and the casting is reduced a small amount by venting—but it is not totally eliminated. No matter what, a small loss of total seating always exists! Therefore, the dentist is challenged to keep this loss to a minimum. He may do so just as effectively without a vent (1) by using a cement of low film thickness; (2) by using a cement mixed to a proper thin consistency on a cool slab in a cool atmosphere; (3) by applying sufficient force during seating, and maintaining the force until setting occurs; and by (4) using a cement of low viscosity and surface tension.

There are shortcomings associated with the use of a crown vent other than the obvious need to repair the hole after final cementation. For example, a thin mix of cement applied to the crown may flow out of the vent before seating; after seating, it may flow out of the hole even more and make for a sloppy and obscure field. Also, as with a copper band that is open at both ends, the cement within is not condensed at the gingival area. Density and a condensed seal in this area are critical to success.

To contend with this problem, the vent can be corked with a well-fitting wire or cast plug until just prior to total seating, when the cork is removed to negate hydraulic resistance to seating and the seating is refined. The metal cork can then be replaced in the vent while the cement is still soft. After setting has occurred, the cork is ground flush with the crown contour, and the margins are burnished.

A Break in the Brake Line

Automotive braking power may be obtained by a practical application of a well-known principle in hydrostatics—that a pressure exerted on any part of the surface of a liquid is transmitted undiminished to every part of the liquid and in all directions. When the fluid in an automotive brake line escapes through a break in the system, hydraulic pressure is negated, and the brake foot-pedal is easily pressed down to the floorboard with no resistance. Similarly, full crowns are also pressed down into place easily and completely when the usual hydraulic kickback is eliminated by a vent. The *viscosity* of zinc phosphate cement is a prime contributor to the hydraulic problem, and much of the research and writing on venting deals exclusively with this cement.[11, 12] In contrast, alumina EBA cement has minimal viscosity and very low surface tension, and crowns cemented with this cement go into place easier and more completely. Venting is not necessary. To repeat—venting is usually only necessary when using zinc phosphate cement. Its benefits are less clinically significant with alumina EBA cement.

There are biologic considerations inherent to the hydrodynamics engendered in the cementation of a fixed restoration. For example, local lateral pressures against the thin dentinal walls of the preparation are determined by the laws of fluid dynamics. These pressures against vital tooth structure may cause pain and contribute to irreversible pulp damage. Hydraulic pressure may drive bacteria or phosphoric acid cement deeper into the dentinal tubules or the pulp. A zinc oxide and eugenol cement may mask the effects of hydraulic pressure by its pain-obtunding ability, but in many instances pain will ensue despite the use of this cement.

Pressures caused by fluid dynamics may also be concentrated on the inner walls of a porcelain crown during cementation, causing it to fracture at once, or initiating strains in the porcelain that will ultimately relax into breakage.

Internal Relief

If some of the inside of the gold crown is removed, there is more room for cement, and the escape of cement is facilitated. The hydraulic pressure created during the cementation procedure is also reduced, and the resultant thicker film of cement improves the insulation of the pulp to thermal changes. Internal relief of a casting may be obtained by grinding, by chemical etching agents, or by electrochemical etching procedures. The integrity of the margins should be respected during grinding, and protected with a layer of wax or lacquer when chemical etching agents are used. Electrochemical etching procedures remove gold rapidly; however, it is questionable as to how much protection the margins require.

The dentist should be concerned about all possible escapeways for the cement trapped between the abutment preparation and the inside walls of the crown during the cementation procedure. This concern should influence the taper and contour of the abutment preparation, the selection and manipulation of the cement, and possibly the utilization of internal relief, grooves, channels, and vents. It should be noted that vents will be more effective if located on the occlusal surface rather than on the lingual or buccal surface. Theoretically, the best location of the vent to provide the most effective escape of cement is in the center of the occlusal surface. However, a location on the mesial-lingual cusp or the mesial-buccal cusp provides good access for manipulation when cementing a crown, and provides a more suitable area for cutting and burnishing the pin flush with the crown than one in the depth of the central fossa.

The Vented Socket

Another interesting dental application of venting to dissipate hydraulic pressure is in the reimplantation of avulsed teeth. The endodontically treated tooth when replaced in its socket in the mouth tends to slowly extrude from the socket, owing to the hydraulic forces confined therein. The original seating may not be obtained.[13] A vent to release the hydraulic pressure that may extrude the tooth will allow complete and passive seating in the socket. The vent is established through mucosa and bone at the apex of the socket[14] (Fig. 9–2).

Venting

In summary, crowns and bridges do not seat easily and accurately when cement is placed. Regardless of film thickness, or the consistency of the cement, crowns and bridges do not seat totally when placed into position in the mouth. Hydraulic kickback and the force required to squeeze out all the unnecessary cement causes a resis-

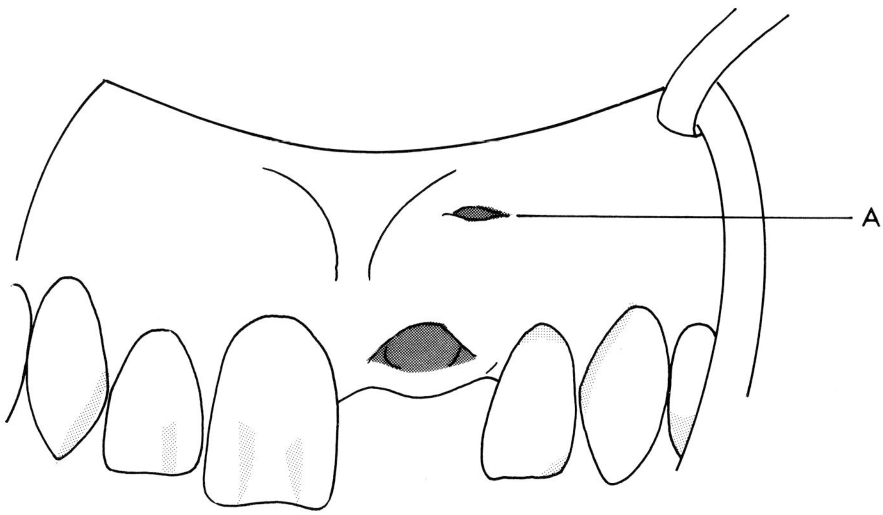

Figure 9–2 Prior to the reimplantation of an avulsed central incisor, a vent (A) is made at the apex of the socket. This will help to negate hydraulic resistance to the complete seating of the tooth. An incision is made through the mucosa and a round bur is used to perforate the bone.

tance to seating. No cement allows complete seating of the casting. Faulty seating results in a disturbed occlusion which needs immediate adjustment for comfort. Venting the casting is an attempt to offset this. It improves the accuracy of the fit of the casting. A crown in high occlusion may result in the following:

1. a tooth sensitive to pressure.
2. hypersensitivity to thermal changes.
3. destruction of the alveolar process, not only on the crowned tooth but on the opposing tooth as well.

Although venting may not be necessary with alumina EBA cement, it may be helpful when zinc phosphate cement or other viscous cements are used and the abutment teeth are long and have little taper. Venting may help to accomplish the following:

1. Allow escape of cement.
2. Permit better seating.
3. Prevent occlusal elevation.
4. Diminish postoperative pain due to pressure of cement on dentinal tubules.
5. Maintain tooth-to-tooth contact areas.
6. Prevent alteration of marginal accuracy.
7. Reduce the filtration factor.

REMOVAL OF EXCESS CEMENT

The various luting agents for the final cementation of fixed restorations cause different problems in the removal of excess cement. The retention of a tiny spicule of excess zinc phosphate cement may cause gingival irritation, and may harbor debris and plaque. With this cement every speck of excess must be removed fastidiously. In doing so, the dentist must take special care not to scratch the polished surfaces of the restoration with sharp instruments. A scratched casting will not be as sanitary as a polished one. Unlike zinc phosphate cement, alumina EBA cement does not require the meticulous removal of excess material. Large interproximal pieces of cement should be removed immediately, as should other fragments located near or in contact with the gingival tissues. However, films or smears of this cement (usually on the lingual surface) may be allowed to remain. If the dentist attempts to remove this excess cement with sharp metal instruments, highly polished surfaces may become scratched. If the excess alumina EBA cement is left alone, it will self-destruct (remove itself) in a day or so through food abrasion and thermal changes and possible enzymic or microbiologic activity. However, excess cement containing eugenol must be removed from an acrylic resin surface as completely and as quickly as possible to prevent subsequent damage to the resin.

Plastic cements, acrylic or polycarboxylate, require special considerations in the removal of excess. Excess plastic cements should be removed before the resins approach the rubbery stage of partial polymerization, or some of the cementing material may be inadvertently pulled out from under a margin, leaving a void or a rough edge, or both, and causing poor sanitation and periodontal health. After complete hardening, excess resin cement may have to be ground away; this is difficult, especially interproximally, and may result in rough and unsanitary areas.

One of a number of silicone greases* is recommended as a practical aid in the removal of excess cement. *Before cementation,* the fixed bridge or splint is covered with a film of silicone grease. A small amount is placed in each interproximal space and a thin film is smeared on the buccal and lingual surfaces. *Caution*! Keep the silicone grease away from the margins and be careful not to push any of this lubricant into the insides of the castings while handling. Do not use abolene oil or mineral oil as a lubricant. Any material with mobility may flow where it is not wanted. Petroleum jelly, carding wax, and other agents have been used to facilitate the removal of excess cement, but silicone grease is more effective.

REFERENCES

1. Myers, G. E.: Status report on zinc oxide-eugenol and modified cement. J. Am. Dent. Assoc. *16*:1053, 1968.
2. Gilson, T. D., and Myers, G. E.: Clinical studies of dental cements: IV. A preliminary study of a zinc oxide-eugenol cement for final cementation. J. Dent. Res. *49*:75, 1970.
3. Jorgensen, K. D., and Holst, K.: The relationship between the retention of cemented veneer crowns and the crushing strength of the cements. Acta Odont. Scand. *25*:355, 1967.

*Opotow Dental Silicone, Teledyne Dental, Palo Alto, CA 94304. RM Silicone Grease, Rocky Mountain Dental Products Company, Denver, CO. ProCem Silicone, Professional Products Company, San Diego, CA 92112.

4. O'Brien, W. J.: Capillary action around dental structures. J. Dent. Res. *52*:544, 1973.
5. Going, R. E.: Microleakage around dental restorations: A summarizing review. J. Am. Dent. Assoc. *84*:1349, 1972.
6. Phillips, R. W., et al.: Adaptation of restorations in vivo as assessed by Ca^{45}. J. Am. Dent. Assoc. *62*:9, 1961.
7. Norman, R. D., Swartz, M. L., Phillips, R. W., and Virmani, R.: A comparison of the intraoral disintegration of three dental cements. J.A.D.A. *78*:777, 1969.
8. Richter, W. A., and Ueno, H.: Clinical evaluation of dental cement durability. J. Prosthet. Dent. *33*:294, 1975.
9. Osborne, J. W., et al.: Solubility and disintegration of luting cements in vivo. I.A.D.R. Abstract No. 517, 1976.
10. Swartz, M. L., Sears, C., and Phillips, R. W.: Solubility of cement as related to time of exposure in water. J. Prosthet. Dent. *26*:501, 1971.
11. Cooper, T. M., et al.: Effect of venting on cast full crowns. J. Prosthet. Dent. *26*:621, 1971.
12. Jones, M. D., Dykema, R. W., and Klein, A. I.: Televison micromeasurement of vented and non-vented cast crown marginal adaptation. Dent. Clin. North Am. July, 1971, p. 663.
13. Lewis, T. M., and Dow, P. R.: Replantation of an avulsed permanent central incisor—case report. J. Dent. Child. *31*:103, 1964.
14. Freedman, G. L., and Hooley, J. R.: Immobilization of anterior alveolar injuries with cold-curing acrylic resins. J. Am. Dent. Assoc. *76*:785, 1968.

ten

Cavity Varnishes, Liners, and Bases

Many persons might have attained wisdom had they not assumed they already possessed it.

Unknown

Varnishes, liners, bases, primers, cleansers, sealers, tooth conditioners, etching solutions, and adhesion boosters increasingly crowd the cabinet shelves in the dental office. The use, abuse, and proliferation of these materials have led to confusion as to which to use, and where. Only a few of these materials are actually needed in crown and bridge therapy. Cavity *varnish* may be applied as a very thin film to protect an abutment preparation from irritating acid materials, or to protect a newly placed cement margin. A cavity *liner* is used as protection against the untoward effects of a composite resin filling material used to repair an abutment tooth, or in a deep area suspected of pulpal exposure. It is also indicated for use under composite resin cement. A *base* material is used as a thick layer at the bottom of a deep cavity to encourage recovery of the injured pulp and to protect the pulp from a variety of insults. It may also be used to completely fill a concavity or an undercut in a tooth being prepared for a crown, so that a proper retentive contour can be obtained. Etching solutions may serve as adjunctive aids in some restorative procedures. The primers, cleansers, sealers, tooth conditioners, and adhesion boosters are not needed for any practical purpose in crown and bridge therapy.

Cavity varnishes, liners, and bases are essentially protective coatings for vital tooth structure that has been prepared for a restoration. The copal type cavity varnish is effective in improving the marginal seal of restorative materials. Varnishes, liners, and bases have been used to provide insulation against thermal and galvanic changes. This utilization, however, is dependent on the thickness of the layer of this material against the tooth structure to be insulated. The copal type varnish forms a film that is too thin to supply insulation against thermal change. Attempts have also been made, with limited success, to provide various types of medication and antibacterial or anticariogenic activity to prepared tooth structure by use of varnishes, liners, or bases of appropriate formulations. Varnishes, liners, and bases, therefore, may be utilized for (1) protection against deleterious agents; (2) improving marginal seal (varnishes only); (3) insulation (depending on thickness); and (4) therapy.

VARNISHES

A typical cavity varnish is composed of a resin dissolved in a volatile solvent. When applied to tooth structure, the solvent evaporates and the resin remains as a somewhat incomplete film of plastic. This semipermeable resin membrane permits the passage of some types of ions but restricts the passage of others. Copal and synthetic resins are typical plastics used, and ether, acetone, and chloroform are typical solvents in a cavity varnish. Although chlorbutanol, thymol, eugenol, and even fluoride are utilized in some varnishes for medicinal value, cavity varnishes possess no enduring bacteriostatic properties. Cavity varnishes do not inhibit caries, and the addition of thymol causes no antibacterial effect and serves no useful purpose.[1]

It is usually difficult to obtain an intact layer of varnish, because there is a tendency for small holes to form as it dries. For this reason, two or three thin coats should be applied. The objective of the multiple layers of varnish is not to build up a thick layer, but to fill in the holes and provide a more complete coating for greater protection of the underlying tooth structure. The ability of a cavity varnish to block acid penetration depends on the continuity of the film formed; therefore, cavity varnishes will *reduce* but not totally prevent the penetration of the constituents of acid-containing cements into dentin.[2] Copal varnish does not have the same effect when applied in thick layers as in thin layers. Although a thin film may prevent microleakage, a thick layer may decrease the integrity of the marginal seal because of its inability to flow out over the tooth surface and wet it. Varnishes become thicker when the solvents evaporate, and they evaporate quickly. Therefore, bottles should be tightly capped when not in use, and the time of opening should be minimized. *Varnish should be thin.* If it thickens it should be thinned with a solvent. What seems thick to one dentist, however, may seem thin to another, and since there is no precise way to measure this characteristic of varnishes, it is safer to stay on the thin side, as the danger lies in having the varnish too thick.[3] In crown and bridge therapy a thick film of cavity varnish applied to a prepared abutment tooth may limit complete seating of a crown by taking up some of the room required for the film thickness of the cementing agent. Also, in a short preparation with questionable retentive form even a thin film of cavity varnish may decrease retention by filling in some of the ultra-small discrepancies that would otherwise be penetrated by the cement.

Zinc phosphate, silicophosphate, and polycarboxylate cements are more sensitive to *early* contact with moisture than they are to *later* contact; that is, they are more soluble before complete setting and a few minutes after setting than they are the next day, week, or month. In fact, the longer the time lapse between mixing the cements and contact with water, the lower the solubility of these cements.[4] For this reason, it is desirable to protect the cement line with these materials immediately after the cementation of crowns, bridges, and inlays. This is done by applying a coating of a water-impervious agent such as copal varnish on the margin areas of these restorations after excess cement is removed, and before moisture is contacted. It is interesting to note that the initial placement of a phosphoric acid cement in the mouth requires a "sandwich of the cement" between two layers of cavity varnish; one layer to protect the tooth from the cement, and the other to protect the cement from oral fluids.

A cavity varnish is contraindicated prior to the placement of a zinc oxide and eugenol cement.

Although a layer of varnish will reduce the diffusion of acid from zinc phosphate or silicophosphate cement into dentin, it should never be used *under* a zinc oxide and eugenol cement. The biologic benefits of zinc oxide and eugenol are obtained only by intimate contact with bare tooth structure. A film of cavity varnish would block off and deprive the dentin of these benefits. The same consideration applies to the utilization of calcium hydroxide; however, after a base or lining of zinc oxide and eugenol or calcium hydroxide is placed in a deep portion of a tooth, this base or lining and the rest of the cavity may then be covered with an application of cavity varnish. In this manner the base in intimate contact with the deep dentin aids the pulp, and the varnish decreases microleakage.

Abutment preparations should not be coated with cavity varnish prior to contact with self-curing acrylic resin. The reaction is uncertain. The monomer liquid of the resin may dissolve the varnish film, or the solvent in the varnish may react with or soften the resin.

CAVITY VARNISH DOES NOT PROVIDE

1. An antibacterial effect
2. Thermal insulation
3. Electrical insulation
4. Therapy
5. Anticariogenic activity

CAVITY VARNISH DOES PROVIDE

1. A barrier to irritants
2. Improved marginal seal
3. Protection against discoloration
4. Protection against desiccation

The following are some typical cavity varnishes.

Copalite (H.J. Bosworth Company, Chicago, IL)
S.S. White Cavity Liner and Varnish (S.S. White, Phila., PA)
Handi-liner (Mizzy, Incorporated, New York, NY)
Caulk Varnish (L.D. Caulk Company, Milford, DE)

LINERS

Cavity liners are aqueous or volatile organic liquid suspensions or dispersions of zinc oxide or calcium hydroxide that can be applied to dentin in a thin film. They are painted or flowed over the tooth structure needing protection, or applied with a needle applicator. The solvents evaporate, and the film residue dries quickly and protects the underlying dentin and pulp. Since the lining is basic, it tends to neutralize the free acid of zinc phosphate and silicophosphate cements. Calcium hydroxide stimulates the formation of secondary dentin, and in a thicker paste form is the material of choice to cover exposed portions of the vital pulp.

A cavity liner is usually used to cover both the walls and the floor of a cavity preparation, while a cement base is generally used to cover just the floor. Cavity liners are used for the following reasons:

1. To modify undesirable physical properties and biological characteristics of certain restorative materials such as unfilled and composite resin and phosphoric acid cements.
2. To protect pulpal tissue from physical and chemical injury.
3. To supply therapy to injured pulpal tissue.
4. To kill microorganisms.

Cavity liners should not be allowed to remain on margins no matter what final restorative material is placed. Calcium hydroxide is readily soluble in the oral fluids.[5]

Among the popular proprietary products available to the dentist are the following suspensions of calcium hydroxide:

Chembar—L.D. Caulk Company, Division of Dentsply International, Incorporated. Stated to contain calcium hydroxide, 6 per cent; zinc oxide, 6 per cent, suspended in a chloroform solution of a resinous material.

Hydroxyline—George Taub Products. A suspension stated to contain calcium hydroxide, 30.4 per cent, with methyl methacrylate polymers, 29.1 per cent, in methyl ethyl ketone.

Hypo-Cal (brand of calcium hydroxide paste)—Ellman Dental Manufacturing Company, Incorporated. Stated to contain calcium hydroxide, 40 per cent; barium sulfate, 10 per cent, suspended in an aqueous hydroxyethylcellulose solution.

Pulpdent Cavity Liner (brand of calcium hydroxide suspension)—Pulpdent Corporation of America. Stated to contain calcium hydroxide, 8.7 per cent, suspended in an aqueous methyl cellulose solution.

Calcium hydroxide is available in suspension for use as a pulp dressing or as a lining for dentin and in a paste for use as a cement base or a pulp capping material. Calcium hydroxide is available in various forms, some that set by air-drying alone and have a long setting time, and others that set by a self-setting mechanism and have a shorter setting time. Hydrex, MPC, and Dycal set like a cement with a chemical reaction. Examples of the various forms of calcium hydroxide are listed here.

1. Powder and liquid—Caldrium*
2. Liquid suspension—Hydroxyline,** Hypo-Cal†
3. Paste—Pulpdent‡
4. Base and catalyst—Dycal,§ Hydrex,|| MPC||

A Liner to Kill Microorganisms

Recent research[6, 7] has shown that the contraction of various restorative materials results in a space between the tooth structure and the restoration that usually contains a dense accumulation of bacteria. This has been pointed to as the cause of inflammation of the pulp. The bacteria may have been present on the walls before the restoration was placed, or they may have entered the space from the mouth through leakage after placement. An antibacterial cavity lining material, Tubulitec,¶ has been suggested to eliminate bacteria before the placing of the restoration. The design of the Tubulitec liner is based on the liner tested and reported by Zander, Glenn, and Nelson[8] in 1950. They found that a liner of polystyrene in chloroform with calcium hydroxide and zinc oxide could form a chemical and physical barrier to prevent irritation of the pulp if used under zinc phosphate, silicate, or silicophosphate cements. This liner became the commercial product Chembar. The original composition modified by the addition of an antiseptic, dithymol diiodide and a fluorine salt, calcium monofluorophosphate, is now available as the liner called Tubulitec. It has been shown to offer protection under several restorative materials, and has prevented bacterial growth on the tooth structure under these materials.[9, 10]

Recently, however, some doubt has been cast on the ability of an antiseptic or a fluorine salt to emanate from a hardened, dry resin film sufficiently to benefit the area of the interface. Accepted Dental Therapeutics (35th Ed.) states that dithymol diiodide is principally thymol iodide or thymol iodine, and is an antiseptic used chiefly as a dusting powder. Tubulitec depends upon this agent for its bacteriostatic action. It should be noted that thymol iodide is an old dental

*Teledyne Dental, Elk Grove Village, IL 60007.
**George Taub Products, Jersey City, NJ 07306.
†Ellman Dental Manufacturing Company, Incorporated, Hewlett, NY 11557.
‡Pulpdent Corporation of America, Brookline, MA 02147.
§L.D. Caulk Company, Milford, DE 19963.
||Kerr Manufacturing Company, Romulus, MI 48174.
¶Buffalo Dental Manufacturing Company, Brooklyn, NY 11207.

medication that has decreased in use over the years and is not looked upon as the epitome of efficacy in bactericidal activity. Although it is listed in National Formulary, tenth edition (NF X), and its use as an antibacterial agent noted therein, it is not listed in the current National Formulary, fourteenth edition (NF XIV). The Martindale, Ed. 26, The Extra Pharmacopoeia, London, The Pharmaceutical Press, 1973, states: "Thymol iodide is insoluble and has little or no antiseptic action. . .". It also states that thymol iodide is incompatible with alkalis and metallic oxides. Nevertheless, when dissolved in the chloroform solvent of Tubulitec, thymol iodide may provide just the optimum small amount of antiseptic action necessary to be effective against microorganisms without harm to the pulp, as suggested in the section of Chapter 2 dealing with drugs and medicaments.

Regardless of other considerations, Tubulitec provides as effective pulp protection as any other chloroform-contained cavity liner. It is best if used in *multiple layers* under a composite resin filling material.

A simple zinc oxide and eugenol formulation may be used in a thin film as a cavity liner. A recent study[14] suggests that the bacteria in a debris layer under a zinc oxide and eugenol cement may not survive and increase in number to an extent that may be detected histologically.

BASES

Compared to a thin layer of varnish or liner, a base is a relatively thick layer of dental cement placed in intimate contact with cut tooth structure prior to covering with a permanent restoration. A base may aid in the recovery of an injured pulp and also protect it from thermal, galvanic, and mechanical annoyance. A base also provides some protection against microleakage, the irritating ingredients of some restorative materials, and bacterial invasion. "Patching" or restoring a prepared abutment tooth to proper form may also be accomplished with a cement base material.

Materials commonly used as a cement base are as follows:

1. Zinc phosphate cement
2. Zinc oxide and eugenol cement
3. Calcium hydroxide mixtures
4. Polycarboxylate cement

All of these materials, in the thickness generally utilized, will insulate the pulp from thermal shock. Some of these bases are *stronger* than others. One provides more *pulp sedation* than the others. One is preferred for placement over small *pulpal exposures* or where one is suspected to exist. One is more *adhesive* to tooth structure than the others. Cement bases, therefore, are selected according to these requirements. Other considerations are biologic compatibility with the pulp, and the type of reconstructive material utilized. For example, acrylic resin temporary crowns will not polymerize over a zinc oxide and eugenol base.

Various cements meet various requirements as protective and palliative bases underneath restorations in deep cavities. It should be noted that a base is usually placed only on the floor of a cavity and not on the margins. In crown and bridge procedures, however, the base may completely fill the cavity or the discrepancy in an abutment preparation.

REQUIREMENT	CEMENT
Strength (but most irritating)	Zinc phosphate
Strength (but not irritating)	Polycarboxylate, zinc oxide and eugenol
Pulp sedation	Zinc oxide and eugenol
Pulp exposure	Calcium hydroxide
Adhesion	Polycarboxylate

Bases in Crown and Bridge Therapy

An abutment crown preparation requires the removal of a large amount of tooth structure. Therefore, for the biologic welfare of the tooth it would be better to avoid the use of zinc phosphate cement as a base because of its acidity and irritational effects at close range to the pulp. Where a base material is required in a deep portion of a prepared abutment tooth, polycarboxylate cement should be used. This cement is strong, adhesive, and non-irritating to the pulp, and may be smoothed to a fine, hard surface that is level with the remaining tooth structure. No other cement will adhere to prepared tooth structure as effectively, and the dentist need not be concerned about the base loosening or falling off during subsequent manipulative procedures. All other base repair materials depend totally on mechanical undercuts for retention. Polycarboxylate cement does not. It should be noted that the creation of undercuts on a tooth reduced to abutment form may be hazardous as far as pulp exposure is concerned.

When pulp sedation is required for a painful tooth, a small amount of fast-setting zinc oxide and eugenol cement may be placed before the application of the polycarboxylate cement. No other material can soothe and sedate prepared tooth structure as well. Similarly, if a pulpal exposure is suspected, calcium hydroxide paste is placed beneath the polycarboxylate cement. Capping with calcium hydroxide is the preferred treatment for pulpal exposures.

Prepared abutment teeth may also be restored to proper form with composite resins (see Chapter 2). However, the vital tooth structure underlying this material must be protected by calcium hydroxide or, if sedation is required, zinc oxide and eugenol cement.

Materials Suggested for Cement Bases

Polycarboxylate cement
  Durelon—Premier Dental Products Company

P.C.A.—S.S. White Company
Zopac—Lorvic Company
Zinc oxide and eugenol cement
Temrex Cement—Interstate Dental Company
Cavitec—Kerr Manufacturing Company
Alumina EBA—Opotow Dental Manufacturing Company
Calcium hydroxide cement
Dycal—L.D. Caulk Company
Hydrex—Kerr Manufacturing Company
MPC—Kerr Manufacturing Company

Practical Considerations

1. Use a copal type cavity varnish under zinc phosphate cement, silicophosphate cement, and amalgam.
2. Use a calcium hydroxide liner under composite resins.
3. To cover minute pulp exposures use a thick layer of calcium hydroxide.
4. Do not cover abutment preparations completely with a lining of calcium hydroxide.
    a. Marginal areas will wash out, owing to the solubility of the calcium hydroxide.
    b. Thin films of zinc phosphate and silicophosphate cement will be neutralized and weakened by the acid-base reaction.
    c. The sedative effect of zinc oxide and eugenol will be blocked off.
5. Polycarboxylate is the best (most adhesive) cement base with which to fill small cavities in abutment preparations and to restore proper form and contour.
6. No other base material can sedate painful tooth structure or reverse pulp damage as well as zinc oxide and eugenol.
7. Margins in prepared tooth structure and margins of cemented crowns may both benefit from the application of a cavity varnish (i.e., amalgam filling and zinc phosphate cementation), which provides protection against microleakage and also against the early dissolution of the cement line.
8. At close range to the pulp, varnish and base solvents may be chemically irritating and injurious because of thermal shock from rapid evaporation.
9. Dycal, MPC, and Hydrex are protective bases of calcium hydroxide that do not require the additional support of a cement. Although they contain calcium hydroxide and various other ingredients, they still provide the desired effect on the pulp.
10. Cavity varnish may contribute to the reduction of the interface gap between tooth structure and restorative material.
11. A zinc oxide and eugenol base material that forms a portion of a wall of a prepared abutment tooth should be covered with a few layers of cavity varnish prior to making an impression with a polysulfide polymer. Otherwise it will retard the setting of the rubber impression material and cause a rough and granular area of contact. The

eugenol component inhibits the polymerization of the polysulfide rubber impression material.

12. If desiccation of tooth structure precedes the introduction of any base, the pulpal reactions will be more severe than if drying was accomplished in moderation.[11]

13. Copalite should not be allowed to contact the gingival tissues. It has been shown that Copalite may be irritating to mucous membranes, causing inflammation and ulceration.[12]

14. Zinc phosphate cement is much more soluble in the first ten minutes after setting than 24 hours later. Therefore, the margins of cemented restorations should be coated with a copal type cavity varnish to prevent early dissolution of the cement.

15. A cavity varnish under a restorative material cannot be depended upon to protect against galvanic shock in the mouth.

16. A cavity varnish should not be used in the very deep areas of a tooth because chloroform or ether is irritating at this proximity to the pulp. As a safety measure for pulpal health, calcium hydroxide should be placed in the deepest area and then the cavity varnish applied.

17. A single thin layer of the liner Tubulitec does not give enough protection beneath some composite resin materials. A double application of this liner is required for complete protection.[13]

SUMMARY

Varnishes, bases and liners are interchangeable to some extent. It is important, however, to remember the following:

1. Only the copal type varnish should *remain on a margin* exposed to the oral environment; other varnishes, bases, and liners should not.

2. Only a base or a thick liner will provide insulation; no type of varnish or thin liner will do so.

3. Cavity varnish should not be applied to tooth structure *under* zinc oxide and eugenol cement or calcium hydroxide. But a film of copal type varnish may be applied *over* these materials.

4. Of all the bases and liners, zinc oxide and eugenol cement is *the only one that will relieve pain* with anodyne action and sedation.

5. Zinc oxide and eugenol cement should not be used as a base where unfilled acrylic resin is to be polymerized. It will inhibit the polymerization.

6. Many of the popular brands of composite resin will polymerize in the presence of zinc oxide and eugenol, and these resins may be used over zinc oxide and eugenol cement for the repair of an abutment tooth that is painful or sensitive.

7. Calcium hydroxide is water soluble and therefore cannot be used at the gingival margins of a restoration. It is important to remember also that it does not provide sedation of tooth structure.

As far as the dental pulp is concerned, the best varnish, liner, or base is *dentin.* In this case, the thicker the better. As far as the dentin is concerned, a thin wall needs protection. Varnishes, liners, and bases are utilized where necessary to provide this protection against thermal or mechanical shock and from chemical or bacterial irritants.

REFERENCES

1. Phillips, R. W., Swartz, M. L., and Norman, R. D.: Materials for the Practicing Dentist. St. Louis, C. V. Mosby Company, 1969. p. 16.
2. Swartz, M. L., et al.: Role of cavity varnishes and bases in the penetration of cement constituents through tooth structure. J. Prosthet. Dent. *16*:963, 1966.
3. Johnston, J. F., Phillips, R. W., and Dykema, R. W.: Modern Practice in Crown and Bridge Prosthodontics. 3rd ed., Philadelphia, W. B. Saunders Co., 1971, p. 362.
4. Swartz, M. L., Sears, C., and Phillips, R. W.: Solubility of cement as related to time of exposure in water. J. Prosthet. Dent. *26*:501, 1971.
5. Phillips, R. W., Swartz, M. L., and Norman, R. D.: Materials for the Practicing Dentist. St. Louis, C. V. Mosby Company, 1969, p. 26.
6. Brännström, M., and Nyborg, H.: Cavity treatment with a microbicidal fluoride solution: Growth of bacteria and effect on the pulp. J. Prosthet. Dent. *30*:303, 1973.
7. Vojinovic, O., Nyborg, H., and Brännström, M.: Acid treatment of cavities under resin fillings: Bacterial growth in dentinal tubules and pulpal reactions. J. Dent. Res. *52*:1189, 1973.
8. Zander, H. A., Glenn, J. F., and Nelson, C. A.: Pulp protection in restorative dentistry. J. Am. Dent. Assoc. *41*:563, 1950.
9. Brännström, M., and Nyborg, H.: Pulpal protection by a cavity liner applied as a thin film beneath deep silicate restoration. J. Dent. Res. *50*:90, 1971.
10. Brännström, M., and Nyborg, H.: The presence of bacteria in cavities filled with silicate cement and composite resin materials. Swed. Dent. J. *64*:149, 1971.
11. Langeland, K.: Prevention of pulpal damage. Dent. Clin. North Am. October, 1972, p. 709.
12. Kaminski, E. J., et al: *In vivo* toxicity of cavity liners to mucous membranes. J. Dent. Res. *54*:125, Abstract No. 323, 1975.
13. Brännström, M., and Nyborg, H.: Protective effect of liner applied as a thin film beneath deep composite resin fillings: Histologic investigation. Odont. Rev. *24*:335, 1973.
14. Brännström, M., and Nyborg, H.: Pulp reaction to a temporary zinc oxide/eugenol cement. J. Prosthet. Dent. *35*:185, 1976.

eleven

Biologic Evaluation of Fixed Restorations

One of the essential qualities of the clinician is interest in humanity, for the secret of the care of the patient is in caring for the patient.

W. Peabody

TEMPORARY CEMENTATION, FACT OR FANCY

The final cementation of a fixed partial denture should be accomplished only after biological compatibility has been verified to some degree. The insertion of the restoration for a trial period is helpful in determining the reaction of the host. This tentative placement to assay tissue reactions, accuracy of fit, occlusal relationships, contact points, and esthetics is termed temporary cementation.

Temporary cementation with zinc oxide and eugenol will prevent the pulpal injury that may occur with a phosphoric acid cement, will relieve pain by its anodyne action, and will permit the formation of secondary dentin.[1]

The philosophy of temporary cementation is looked upon more favorably today for many reasons, the most important being that abutment teeth seem to be less sensitive to irritation from zinc phosphate cement if they are sedated over a period of time with an anodyne temporary cement. Ewing[2] has pointed out that restorations may be cemented temporarily for periods of many months, or possibly years, provided that they are examined periodically. Kazis and Kazis[3] observed that temporary cementation of restorations over an extended period is extremely beneficial and that immediate and permanent cementation of extensive restorative work should be avoided. McCracken[4] notes that restorations have been removed after intervals as long as three to five years without evidence of leakage or deterioration of zinc oxide and eugenol cements, and suggests postponing the final cementation of fixed restorations until evidence of the success of the restoration can be evaluated.

The biologic evaluation of a fixed partial denture is accomplished by temporary cementation. Current experience and observations, however, indicate that temporary cementation should be of limited duration and not for extended periods of time as suggested above. The time allotted to verify biologic compatibility (temporary cementation) should be *just long enough to determine the reaction of the host.* What is the length of time required to evaluate a fixed bridge prior to final cementation? In other words, how long is temporary cementation? A day? A week? A month? The factors influencing this decision are the amount of abutment retainers and pontics, the length of the span, and the position of the pontics (i.e. cantilever). A simple three unit fixed bridge (only one pontic) may be effectively evaluated over a temporary cementation period of approximately five days. A more extensive fixed bridge should have a trial cementation of a week to 10 days. A full arch splint may be evaluated for about two weeks. No more time is necessary. A non-setting cement may be the ideal material for most full arch splints. However, these cements do not function effectively for much longer than two weeks. With very short preparations and with preparations of poor retentive form and with long-span bridges, a cement that provides more retention is indicated. A rule of thumb is that the smaller the fixed bridge the shorter the time period of temporary cementation. The more extensive the bridge the longer the time of evaluation.

TEMPORARY CEMENTATION AND THE SINGLE CROWN

Single crowns should *not* be cemented temporarily for the following reasons:

1. They are difficult to remove prior to final cementation.
2. Removal forces may traumatize the abutment tooth.
3. Removal attempts cause harm to the finish and polish.
4. There is little to learn from the procedure.

A single crown, or a series of single crowns should not be routinely subjected to temporary cementation. After all, the trial insertion is only meant to provide information so that the dentist may assess and adjust accordingly. The temporary cementation of an individual crown provides very little information. Its value should be balanced against the difficulty of removing a single crown when it is cemented securely, the potential for loosening if the crown is cemented weakly, and the need to repolish the scratches and scrapes inflicted during removal instrumentation. There is just not enough to be gained from the routine temporary cementation of single crowns. Also, the usual small, rounded, knoblike extension placed on the lingual surface of a crown to assist in removal is very poorly designed for that purpose. Removal instruments slip off easily and at best transmit torque and abusive pressures to the periodontal attachments. The extension must also be ground off and the area polished prior to final cementation, and this engenders heat that may harm (depolymerize) a resin veneer. By comparison, fixed bridges present interproximal areas that may be engaged by removal instruments. Also, floss or fine wire may be threaded beneath the pontic to aid in removal after temporary cementation.

THE DISADVANTAGES OF TEMPORARY CEMENTATION

Temporary cements are usually formulations of zinc oxide and eugenol that contribute therapy and sedation to the prepared abutment tooth. Notwithstanding these advantages, temporary cementation has certain drawbacks:

1. There is a potential for washout and loosening in the mouth.
2. There is a potential for washout without visible signs of loosening.
3. The removal of excess cement is difficult.
4. The eugenol in the excess cement may harm resin veneers.
5. Restorations may resist removal prior to final cementation.

The difficulty in removal of restorations after temporary cementation is probably the greatest deterrent to its utilization.

The withdrawal of a temporarily cemented restoration is usually associated with the application of force. This is especially true with full-arch splints and other large fixed restorations with many full crown retainers, for these restorations tend to fit the prepared teeth rather tightly, owing to the multiplicity of their tensofrictional grip.

After being tried in the mouth, an extensive restoration may be difficult to remove, even when no cement is applied. If a zinc oxide and eugenol cement *that sets to any degree of hardness* is used for temporary cementation, the restoration may resist removal. The force necessary for dislodgment is traumatic and potentially dangerous. *The dentist may fracture an abutment tooth, the restoration, and his relationship with the patient, all in one fell swoop.* How is he to cope with this problem and reap the benefits of temporary cementation? If retention is adequate, why not allow the patient to wear a fixed restoration temporarily without any cement? Obviously, the leakage of saliva and bacteria between the crowns and the abutment teeth may cause damage to the pulp, painful sensitivity, a bad taste, and an unpleasant odor upon removal. A cement must be used, therefore, if for no other purpose than to provide *a marginal seal.*

A dual problem confronts the dentist. The temporary cement should augment the retention of the fixed bridge and provide a marginal seal to the abutment crowns; at the same time the cement should not be strong enough to make removal difficult. In other words, the temporary cement should hold and seal, and yet allow release on demand. This is a sophisticated requirement for a cementing material. Actually, success is not totally dependent on the temporary cement but on a combination of the cement and the related biophysical factors (see Chapter 7). With favorable biophysical factors, such as long preparations, parallel walls, multiple abutments, and excellent fit, a weak temporary cement should be selected. With less favorable biophysical factors, such as short and tapered preparations and long-span bridges, a stronger temporary cement should be utilized. The dentist should develop his own judgment for the selection of an appropriate temporary cement. This requires that he recognize the biophysical factors involved and be able to evaluate the retentive quality of a fixed restoration and the extent of the occlusal forces to which it will be subjected. This information is then utilized in the selection of a temporary cement of the required compressive strength.

THE SPECTRUM OF CEMENTS AND ITS PRACTICAL APPLICATION

To meet a wide range of clinical needs, zinc oxide and eugenol cements with compressive strengths from zero (nonsetting) to 3500 psi are necessary. In a clinical study of temporary cements,[5] a cement with a compressive strength of 1000 psi most frequently met the requirement of the final prostheses utilized. Also, cements of compressive strengths of 200, 400, 600, 2200, and 3500 psi were required with sufficient frequency to indicate the need for temporary cements over this range of compressive strengths.[5] Stronger temporary cements should not be used for the temporary cementation of completed prostheses. They may be resorted to, however, when necessary (including final cements such as Fynal* and Zebacem*) to retain *problematic acrylic resin temporary bridges (protective coverage).* Here, unfavorable biophysical factors plus the easy deformation of the resin crown retainers allows removal prior to final cementation.

Should the clinician err on the strong side, or the weak has always been a perplexing question. An error in judgment of the prevailing conditions and in the selection of a cement that may be too weak can lead to premature loosening and the sequela of pain or embarrassing loss. On the other hand, selecting a cement that is too strong may bring breakage or resistance to removal, which is equally embarrassing. Weighing all considerations, *clinical experience leads us toward selection of a cement that may be too weak* rather than one that may be too strong.

Many dentists use petroleum jelly as an additive to obtain a weak temporary cement. However, the practice of mixing petrolatum with zinc oxide and eugenol for this purpose has certain shortcomings. Although the mixture may set to a lesser degree of hardness, it still sets hard enough in many instances to make removal difficult. Petrolatum is slightly soluble in eugenol and may limit its therapeutic action. Petrolatum tends to leach out of the cement, it turns rancid, and it absorbs mouth odors. Dental silicone grease, another material utilized for the same purpose, is more effective and has fewer shortcomings. It is highly water repellent and non-toxic, and is mixed with a zinc oxide and eugenol mixture on an empirical basis

---

*L.D. Caulk Company, Milford, DE 19963.

depending on the requirements. The larger the amount used, the weaker the cement. Various other concoctions that have been resorted to by dentists at this stage of restorative treatment include antibacterial ointments, corticosteroid mixtures, zinc ointment, calcium hydroxide mixtures, and various non-eugenol cements. These materials, however, do not provide the biologic benefits of a zinc oxide and eugenol cement—they do not soothe and sedate the prepared tooth structure or contribute a continuous anodyne action. Therefore, the best material for the temporary cementation of final fixed prostheses is a zinc oxide and eugenol cement that has been formulated to be weak enough to allow removal prior to final cementation. How weak should it be? Again, this depends on the biophysical factors involved (Chapter Seven). Retentive, well-fitting restorations may require only a non-setting zinc oxide and eugenol cement to seal and sedate the abutment teeth. In other, less ideal, situations a zinc oxide and eugenol cement that sets to a semihard consistency may be indicated. And in the problem case involving a long-span, or very short abutment preparations, a harder cement should be selected to insure retention. Obviously, more than one type of zinc oxide and eugenol cement may be necessary to fulfill the requirements of temporary cementation, and since the available commercial brands differ in their physical setting as far as hardness is concerned,[6] some setting to a relatively soft state and some setting hard, they are classified as: 1) non-setting cement, 2) soft-setting cement, and 3) hard-setting cement.

Table 11–1 illustrates a practical application of this classification, and shows how it may be applied to the selection of an appropriate cement for a given restoration. This selection is logically governed by the type of restoration and the biophysical factors involved, and is analogous to the selection of a particular casting gold for a given restoration. Soft, burnishable gold is not used for the lingual or palatal bar of a removable partial denture, and, of course, very hard gold is a poor selection for a simple occlusal inlay. Just as one type of gold is not suitable for all dental gold uses, so also, one type of cement is not suitable for all types of temporary cementation.

TABLE 11–1 SELECTION OF CEMENT ACCORDING TO TYPE OF FIXED PARTIAL DENTURE

Fixed Prosthesis	Temporary Cementation (*Zinc oxide/eugenol*)	Final Cementation
Multiple unit bridge or full-arch splint	Non-setting cement	Alumina EBA cement* Zinc phosphate cement
Short-span bridge	Soft-setting cement	Alumina EBA cement
Long-span bridge or cantilever bridge	Hard-setting cement	Zinc phosphate cement** Alumina EBA cement

*Preferred because of ample working time and biologic values.
**Preferred because of high strength properties.

THE DEVELOPMENT OF NON-SETTING ZINC OXIDE AND EUGENOL CEMENT

Zinc oxide and eugenol cement may be modified by additives to retard and inhibit hardening.[7,8] An example of a non-setting formulation is as follows:

Zinc oxide (USP) with 1 per cent propyl paraben	0.2 gm
Eugenol (USP)	0.25 ml
Silicone grease	0.57 gm

Results of similar formulations utilizing commercial brands of zinc oxide and eugenol may differ because of variations in composition. However, trial mixes of these cements with various amounts of silicone grease will reveal an appropriate consistency for the temporary cementation of multiple-unit fixed restorations. Approximately 1 per cent of methyl- or propylparaben should be added to the mixture. The high water repellency of silicone grease makes it especially valuable as a sealing agent. It is an inert, nontoxic, and highly stable material. Examples of dental silicone grease are as follows:

R.M. Silicone Grease, Rocky Mountain Products
Opotow Dental Silicone Grease, Teledyne Dental
Masque, H. J. Bosworth Company

Solvents for silicone grease are xylene, mineral spirits, perchloroethylene, and lacquer thinners.

Methyl- and propylparaben (methyl- and propylparahydroxybenzoate)* are neutral esters of parahydroxybenzoic acid and are fine white powders that show marked bacteriostatic and fungistatic activity at low concentrations against a wide variety of microorganisms. They are nontoxic and soluble in eugenol. Since the use of an antibacterial agent may cause the surface of the dentin to be an unsuitable locale for bacterial proliferation when exposed to seepage of saliva, the parabens are added to enhance this property of the eugenol (Fig. 11–1).

A small amount of methyl- or propylparaben (approximately 1 per cent) added to the usual mix of zinc oxide and eugenol employed in temporary cementation will increase the plasticity of the mix and upgrade antibacterial properties.

Clinical Observations with Non-setting Zinc Oxide and Eugenol Cements[9]

1. The functional forces of the oral environment improved the original seating of the castings.
2. The removal of restorations was facilitated.
3. On removal, crowns did not have an unpleasant odor.
4. Abutment teeth were not unduly sensitive to air.

---

*Opotow Crown and Bridge Paraben, Teledyne Dental.

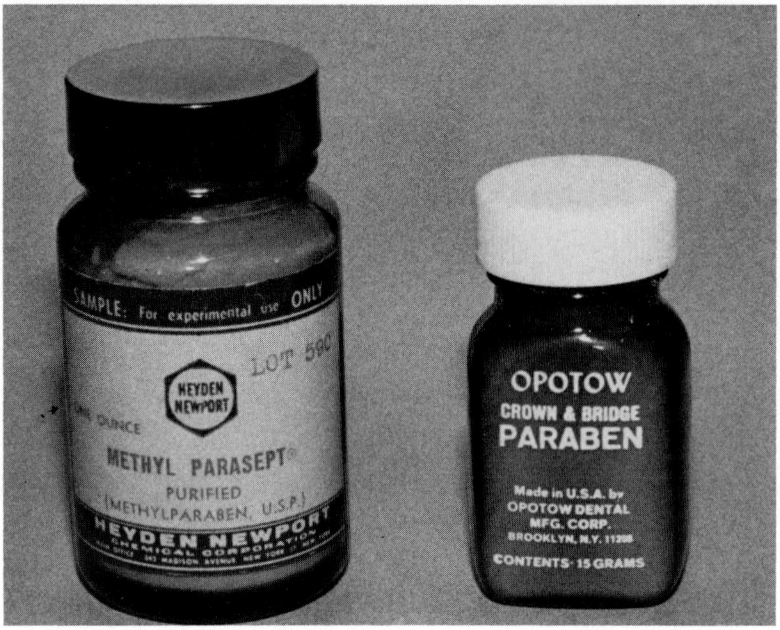

Figure 11–1 Methylparaben, USP and a combination of methyl- and propylparaben supplied as crown and bridge paraben. These chemical agents added to a mix of zinc oxide and eugenol temporary cement will increase antibacterial properties.

5. After removal the cement was difficult to clean from tooth and casting.
6. Sealing ability was only partially effective.

THE FIRST TRULY NON-SETTING CEMENT

The zinc oxide and eugenol cements modified with silicone grease to act as non-setting cements were only partially effective in providing a marginal seal; also, they would harden to some degree depending on the time in use. They were not truly non-setting cements in that they did not seal and yet maintain their original soft consistency over an extended period of time. A new temporary cement called Trial* (Fig. 11–2), zinc oxide and eugenol in an elastic base (silicone rubber), has been developed to allow easy and non-traumatic removal of multiple-unit fixed bridges and splints after evaluation in the mouth for *trial periods of up to four to six weeks.* Trial cement provides a soft, flexible, water repellent, medicated material with the biologic virtues of zinc oxide and eugenol. This cement does not set hard. It is classified as a "non-setting" cement. It produces a thin film or gasket of rubber-like material (Fig. 11–3) that seals fixed bridges in the mouth over a *trial* period and yet allows for *easy and non-traumatic removal* prior to final cementation. It is

*Teledyne Dental, Elk Grove Village, IL 60007.

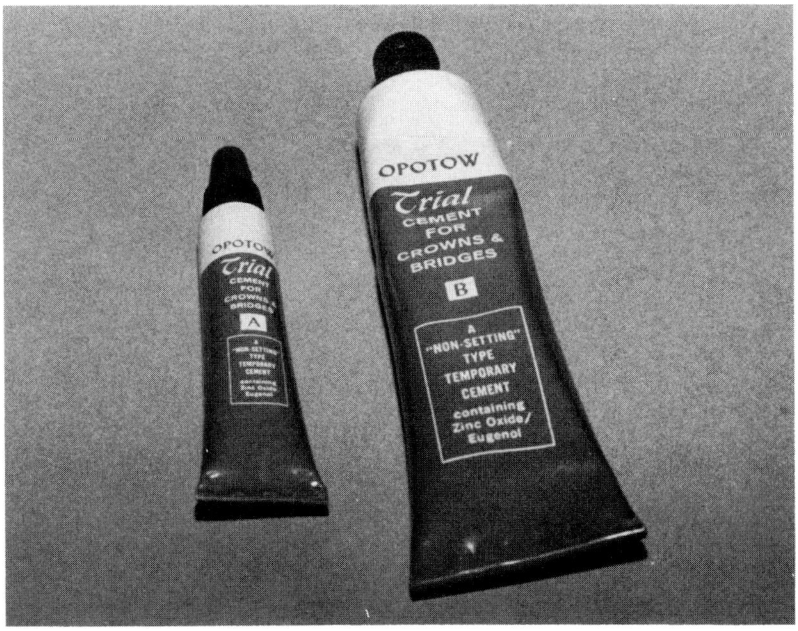

Figure 11–2 A non-setting cement that supplies a flexible, water repellent film containing zinc oxide and eugenol.

especially suitable for the temporary cementation of porcelain-over-metal bridges, multiple-unit fixed restorations, full arch splints, and the superstructure components of telescope-type restorations. Also, owing to its flexibility, it very effectively maintains seal and sedation

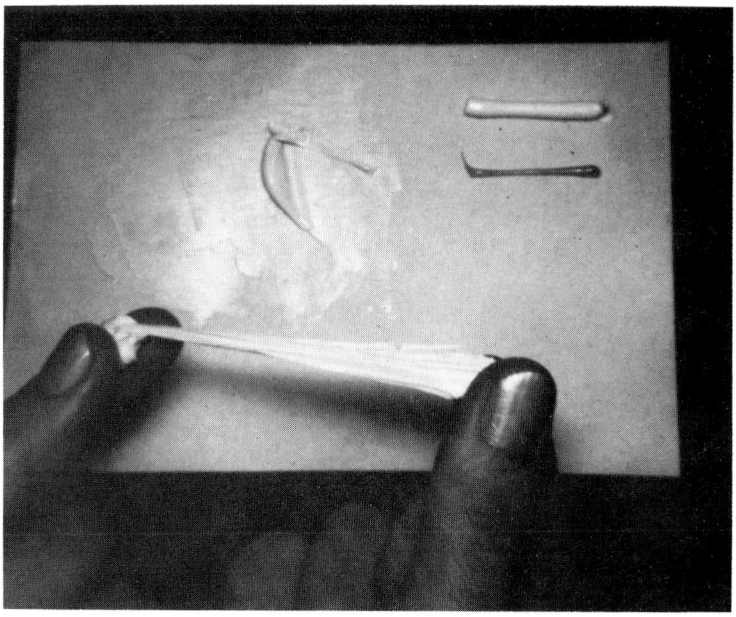

Figure 11–3 The non-setting rubbery material makes temporary cementation for biologic evaluation a trauma-free procedure.

while *allowing the slight repositioning of abutment teeth necessary for non-binding final cementation.*

Since Trial cement supplies *little or no retention,* it should not be used for all temporary cementation procedures, but only where retention is inherent to the multiple crown-tooth couplings. In the temporary insertion of cantilever or large-span bridges, for example, in which retention is a most important factor, a harder-setting temporary cement should be used. As the need for retention increases, a harder-setting temporary cement is needed. The biophysical factors that influence retention are discussed in Chapter 7, and these should be reviewed and considered prior to the selection of a temporary (or final) cement.

Practical Considerations with Trial Cement

1. The rubber-like film developed by this cement probably seals because of its water repellency and compressibility. However, it is not sticky or adhesive to any degree. It may be peeled away from any mixing surface (glass, paper, or countertop) and also from the inside of the crowns after removal.

2. Excess cement should be wiped away immediately after seating a restoration and before it becomes flexible, otherwise removal of the excess cement is more difficult because the rubbery particles spring back to position and resist removal. If extra care is not extended to the meticulous removal of subgingival excess, marked gingival displacement will occur.

3. The inside walls of the crowns should be *dry* before application of the cement. The abutment preparations should also be *dry.*

4. After the term of evaluation, a fixed bridge may be removed by simply grasping it with a gauze square held between the fingers and pulling in an opposite direction to the path of insertion.

5. It is not necessary to wait for this cement to set on the mixing pad or in the mouth. After removal of the excess cement the patient may be dismissed.

6. To delay the setting time to allow placement in multiple-unit bridges, add a *single* drop of eugenol to the mix.

7. In contrast to most zinc oxide and eugenol cements (especially the powder-liquid type, which have a very long shelf life), Trial cement may not have a long shelf life, and the catalyst may harden in the tube when low temperatures prevail. Hardened tubes should be warmed slightly and a test mix made before utilization.

TEMPORARY CEMENTS

The many proprietary zinc oxide and eugenol cements available reflect large differences in strength properties. Most when set provide a relatively weak mass of zinc oxide and eugenol. Some, such as Temp-Bond and Scutabond, have a third component, a modifier, which may cause an even weaker end result. The more modifier added to the mixture, the weaker the cement. This is a very useful concept, especially if the amount of modifier is adjustable to the biophysical factors involved (Figs. 11–4 and 11–5).

Examples of temporary cements used to maintain fixed prostheses in the mouth over a trial period are as follows:

Non-setting Temporary Cements

Zinc oxide, USP and eugenol, USP with silicone grease and parabens

Trial Cement, Teledyne Dental, Opotow-Getz Division

Soft-setting Temporary Cements

ZOE 2200, L.D. Caulk Company

Interstate Temporary Cement, Interstate Dental Company

Buffalo Temporary Cement, Buffalo Dental Manufacturing Company

Temp-Bond, Kerr Manufacturing Company

Opotow Temporary Cement, Teledyne Dental, Opotow-Getz Division

Moyco ZRE Cement, J. Bird Moyer Company, Incorporated

Scutabond, Premier Dental Products Company

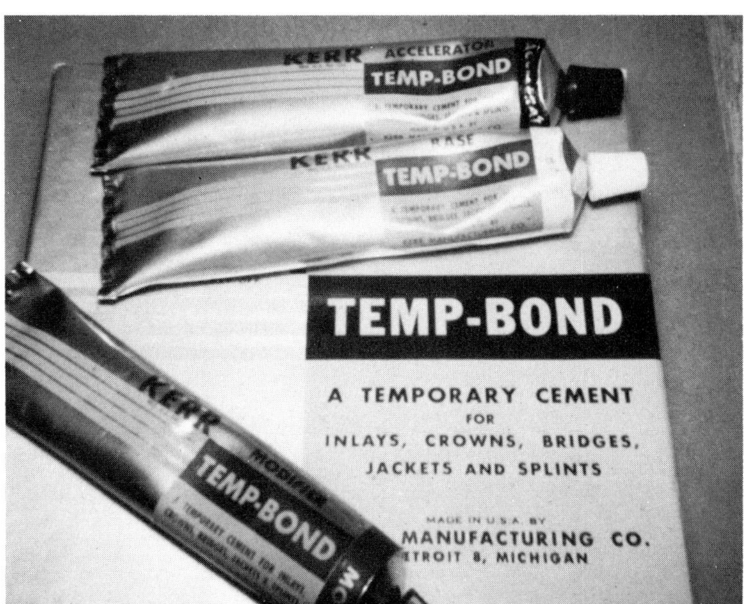

Figure 11–4 By varying the amount of modifier the hardness of this temporary cement may be controlled. It provides a choice of strength to influence retention or ease of removal.

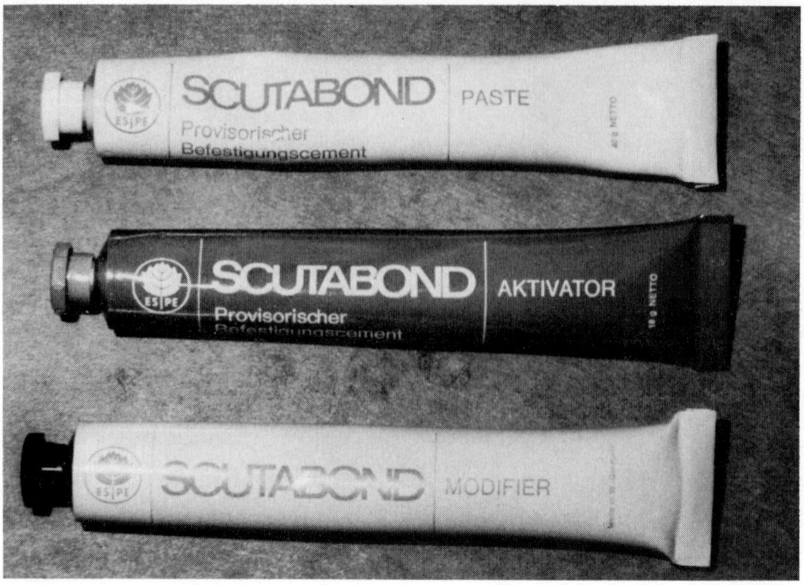

Figure 11–5 A zinc oxide and eugenol temporary cement with a modifier that reduces the strength of the cement when added to the mix.

Hard-setting Temporary Cements

TemPak, Westward Dental Products Company
Temrex Cement, Interstate Dental Company

The holding ability of a temporary cement depends on its compressive strength, hardness, film thickness, dryness, *and what it is holding.* Is it retaining hard metal or soft resin? Couple these considerations with the biophysical factors that govern retention (Chapter 7), and it becomes quite evident that the selection of a temporary cement for a given restoration is indeed similar to the selection of a particular casting gold for a given type of restoration. If abutment preparations are long, walls are parallel, and there is little or no span, temporary cementation with a hard-setting cement may make subsequent removal difficult, and hazardous if teeth are fragile and old. A soft-setting cement should be selected. On the other hand, if retentive form is questionable, the preparations short, and the span long, a soft-setting cement may not be retentive enough, and premature loosening may occur. A hard-setting cement would be more appropriate in this instance. There are also challenging conditions of retention such as the cantilever bridge, unfavorable occlusion, noxious habits of clenching and bruxism, and the overly long-span bridge. Successful retentive temporary cementation for these conditions may be accomplished only by selecting a very-hard–setting cement.

It should be noted that there is an important line of separation between the temporary cementation of temporary protective coverage such as acrylic resin crowns and bridges and the temporary cementation, actually "trial" cementation, of final prostheses. The cementation of the acrylic resin is to "retain" and "protect," while that of the metal or porcelain is to "evaluate." Because different cementing materials are required, it is important to select the correct one for the appropriate purpose. Because of basic physical differences in rigidity and resistance to deformation, a cement that is temporary when used with an acrylic restoration may inadvertently be a final cement when used *with a metal restoration;* and a final cement with metal may be utilized as a temporary cement with the *more flexible acrylic restoration* when certain biophysical factors prevail. For example, a final zinc oxide and eugenol cement such as alumina EBA may be used to retain protective acrylic coverage to prepared abutment teeth that are very short and of poor retentive form, and where a large-span bridge is planned. However, many of the temporary cements used to retain acrylic resin provisional coverage may *set too hard* to be suitable for the trial cementation of well-fitting final crowns and bridges. Here, it is of the utmost importance to select a cement that will allow removal without the dangerous application of undue force.

A temporary cement should be selected that will allow easy and non-traumatic removal of fixed bridges after evaluation in the mouth for a trial period.

REMOVAL OF RESTORATIONS AFTER TEMPORARY CEMENTATION

Temporarily cemented fixed bridges are removed prior to final cementation with selected hand instruments, the reverse mallet crown remover, and dental floss. Removal accomplished with hand instruments is more desirable than with the reverse mallet. Orban type dulled hoe scalers Nos. 5 and No. 6 are very effective for the removal of fixed restorations that have been cemented temporarily (Fig. 11–6). The appropriate instrument is applied at the gingival margin of the buccal or lingual surface and the crown is lifted off. Just enough pressure may be necessary to slightly spring the crown. It may be necessary to apply the instrument first to the buccal surface and then to the lingual surface a number of times before the bridge lifts off. It may also be necessary to alternate the application of the instrument from one end of a bridge to another until loosening occurs.

Multiple unit splints, and bridges with many abutments, may be difficult to remove with hand instruments. Retention of these crowns is especially enhanced by the multiplicity of their tensofrictional grip. *Gentle taps* with a reverse mallet at each end and in the middle may be necessary for removal. The operator should be *keenly aware of the potential for fracture* of an abutment tooth when a reverse mallet is used with too much force.

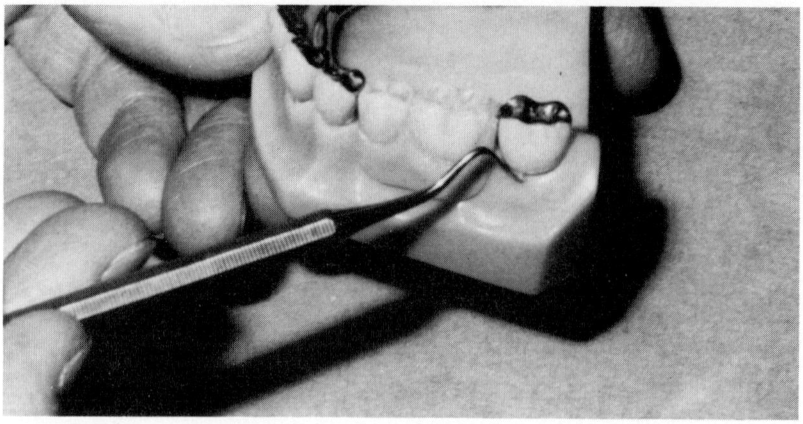

Figure 11–6 A dulled hoe scaler is very effective for the removal of a temporarily cemented crown if it is placed as illustrated at the gingival margin of the buccal surface of the crown.

No matter what method of removal is used certain precautions may be necessary:

1. A gauze square should be placed lingual to the fixed bridge to help engage it during removal and to prevent it from slipping back into the patient's throat.
2. Waxed dental floss may be threaded beneath and around the bridge at two different areas (mesial and distal) and joined and twisted outside of the mouth to entrap the bridge and prevent it from springing into the throat or outside the mouth. Tugging on dental floss entwined around a temporarily cemented bridge is also a method of removal (Fig. 11–7).

Crowns when removed from the mouth usually retain the film of temporary cement. The removal of the adherent cement is accomplished very effectively with Jel-Sol,* a solution designed specifically to remove zinc oxide and eugenol type temporary cements from prostheses. The restoration is placed in a wooden-handled porcelain casserole dish containing Jel-Sol solution. The dish is placed over a Bunsen burner, the solution is brought to a boil, and the flame is turned off. After 10 minutes in the solution, the restoration is removed and all of the cement is washed and brushed out in tap water. It may now be dried, adjusted if necessary, and polished prior to final cementation.

PSYCHOLOGICAL CONSIDERATIONS

A new and "strange" fixed restoration placed in the human mouth elicits a variety of responses. It becomes a curiosity to the

*J. F. Jelenko & Company, Incorporated, New Rochelle, NY 10801.

tongue, an awareness to the lips and cheeks, the cause of extra salivation, a speech modifier, a trap for food, and the cause of a variety of subconscious fears. When a fixed partial denture is initially installed in the oral environment it is often comforting to the patient to know that the restorative therapy has not been abruptly finalized and that modifications and adjustments can still be accomplished. The patient should be informed that the fixed therapeutic measure placed in the mouth will be removed and modified if necessary after a period of evaluation and trial function.

The patient and the prosthesis are allowed to develop a togetherness, an intimacy that will yield clues to the adjustments required to further enhance the relationship. A mutual adaptation and adjustment occurs. Ultimately, not only a bridge but a biologically adjusted relationship will be cemented. In the meantime the door is not closed to further therapy. The patient is comforted to know that in case of pain and discomfort the restoration may be removed, and that any manifestation of fear or subconscious rejection of the foreign body may be dealt with. At the same time psychologic benefits accrue to the dentist. He has reached the homestretch of his therapeutic endeavor without committing himself. Trial insertion allows him the opportunity to evaluate his accomplishment and to make improvements if necessary. He may feel more artistic at some future date. With the passage of a short period of time he may recognize and contend with mechanical, biologic, esthetic, or preventive considerations that were overlooked. Stress, worry, and concern for successful therapy may now be less intense.

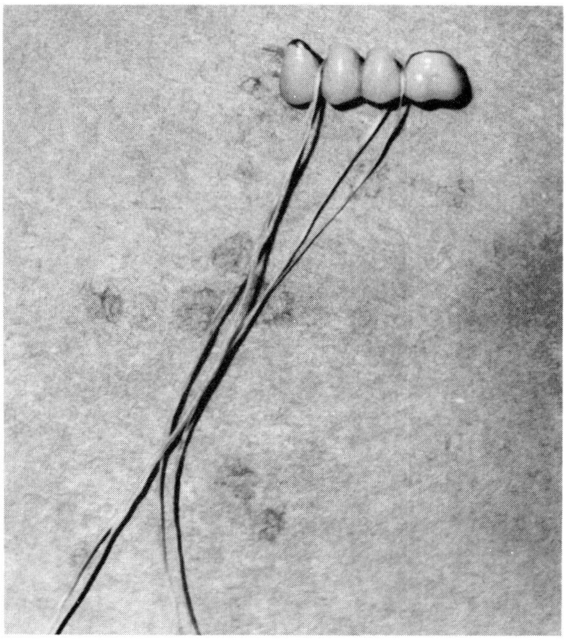

Figure 11–7 Dental floss applied to the interproximal spaces of a temporarily cemented fixed bridge will aid in removal and control its movements after removal.

A SUMMARIZING REVIEW OF TEMPORARY CEMENTATION

OBJECTIVES

1. To assess the accuracy of fit and contact points
2. To verify occlusal relationships
3. To evaluate esthetics
4. To assay tissue reactions to pontics and margins
5. To allow for minute repositioning of abutment teeth, improved seating, and a more passive final cementation
6. To condition the abutment teeth to minimize pulpal reaction from a phosphoric acid cement
7. To learn the potential for sanitation and the patient's ability to maintain oral hygiene, and the need to modify spaces for the access of dental floss and oral hygiene devices

TEMPORARY CEMENT REQUIREMENTS

1. Provide a marginal seal
2. Provide sedation and protection from pain
3. Provide retention and yet allow non-traumatic removal

TEMPORARY CEMENT SELECTION (ACCORDING TO THE REQUIREMENTS OF THE BIOPHYSICAL FACTORS)

1. Non-setting cement for long, retentive-shaped preparations, multiple abutments, and most porcelain-over-metal bridges
2. Soft-setting cement for short-span bridges
3. Hard-setting cement for long-span and cantilever bridges

TIME INVOLVED IN TEMPORARY CEMENTATION

1. Short-span bridge—five to 7 days
2. Long-span bridge—seven to 10 days
3. Full arch splint—10 to 14 days
4. Combination of fixed bridge or splint and removable partial denture—14 days

PRACTICAL CONSIDERATIONS FOR TEMPORARY CEMENTATION

1. In temporary cementation procedures the crowns *should not be filled* with cement before placement. Only the internal walls

of the crown should be lined with a film of cement. To determine how much cement to use the dentist must estimate how much the fit of the crown has been modified by internal relief, the thickness of lacquer applied to the abutment die, and the accuracy of the fit of the casting.

2. Non-eugenol cements do not obtund pain or provide the desired sedation of prepared tooth structure.

3. Abutment preparations should be lightly dried to show no visible signs of moisture. Do not dehydrate. A *properly dried* abutment preparation allows better retention and *more positive palliative action.* Immediately after cementation dryness need not be maintained. Water and saliva will not interfere with the set. A warm water rinse will accelerate the set.

4. The zinc oxide and eugenol temporary cements of the powder-liquid type have an unlimited shelf life. The liquid component (eugenol) is usable and just as effective if its color has changed to dark yellow or brown. No aspect of spatulation is critical. The powder may be added to the liquid at any rate of speed, utilizing any size of increment. In fact, all the powder may be incorporated into the liquid at once. A thick mix sets fast; a thin mix sets slowly. Any mix will set faster in a warm or humid room.

5. A record should be kept of the temporary cement selected for the trial insertion of a fixed restoration. If a bridge is to be replaced in the mouth for a further period of evaluation, selection of the temporary cement for this installation should be based on the difficulty encountered in removal. If the restoration was loose, or very easy to remove, a stronger temporary cement than the original should be selected for the next trial cementation; conversely, if the restoration was difficult to remove, a weaker cement may be indicated for subsequent cementation.

6. For short preparations, where retention may be questionable, a stronger temporary cement such as Temrex Cement should be used. Bear in mind, however, that a strong temporary cement should be used with caution on long preparations that carry well-fitting metal crowns because of the difficulty of removal.

7. There is a need for the protection of acrylic resin surfaces that may be contacted by excess zinc oxide and eugenol temporary cement. Although silicone grease is recommended for this purpose, clinicians have used petrolatum, carding wax, and Albolene oil. These agents should be kept away from the margins. Regardless of the protective film utilized, the eugenol component may still penetrate and attack the acrylic resin veneer and predispose it to discoloration. A phenolic compound of any type has a deleterious effect on acrylic resin and tends to depolymerize it. Therefore, any excess of zinc oxide and eugenol

cement that flows out over an acrylic resin veneer should not be allowed to remain until it hardens; it should be wiped away with a cotton roll or gauze immediately after complete seating of the restoration. This will *minimize the time of contact of the excess cement and the acrylic resin,* and therefore limit the deleterious effect on the resin, since it is related to *the length of time cement and resin are in contact.* Poor technique that allows delayed removal of the cement or hardening of the cement prior to removal from the external surfaces of the resin will increase the potential for discoloration.

SUMMARY

The biologic evaluation of a fixed partial denture is accomplished by temporary cementation. Temporary cements are usually formulations of zinc oxide and eugenol and contribute seal and sedation to prepared tooth structure. The greatest deterrent to the utilization of temporary cementation has been difficulty in removal prior to final cementation. The withdrawal of a temporarily cemented restoration is usually associated with the application of force that has the potential for injury to teeth, tissues, and restoration. With the advent of new cements and concepts, however, many of the problems of temporary cementation have been resolved. Temporary cementation should be of limited duration and not for extended periods of time. The time allotted to verify biologic compatibility (the time of temporary cementation) should be just long enough to determine the reaction of the host. As a rule of thumb, the smaller the fixed bridge the less the time of temporary cementation; the more extensive the bridge the longer the time of evaluation. Single crowns should not be cemented temporarily unless meaningful information can be derived from the procedure. Temporary cements should be selected for a given restoration according to the biophysical factors involved.

REFERENCES

1. Massler, M.: Pulp protection and preservation. Pract. Dent. Monog. January 1958, p. 47.
2. Ewing, J. E.: Temporary cementation in fixed prosthesis. J. Prosthet. Dent., *5*:388, 1955.
3. Kasis, H., and Kasis, A. J.: Complete Mouth Rehabilitation Through Crown and Bridge Prosthodontics, Philadelphia, Lea & Febiger, 1956, p. 363.
4. McCracken, W. L., Partial Denture Construction; Principles and Techniques. St. Louis, C. V. Mosby Co., 1960, p. 282.
5. Gilson, T. D., and Myers, G. E.: Clinical studies of dental cements. III. Seven zinc oxide-eugenol cements used for temporarily cementing completed restorations. J. Dent. Res. *49*:14, 1970.
6. Swartz, M. L., Phillips, R. W., Norman, R. D., and Oldham, D. F.: Strength, hardness and abrasion characteristics of dental cements. J. Am. Dent. Assoc. *67*:367, 1963.
7. Horn, H. R.: Non-setting zinc oxide and eugenol cements. J. Dent. Res. *40*:775, 1961.
8. Roydhouse, R. H.: Materials in Dentistry. Chicago, Year Book Medical Publishers, 1962, p. 175.
9. Horn, H. R.: The cementation of crowns and fixed partial dentures. Dent. Clin. North Am., March 1965, p. 65.

twelve

The Final Cementation of Crowns and Bridges

Ideals are like stars; you will not succeed in touching them with your hands. But like the seafaring man on the desert of waters, you choose them as your guides, and following them you will reach your destiny.

Carl Schurz

Cementation is the process by which a restoration is attached to natural teeth by means of a cement. In reality it is a "wedding ceremony" aimed at fulfilling the physiologic objectives of a fixed restorative procedure. Cementation requires meticulous care and planning. An impression or casting that is not suitable may be remade, but the damage caused by faulty cementation is irreversible. It must be accommodated. *Faulty technique, poor timing, and lack of essential preparation may undermine all previous mechanical accomplishments.* Fit, function, and esthetics may be lost.

The abutment preparation is actually the first step in the cementation procedure. At this time, the length, taper, and shape of the tooth are influenced by the operator's knowledge of the pertinent biophysical factors related to the fixed prosthesis and the involved oral environment. Modifications are made according to the recognition of these factors.

The most effective cementation procedure, utilizing the most ideal cement, may still initiate undesirable changes. Cementation may change comfort to pain. It may alter occlusal and marginal relationships and bring on other conditions such as hydraulic phenomena, pulpal injury, and the loss of contact points and esthetics. The dentist is challenged to keep these changes to a minimum by the proper selection and manipulation of an appropriate cement.

THE BIOLOGIC INSTALLATION OF CROWNS AND BRIDGES

In past years crowns and bridges were fabricated by a series of technologic procedures and the mechanical end-results routinely cemented into the mouth with an irritating acid cement. This was essentially a mechanical accomplishment. In today's dentistry, with its increasing concern for biologic considerations, a biologic installation of a fixed restoration is more desirable. What is a biologic installation? It is one in which:

1. The biophysical factors related to retention are recognized and modified if necessary to be favorable to positive retention and longevity.
2. Biologic compatibility has been verified by temporary cementation.
3. The final cementing material meets biologic requirements. The biologic requirements of an ideal final cement are as follows:
    a. Pulpal tolerance – soothing, sedating, and non-irritating to the pulp.
    b. Tissue tolerance.
    c. Ability to initiate reparative dentin.
    d. Antibacterial and anticariogenic properties.

Selection of a Final Cement

One of the most provocative areas of concern in crown and bridge therapy is the selection of an appropriate dental cement for the final cementation of the restoration.

In past years a dentist selecting a final cement was primarily concerned with two guidelines, both dealing with the cementing material – strength and "adhesion." Today, considerations for the selection of an appropriate cement are far more extensive and encompass biologic, biophysical, and esthetic factors.

The selection of a final cement is no longer based only on the physical properties of the various cementing materials and their special characteristics. The dentist must now consider the sensitive prepared abutment tooth that is painful to touch or contact with air. He should take into account patients' noxious habits of bruxism and clenching, and dietary habits that involve the use of chewing gum, candy and carbonated beverages. Also to be considered are esthetics and the need for translucency, the non-vital abutment tooth, the challenging design of a cantilever or a long-span bridge, and the very short abutment preparation and the one with poor retentive form. The patient's medical history is meaningful in the selection of a final cement, for allergenic reactions, respiration (diabetics may breathe acetone), medications, and regurgitation must be considered.

The proper cement for a particular cementation should be selected only after due consideration of the following factors:

1. The biophysical factors for retention.
2. The biologic factors of pain, sensitivity, vitality, tissue tolerance, and antibacterial and anticariogenic activity.
3. The medical history – allergy, diabetes, peptic ulcer.
4. Dietary habits – chewing gum, candy, soda.
5. Noxious habits – bruxism, clenching, tongue thrusting.
6. Esthetics – translucency.

THE OUTSTANDING FEATURES OF SOME FINAL CEMENTS

Zinc phosphate cement—strength, low film thickness

Silicophosphate cement—strength, anticariogenic value, and translucency

Alumina EBA cement—biologic values, working time

Polycarboxylate cement—adhesive and biologic values

Composite resin cement—strength, insolubility, and translucency

These features are related to the special requirements of a final cementation procedure as follows:

Translucency—silicophosphate and composite resin cement

Anodyne action—Alumina EBA cement

Pulp compatibility—Alumina EBA and polycarboxylate cement

Strength—composite resin, silicophosphate and zinc phosphate cement

Insolubility—composite resin and silicophosphate cement

Anticariogenic value—silicophosphate cement

SELECTION ACCORDING TO REQUIREMENTS

The selection of a cementing material is made according to characteristics or features that meet special requirements. Here emphasis is placed on the unique characteristics of specific cements. For example, if retention is a special problem, or if adhesion, translucency, or a good pulpal effect is of prime importance, the following cements are indicated:

Retention—composite resin cement. Example, Epoxylite CBA 9080*

Pulpal effect—alumina EBA cement. Example, Zebacem cement**

Adhesion—polycarboxylate cement. Example, Durelon cement†

Translucency—silicophosphate cement. Example, Fluoro-Thin,‡ and Lucent**

---

*Lee Pharmaceuticals, South El Monte, CA 91733.
**L. D. Caulk Company, Milford, DE 19963.
†Premier Dental Products Company, Norristown, PA 19401.
‡S. S. White Dental Products, Philadelphia, PA 19102.

TABLE 12–1 SELECTION OF FINAL CEMENT ACCORDING TO TYPE OF FIXED PROSTHESIS

Fixed Prosthesis	Final Cement	Reason for Selection
Full arch splint	Alumina EBA cement	Ample working time
Short-span bridge	Alumina EBA cement	Biologic values
Long-span bridge	Zinc phosphate	Strength
Cantilever bridge	Zinc phosphate	Strength
Porcelain jacket	Silicophosphate	Translucency
Metal crown (short)	Zinc phosphate	Strength
Metal crown (long)	Alumina EBA cement	Biologic values
Splint (no pontic)	Alumina EBA cement	Biologic values

The selection of a final cement according to the type of prosthesis, and the reason for the selection is shown in Table 12–1.

Final Cements for Posts and Cores

For the optimum retention of posts and cores the following cements are listed in the order of preference:

POST	CEMENT
Stainless steel	1. Polycarboxylate cement 2. Zinc phosphate cement 3. Composite resin cement
Gold	1. Zinc phosphate cement 2. Polycarboxylate cement 3. Composite resin cement

SEQUENCE OF PREPARATION FOR CEMENTATION PROCEDURE

1. Preparation of Fixed Restoration

The prosthesis is evaluated in the mouth for fit, contour, contacts, esthetics, and occlusion. Check for sharp edges on the margins or the tissue-facing surfaces of pontics. Rubber-wheel and polish away knife-edge margins. Roughen the inside walls of metal castings to upgrade retention. Modify where necessary, repolish, clean, and *dry* the restoration. A drying agent may be used inside crowns (Cavilax* or Cavidry**), but not on vital abutment teeth (Fig. 12–1). Lubricate the interproximal spaces and acrylic resin veneers with silicone grease. Keep the silicone grease away from the margins. Do not use oil or any material that may inadvertently flow over the margins. Black or red carding wax may be helpful for this purpose in some instances.

---

*Premier Dental Products Company, Norristown, PA 19401.
**Parkell, Farmingdale, NY 11735.

2. Preparation of Patient

If saliva is copious or there is a problem in controlling salivation, administer an antisialogogue (methantheline bromide, 50 mg) 45 minutes before cementation. Another effective drug for this purpose is Pro-Banthine,* 15 mg, which has fewer side effects. This should be taken 30 minutes before the procedure. These drugs should be prescribed *only for excessive salivation and not routinely*. They are contraindicated for the patient with prostatic hypertrophy, glaucoma and cardiac conditions. If the patient has a cold, is recovering from a cold, or has a sinus condition, a nasal mucosa astringent will help to clear nasal passageways and improve breathing while the mouth is kept open and dry. This is an important consideration when it is estimated that 90 per cent of the population suffers from some sort of nasal obstruction.[1] Position the patient's head to receive the seating force of insertion. Apply saliva removal apparatus.

Antisialogogues should be prescribed only for excessive salivation.

3. Preparation of Materials

Select appropriate cement as indicated by biophysical factors. If zinc phosphate cement or polycarboxylate cement is to be uti-

*G. D. Searle & Company, Chicago, IL.

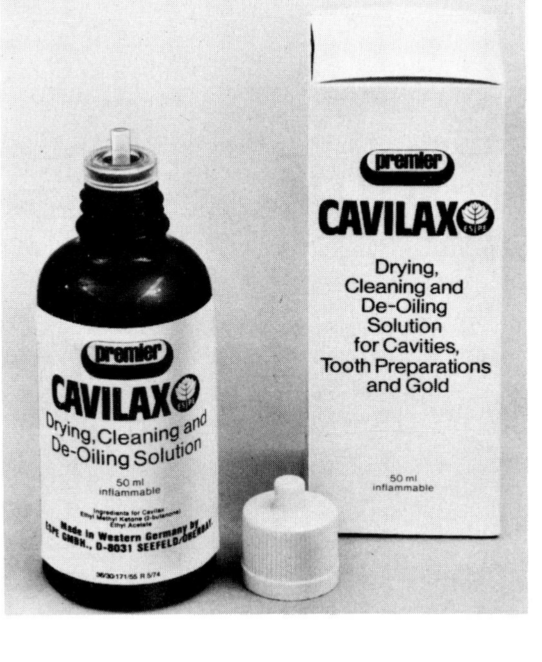

Figure 12–1 A drying agent that will effectively clean and dry the internal surfaces of inlays and gold and porcelain crowns prior to final cementation. The benefits of the application of a drying agent to vital tooth structure must be weighed against the potential for chemical irritation, rapid evaporation with subsequent chill, and the deposition of a residue.

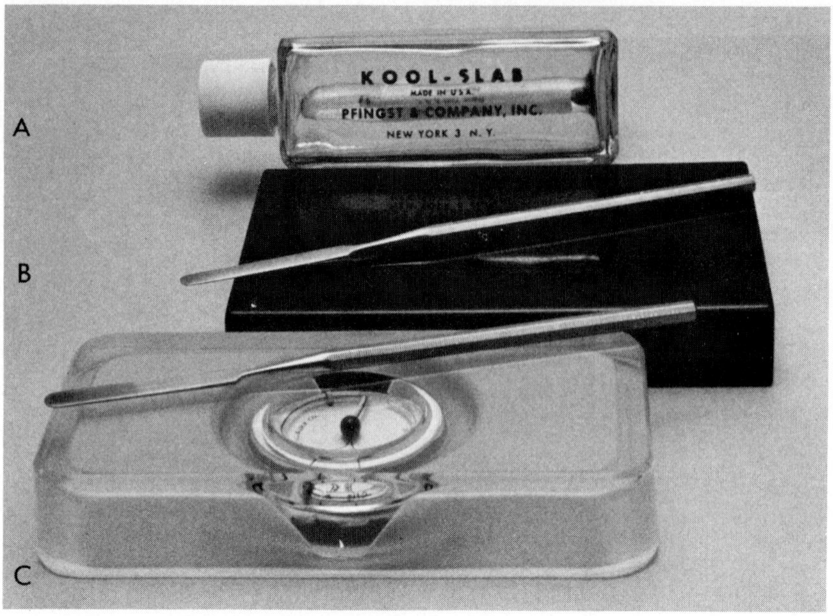

Figure 12–2 Three types of glass slabs used for mixing dental cements. *A*, Kool-Slab (Pfingst & Company, Inc., NY) is a rectangular bottle with a thermometer attached inside. The cement is mixed on its large, flattened surface. The temperature of this slab may be controlled by filling the bottle with warm or cold water. *B*, A black tile slab with a porous underside maintains a cool surface for mixing dental cement. *C*, A solid glass slab with a built-in thermometer (L.D. Caulk, Milford, DE). This slab may be chilled to an appropriate temperature by running tap water over it.

lized, place *powder* on cold, dry glass slab (not below dew point) (Fig. 12–2). Polycarboxylate cement may also be mixed on an appropriate paper mixing pad, but a glass slab is preferred.[2] *Do not place liquid on slab* at this time. If a zinc oxide and eugenol type cement is to be used, both powder and liquid may be placed on the slab at this time. Place mixing spatula and other instruments in readiness. Include an instrument small enough to fit inside the crowns to place cement therein. Prepare the bite block or apparatus to maintain seating pressure during setting of the cement.

4. Preparation of Abutment Teeth

Clear gingival debris and clean meticulously with luke-warm water. If necessary, control seepage or bleeding with 8:100 solution of racemic epinephrine. Isolate and dry prepared teeth with cotton and use warm air in the gingival area sparingly. Do not apply chemical agents—no alcohol, phenol, or silver nitrate. When using zinc phosphate cement, a thin layer of a copal type cavity varnish may be applied, but do not use calcium hydroxide, because it may neutralize and weaken a thin film of acid cement, and it cannot be applied at the margins because it is soluble. No cavity varnish or liner should be used with a zinc oxide and eugenol type final cement. Calcium hydroxide is not insoluble in oral fluids and therefore should not be placed at the gingival margins or it may wash out. The gingival area is the very region that needs protection, perhaps more than the other areas of the abutment tooth.

Proceed as follows:

If zinc phosphate cement is utilized:

1. Place cement liquid on the glass slab (never add a drop of eugenol).

2. Incorporate a small amount of powder to start the mix; note the time.

3. Add additional portions slowly and mix for 90 seconds.

4. Be sure to incorporate the *maximum* amount of powder within the limit of consistency.

5. Spread the mix over a large area of the cooled mixing slab.

6. Fill castings with the resultant thin mix.

7. Apply cement to crevices or irregularities in abutment teeth, and *spin* cement into pin or post holes, if present, with a spiral rotating instrument (Lentulo).

8. Seat the restoration with heavy pressure.

9. Wipe away excess cement.

10. A mallet and an orangewood stick may improve seating.

11. At this time do not wipe away further excess cement.

12. Do verify and check occlusion by a quick closure.

13. Open and wipe away excess cement if necessary.

14. Maintain *pressure* and *dryness* until set. The eventual film thickness depends on the factors shown in Table 9–2.

15. Balance biting pressure on opposite side if possible. Neurophysiologic studies have revealed that when the mandible is moved with heavy pressure against premature occlusal contact there is a sustained stimulation which remains after the stimulus is removed. Practically speaking, when a patient closes with firm pressure on a wooden tongue blade, cotton roll, or orangewood stick during cementation of a crown or a bridge he will continue to close to the side of stronger pressure when the bite block is

removed. Bite blocks should be placed on both sides of the mouth during the cementation procedure so that the patient will be stimulated bilaterally with equal pressure. This may be effectively accomplished by using two Bowen Dental Jacks* or two Medart Inlay Pressure Applicators** (Fig. 12–3).

16. Avoid adjusting the occlusion until the cement is fully set.

17. After the cement has set, remove excess with scaler and floss.

18. Adjust occlusion; torque caused by prematurity may break bond.

19. X-ray area.

20. Instruct in oral sanitation related to the restoration, oral hygiene, and nutrition.

If alumina EBA cement is utilized:

1. Measured amounts of powder and liquid may be incorporated in any manner and at any speed.

2. Do not fill castings; line the inside walls.

3. Seat restoration with heavy pressure.

---

*Bowen & Company, Incorporated, Bethesda, MD.
**Surgident Ltd., Los Angeles, CA 90066.

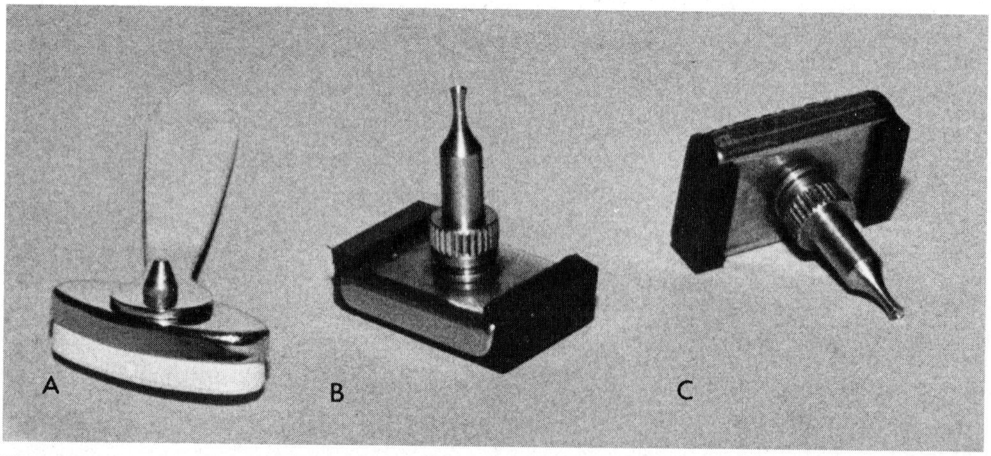

Figure 12–3 Devices used to hold and seat inlays, crowns, or bridges during the cementation procedure by means of the patient's biting pressure. *A*, The Medart Inlay Pressure Applicator has a central bearing point on one side and a removable rubber bite pad on the other. The handle facilitates placement. The central bearing point is placed in the central fossa of an inlay or crown, and the opposing jaw bites on the rubber pad to press the restoration into position and to hold it until the cement sets. *B* and *C*, The Bowen Dental Jack also has a bearing area and a removable rubber biting area. It may be adjusted in length to modify the mouth opening.

4. Wipe away excess cement.

5. A mallet and an orangewood stick will improve seating.

6. Again, wipe away excess cement.

7. Verify and check occlusion.

8. Maintain pressure; dryness is not necessary.

9. Remove excess cement after set.

10. X-ray area.

11. Instruct in oral sanitation related to the restoration, oral hygiene, and nutrition.

12. Caution the patient to avoid heavy pressures for 24 hours. This is very important with zinc oxide and eugenol cements, since the degree of set and hardness increases more slowly than it does with zinc phosphate cements.

Psychologic Considerations for "Final" Cementation

The fixed restoration is the "physical" component of restorative therapy. Its existence and *durability* are governed by underlying biologic and psychologic factors. Other components of restorative therapy cope with these factors. Therefore, when a fixed restoration must be replaced, only the "physical" component is lost. Function, arch maintenance, occlusal repair, and abutment protection are benefits to the dentition that are still provided over a period of time. Also left behind are benefits to the psyche that the restoration supplied in the form of esthetics.

No permanent cementation is really permanent.

No material lasts forever. Every dentist knows the exact connotation of the term "permanent cementation." He may wince at the exact meaning. He knows that owing to the many mechanical, physiological, and psychological factors that are *beyond control,* it is illogical to use the word "permanent." Nevertheless, because the term "permanent cementation" is habitually and commonly used in lectures and literature, it more or less conveys the intended meaning. In the patient's interests, however, it would be more appropriate to designate the insertion of crowns and bridges as "final cementation" for an important psychologic reason. "Final cementation" is less likely to imply a warranty to the patient that the physical component of repair will last forever. The dentist who is in the habit of using the word "permanent" may be totally unaware of the mental conditioning he has triggered in the mind of the patient, who is more than willing to accept the word at its full value. Dentists know that a "permanent" restoration is not actually permanent. Patients may not. The changing of thoughts and attitudes takes time, and it should be recognized that in this case the change should begin with the dentist. He should modify his terminology to cope with the problem. Various dental teachers have presented the problem to the profession.[3–5] Pincus[3] notes, "there is nothing permanent in dentistry." In an article entitled "The myth of permanent dentistry," Barone[4] states that, in the education of the patient, "The first lesson the patient must assimilate is that there is no such thing as permanent dentistry." He further states: "The word *permanent* must be eliminated from the dental vocabulary."

After the preparation of abutment teeth, protective restorations are called "temporary." "Temporary" cement is used for retention and seal. The restorations are removed and replaced as required in subsequent procedures. Each time, the term "temporary" restoration is coupled with the term "temporary" cement. It is inevitable that the word "temporary" will mentally condition the patient to regard the forthcoming prosthesis and the ultimate cementation as "permanent."

The future of crown and bridge prosthodontics is dependent not only on new concepts, techniques, and materials but also on new terminology and psychologic considerations that will provide more harmony and precise understanding in communication with patients. Therefore, the following changes are proposed for the terminology of the future:

1. The temporary crown should be designated as a *protective* crown, a *provisional* crown, or an *interim* crown.
2. The temporary bridge should be termed a *substitute* bridge or a *provisional* bridge.
3. However, the protective, provisional, or interim crown and the substitute or provisional bridge may be cemented with *temporary* cement.
4. Since the true purpose of the *temporary cementation* of a *final prosthesis* is to allow for biomechanical evaluation, it would appear to be more cogent to call it *trial cementation.*

Meanwhile, until a large-scale effort is made to sweep away misleading terminology and establish a new and meaningful communication, it is necessary to continue to use the "habitual" terms in order to be understood.

Practical Considerations for Final Cementation

1. In the cementation of porcelain jackets the dentist should use the "eyes" in his fingertips to detect any sharp edges on the margins. He should recognize that the gingival tissues will find these sharp edges if his fingers do not. Glasslike sharp edges contribute greatly to gingival irritation. Prior to final cementation they should be removed with a porcelain trimming wheel

(PTW)* and the area polished to a high luster with a porcelain polishing wheel (PPW).*

2. The shelf life of resin-type cements such as the polycarboxylate and the composite resin cements is not as good as that of the phosphoric acid and zinc oxide and eugenol cements.

3. If the pressure of mastication is applied to a cemented restoration before the cement sets hard enough to reach an appropriate degree of compressive strength, the cement may be pulverized and break down and solubilize out.

4. Successful final cementation depends on *preparation*. The stage must be set by the sequence of preparation described in this chapter.

5. During the cementation procedure restorations should be seated firmly with finger pressure and then *quickly tapped* with a mallet and orangewood stick into more complete seating before viscosity increases and setting progresses.

6. Because warmth and moisture accelerate the setting of all dental cements, the dentist should not apply the mixed cement to preparations in the mouth, for it may thicken enough to prevent complete seating during the time it takes to apply the cement and to position the restoration in the mouth.

7. Phosphoric acid cements and polycarboxylate cements must not be allowed to contact water in the early stages of setting. Cavity varnish applied to the margins after cementation is one way to cope with this problem. Another method is to leave hardened excess cement in position for a longer period of time before removal. Saliva will then contact the excess cement instead of the critical cement line beneath it.

8. In the cementation of posts it is always a problem to get cement into the depth of the canal prepared to receive the post. A jiffy tube or a Centrix syringe** with a tip that fits well up into the post hole will solve the problem.

9. In a clinical study of dental cements[6] involving a recall evaluation of restorations cemented with a reinforced zinc oxide/eugenol cement and a zinc phosphate cement after a four-to-seven-year interval no significant differences in clinical success were noted between restorations installed with the two cements. Nor was there any significant difference in the incidence of caries on the margins of abutment teeth detected between the two cements.

---

*Dental Development & Manufacturing Corporation, Brooklyn, NY 11204.
**Centrix, Incorporated, Fairfield, CT 06430.

10. The first criterion for selecting a zinc phosphate or silicophosphate cement should be to check whether they are certified as meeting American Dental Association specifications No. 8 or 21.

11. To avoid chemical irritation, dehydration, and the chill of rapid evaporation, drying agents should not be applied to prepared vital teeth. It has been shown recently that drying materials such as Cavidry (Parkell) and Prep-Dry (Lee Pharmaceuticals) *leave a residue on evaporation.*[7]

12. The successful final cementation of fixed prostheses depends upon the rheological (viscous) properties of the cementing material.[8] It should be noted that the viscosity of zinc phosphate and polycarboxylate cement increases with time and temperature.[8]

13. After having been evaluated by a term of temporary cementation, all fixed restorations should be "fixed" in the mouth by final cementation. There are very few indications for prolonged or continuous temporary cementation. There is no cement available that will provide retention and resistance to washing out, and also allow removal when desired. Noncommittal cementation, or the so-called "temporary-permanent" cementation, has been the cause of many completely eroded or decayed abutment teeth.

14. In the course of preparation for final cementation the dentist has his last opportunity to modify and adjust the fixed prosthesis and to attend to other details that will contribute to successful therapy. One important but often overlooked detail is the finishing and polishing of porcelain occlusal surfaces that have been subjected to substantial grindings for occlusal adjustment either before or after final cementation. In either case, the ground porcelain surfaces should be finished and polished to a smooth luster. Rough surfaces collect stains and food particles. Rough, unpolished cusps cannot glide over other cusps in chewing movements. Repolishing is also important to reduce friction and to minimize the abrasive effects on the opposing dentition. Although several methods of poli hing porcelain have been advocated, Trupolish #3, a component of the Dentsply Porcelain Finishing Kit* is especially suited for this purpose[9] both in and out of the mouth (Fig. 12–4). It is important to keep this polish from drying out by adding glycerine or water. It is used on a rag wheel after a rubber wheel and pumice have been applied to the porcelain.

15. Two different types of cement may be used in the final

---

*Dentsply International, York, PA 17404.

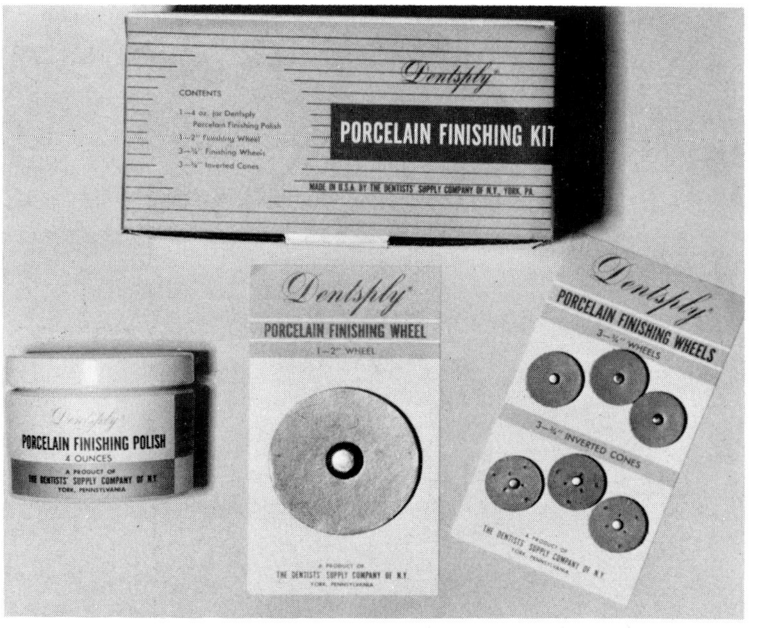

Figure 12–4 The Dentsply Porcelain Finishing Kit contains a polishing agent that is effective in restoring a polished surface to porcelain that has been ground for occlusal adjustment. (Courtesy of Dentsply International, York, PA.)

cementation of a full arch splint or an extensive multiple-unit bridge composed of a series of consecutively splinted abutment teeth and an isolated terminal abutment tooth separated from the splinted segment of the bridge by two or more pontics. A mix of alumina EBA cement is prepared first and applied to each crown of the splinted segment. Without delay, zinc phosphate cement is spatulated and applied to the terminal abutment, and the prosthesis is seated in the mouth. Because terminal abutments usually present a challenge to retention, they require a stronger cement, whereas a series of splinted crowns may readily be retained by a weaker cement, with the additional benefit of biologic compatibility.

16. The term "adhesive" used in an advertisement to describe the nature of a dental cement implies that the cement is adhesive in clinical use. Unfortunately, the term also suggests that the usual mechanical methods of retention are not necessary. This is misleading to the dentist. The Council on Dental Materials and Devices of the American Dental Association recently stated: "No data have been presented to the Council to substantiate the claim of adhesive qualities under clinical conditions for any commercially available restorative materials in dentistry."[10]

SUMMARY

The cementation requirement is the Achilles heel of fixed prosthodontics. Although the fabrication of crowns and fixed partial dentures has been facilitated in recent years by improved tooth reduction apparatus, impression materials and casting procedures, dental cements and insertion procedures have seen relatively little progress in the past century. Cementation remains an unsound link in the chain of fixed restorative procedures. It is a critical maneuver that has the potential to sabotage the most perfect fixed prosthesis. It may cause pain, occlusal disharmony, and marginal discrepancies. Occasionally, crowns and bridges loosen prematurely, despite the use of so-called "permanent" cement. Conversely, restorations cemented with temporary cement are often difficult to remove prior to final cementation.

Despite the luting problems, fixed prostheses are increasingly prescribed to repair and preserve the oral structures. Since cementing media and procedures leave much to be desired, it is necessary to utilize them with the greatest possible skill and knowledge. It may be helpful to recognize and occasionally review the following pertinent philosophies.

1. The cementation procedure and the cements utilized therein are means to fulfill the biologic and physiologic objectives of a restorative process.
2. Fixed restorations are therapeutic measures, not mechanical contrivances.
3. Biological evaluation of restorative dental materials is necessary to assess their effect on the oral structures. Accordingly, an appraisal of a dental cement should take into account not only physical and mechanical properties but also pulpal reaction, tissue compatibility, the formation of secondary dentin, and antimicrobial and anticariogenic properties.
4. The art and science of fixed prosthodontics have matured to the stage where vital cementation procedures should be *based upon research evidence rather than on custom, habit, empiricism, and folklore.*
5. Biophysical factors influence retention and the selection of an appropriate final cement.

The ultimate success of crowns and bridges is substantially dependent on the manner of cementation, the cement utilized, and pertinent biophysical factors related to the structures being luted and the oral environment involved. The dentist is challenged to cement fixed prostheses painlessly and to keep the resultant film of cement to a minimum so that previously established margins and occlusal relationships will not be disturbed.

Some of the problems associated with cementation may be partially resolved with recognition of essential biophysical factors, knowledge of the cementing media, and skill in the handling and applying of the luting agents.

REFERENCES

1. Ogura, J. H.: Study questions function of the nose. J.A.M.A. *203*(3):42, 1968.
2. Smith, D. C : Dental cements. Dent. Clin. North Am. January 1971, p. 29.
3. Pincus, C. L.: Cosmetics – the psychologic fourth dimension in full mouth rehabilitation. Dent. Clin. North Am. March, 1967, p. 71.
4. Barone, J. V.: The myth of permanent dentistry. J. Prosthet. Dent. *28*:43, July 1972.
5. Brecker, S. C.: Clinical Procedures in Occlusal Rehabilitation. Philadelphia, W. B. Saunders Company, 1958, p. 470.

6. Silvey, R. G., and Myers, G. E.: Clinical studies of dental cements: V. Recall evaluation of restorations cemented with a zinc oxide-eugenol cement and a zinc phosphate cement. J. Dent. Res. *55*:289, 1976.
7. Rohr, M. W., and Makinson, O. F.: Residual films from cavity preparation drying materials and a bonding agent. J. Dent. Res. *55*:519 (Abstract 11), 1976.
8. Vermilyea, S., Powers, J. M., and Craig, R. G.: The rheology of a zinc phosphate and a zinc polycarboxylate cement. J. Dent. Res. *55*:B94 (Abstract 129), IADR, 1976.
9. Morrow, R. M., et al.: Evaluation of methods for polishing porcelain denture teeth. J. Prosthet. Dent. *30*:222, 1973.
10. Council on Dental Materials and Devices, Council statement claims related to "adhesion" or to "adhesive" restorative materials. J. Am. Dent. Assoc. *88*:393, 1974.

thirteen

The Reasons For Premature Loosening of Fixed Restorations

We like to continue to believe what we have been accustomed to accept as true, and the resentment aroused when doubt is cast upon any of our assumptions leads us to seek every manner of excuse for clinging to it. The result is that most of our so-called reasoning consists in finding arguments for going on believing as we already do.

Prof. J. H. Robinson

Successful crown and bridge therapy depends on the positive, long-lasting retention of a fixed restorative measure. However, failure of therapy does occur in a small percentage of fixed restorations due to premature loosening after final cementation. Indeed, fixed restorations loosen despite the dentist's efforts to install them securely. And yet, when he wants to remove a cemented restoration, it may resist tenaciously. It is important to focus on the causative factors of premature loosening.

Although the retention of a crown or a bridge depends on many different biophysical factors, only the cement is indicted for the failure of a fixed restoration due to premature loosening. The cement takes the blame. Many dentists consider dental cement to be the sole provider of retention, and give little recognition to the other, equally important, factors that contribute to the retention of a fixed restoration. For example, if abutment teeth are very tapered and not prepared to a retentive form, if the fit of the casting is poor, or if the span of a bridge is too long, no cement can be expected to provide retention that will endure. Indeed, the cement is only an adjunct to retention, not the sole source. Fixed restorations seldom loosen in the mouth; but if they do, it may have *very little to do with the cement* and quite a lot to do with the following causes of premature loosening:

1. Poor Fit of the Casting

Retention depends more on precise fit than on cement. Lack of tensofrictional grip may lead to premature loosening. Also, a cement that fills areas of poor marginal fit is more readily subject to dissolution because there is more surface area of cement open to attack by oral solvents.

Some components of a bridge fit better than others. Occasionally, one abutment will fit well and another will fit poorly. This unfortunate situation must be corrected, for compromise will only lead to failure. If loosening occurs the patient may not be able to discern that something is amiss. Since the patient is not aware of the condition, or of the potential sequelae, in time loosening and possibly other destruction will take place. It is important that the dentist check all fixed bridges for signs or evidence of loosening at subsequent appointments.

2. Inadequate Retention Form

Cone-shaped preparations give little retention even with the best-fitting castings. The required parallelism, grooves, boxes, and pins should be utilized when necessary. Short preparations should have parallel walls. Preparations should be asymmetrical to resist forces of rotation. When a fixed bridge loosens because of abutment teeth with inadequate retention form, the only answer is *a new bridge* on abutment teeth modified to be retentive.

3. Deformation of Abutment Castings

Occlusal pressures may deform thin walls of a casting, causing margins to move away from the preparation. This will occur more readily when the yield point of the casting metal is low. Deformation may occur from masticatory forces, or bruxism and clenching. It may cause the separation of tooth, cement, and casting, leaving an open door for microleakage and loosening.

4. Unfavorable Occlusal Factors

The forces of occlusion may break a cement bond when a premature contact exists or when the opposing occlusal surface (in the opposite arch) is part of a more extensive multiple-unit restoration. The balance of power favors the larger, harder, multi-splinted prosthesis in its repeated impact with a smaller cemented restoration. It is the smaller restoration that gets knocked loose.

5. Caries

Recurrent caries may have a number of causes, including health, habits, heredity, hygiene, and diet factors. Areas of hard tooth structure that are healthy at the time of final cementation may be lost as time passes and caries progresses. The softened, diseased area of a tooth may deteriorate the tensofrictional grip of a casting and allow it to loosen.

Caries may also develop because of gingival recession and increasing marginal leakage. When a poorly designed pontic overcrowds the edentulous space between abutments, the interproximal spaces become too small, and are hard to clean. This predisposes these areas to recurrent caries.

6. Periodontal Conditions

Inadequate splinting, mobile teeth, and periodontal conditions that allow movements associated with torque permit an abutment tooth to move out of its cast retainer.

7. Faulty Cementation Procedure

Utilization of cement that is poorly mixed or at the wrong stage of its consistency, and *failure to dry both casting and tooth* prior to cementation may lead to premature loosening. Also, failure to mix and apply the luting agent and then seat the restoration before the working time of the cement has expired will result in incomplete seating, a raised occlusion, and a predisposition to loosening. Occlusal adjustments by grinding should not be done before the cement is fully set; otherwise, heat and vibrations may damage the unset cement and predispose it to fracture and dissolution. Patients should be given clear instructions to *delay forceful mastication* with newly cemented restorations for a few hours, so that the full strength of the cement may be attained. This is especially important with EBA type cements, for after final setting they gain strength slowly with the passage of time. Here again patients should be cautioned to avoid hard chewing for about six hours.

8. PROBLEMATIC DESIGN OF FIXED RESTORATION

Long-span bridges tend to deflect at each end under pressure. The longer the span, the greater the tendency for deflection and loosening at each end. Any long-span bridge may loosen if retention form, fit, and metallurgical characteristics are not favorable. The cantilever bridge is an engineering problem that poses a special retention challenge. Functional occlusal pressure on the pontic extending out in mid air (cantilevered) may wreak havoc with the retentive bond. All cantilever restorations have a pump-handle effect on the last tooth. The lever action may fracture the cement in the terminal abutment crown and allow caries to form.

9. SOLUBLE OR WEAK CEMENT

Soluble or weak cement may be immediately suspected in the premature loosening of a fixed restoration. Usually the most readily acknowledged causes for loosening involve the physical properties of the cement. However, *much more recognition should be given to the causes listed above.* Since the minimum compressive strength necessary to hold castings has never been determined, a cement of reasonable strength and low solubility should be adequate for the retention of fixed restorations if consideration is given to retention form, fit, occlusion, and effective cementation technique. Also, since solubility is influenced by oral fluids, oral chemistry, diet, and other factors, a particular dental cement may prevail in one mouth and wash out in another.

Practical Considerations to Avoid Premature Loosening

1. Prepare abutment teeth with as much parallelism as the path of insertion will tolerate, with the exception that very tall preparations should be more tapered for better fit and ease of insertion.

2. When taper is unavoidable, try to flatten one wall or add grooves, boxes, or pins.

3. Create parallel walls on short abutment teeth.

4. Reduce occlusal surfaces of posterior teeth and the lingual surface of upper anterior teeth enough to allow for an adequate thickness of coverage.

5. If a casting does not fit well, do not compromise, do it over. Better now than later.

6. Reduce enough tooth structure interproximally to allow for crown walls of adequate thickness and still leave room for the interdental papilla.

7. Evaluate the psychologic makeup of the patient and determine the extent of stresses involved and the possibility of bruxism. When necessary, prescribe dental biofeedback therapy to control bruxism.

8. Eliminate premature occlusal contacts and refine and adjust the occlusion within 48 hours after final cementation.

9. Suggest cutting down sugar intake of all forms, especially candy mints.

10. In an area of bone loss and slight mobility, a bridge abutment must be prepared with special concern for retention or it may loosen from its cast retainer, owing to movements associated with torque and function.

11. Dry the inside walls of crowns with a drying agent such as Cavilax* or Prep Dry.**

12. Dry prepared abutment teeth carefully. Do not overdry. Chemical drying agents are not necessary. Beware of saliva contamination.

13. Do not use cavity varnish that is too sticky or gummy because of evaporation of its solvent, for the surface presented for contact with cement will not be ideal.

14. Timing and rhythm are important in cementation. Do not overextend the spatulation time of any cement. Do not delay the application of the cement after it is mixed. Rehearse the path of insertion so that complete seating may be accomplished without undue delay once the restoration and cement has entered the warm, moist atmosphere of the mouth.

15. Use enough force, and maintain pressure long enough to insure proper seating.

16. Do not grind occlusal surfaces to adjust occlusion *too soon* after the cement hardens. The heat and vibration of grinding may be harmful to the integrity of the cement film at this time.

---

*Premier Dental Products Company, Philadelphia, PA 19107.
**Lee Pharmaceuticals, South El Monte, CA 91733.

fourteen

Removal of Restorations After Final Cementation

To look at his picture as a whole, a painter requires distance; and to judge of the total scientific achievement of any age, the standpoint of a succeeding age is desirable.

John Tyndall

The removal of cemented crowns and fixed partial dentures may be required because of wear, breakage, caries, partial loosening (one or more abutments), inadequate esthetics, periodontal conditions, and occlusal changes. Fixed bridges are also removed when the restorative therapy requires more pontics or abutments or when splinting of additional teeth is necessary.

Although restorations may loosen prematurely, they never seem to loosen when it is necessary to remove them. There is no way to remove permanently cemented crowns and bridges lightly, politely, and pleasantly. Indeed, the most successful removal is an unpleasant experience for both dentist and patient. Removal requires the application of force. This force is traumatic and may involve cutting, torque, torsion, and bending. There is a great potential for damage to the prepared abutment teeth and the surrounding soft tissues.

The prime consideration in the mind of the dentist attempting to remove a cemented fixed restoration is the preservation of the underlying abutment teeth.

The dentist should precondition himself and the patient to the challenging nature of the removal procedure. Since force must be utilized, it should be carefully controlled and be applied with sensitivity. As incongruous as it may seem, force should be applied delicately. The dentist is challenged to remove fixed retainers without fracturing the whole or part of an abutment tooth, and without harming the pulp or gingival tissues.

Removal procedures are loaded with psychologic as well as physical problems. The failure of a restorative treatment is the issue. Time, money and teeth are lost by the failure; and regardless of the fact that the fixed restoration is removed successfully, the memory lingers on. Mental pain may overshadow the physical aspects of this stressful situation. The dentist should be careful not to compound the issue with an inadvertent fracture or soft tissue injury. Every effort should be made to minimize the inescapable trauma involved in the removal of cemented restorations.

Removal usually results in damage to the fixed prosthesis. Although some fixed restorations are removed more easily than others, there is very little chance that a cemented restoration can be removed without some physical alteration. For example, a crown may be slit vertically, or have a hole made on the occlusal surface, or be deformed by twisting, torque, and pressure. The end result of the removal is divided into two categories: 1) a usable prosthesis, in which case the restoration may be repaired and recemented; or 2) an unusable prosthesis, in which case the restoration is destroyed by removal. The dentist's objective may be in either of these categories. There are occasions when it is necessary to salvage the prosthesis because of health, time, or economic factors. However, this is not always possible. In most instances the prosthesis is not usable after removal. It is destroyed for the welfare of the underlying structures. Usually both dentist and patient are resigned to the sacrifice of the restoration in order to allow new crown and bridge therapy. In either instance, the prime consideration is to preserve the abutment teeth. This statement is repeated for emphasis: *the prime consideration is to preserve the abutment teeth.*

Factors that Influence Removal

Dentists who are eager for an easy and effective way to remove fixed restorations are often victimized by a sales pitch for some contrivance, device, or apparatus that promises to accomplish the removal. This promise is seldom kept. Instead, the dentist now has an addition to the increasing number of ineffective gadgets gathering dust on his supply shelf. He can avoid or minimize this situation by recognizing that the use of devices for removal and all other methods of removal are governed by the following factors:

1. Location of the restoration
2. Number of abutments
3. Thickness of castings
4. Restorative materials
5. Pulpal conditions
6. Carious dentin
7. The cement used
8. Age, brittleness, and retentive form of the preparation
9. Other biophysical factors (see Chapter 7)

ABUTMENT CROWN REMOVAL

Hammering, reverse malleting or forceps of any kind should not be used to remove cemented crowns and bridges, or partial or complete fracture of a tooth may result. Cemented crowns, single, splinted, or bridged, may be removed by 1) the slit, or 2) the hole.

The Slit

In the early days of dentistry, when thin-walled gold shell crowns were placed, removal was accomplished with a forceps designed to slit one wall of the cemented crown. After slitting, spreading the halves allowed easy removal. In today's dentistry, cast gold crown walls are thicker and stronger and cannot be slit by hand. Nevertheless, the approach to the removal of the cemented crown is still the same. Now, the buccal (occasionally the lingual) surface is slit in a vertical direction with a 701 carbide bur in a high-speed handpiece. In like manner, a small, thin diamond stone is used for porcelain and porcelain-over-metal crowns. The vertical slit is initiated at the gingival third of the tooth and progresses to the occlusal surface. It should include all the occlusal surface if the crown is tall, less if it is short. If a fixed bridge or splint is being removed, each abutment crown is slit. However, care must be exerted to make each vertical cut parallel to the vertical cut on the other abutment(s), as shown in Figure 14–1.

When the carbide bur penetrates the gold and touches the underlying tooth structure, a groove is created on the surface of the tooth. This groove should be parallel to the path of insertion of the crown and also of other crowns involved. It is virtually impossible to cut through a crown of any material without making an indentation into the underlying tooth structure. The groove that results should be

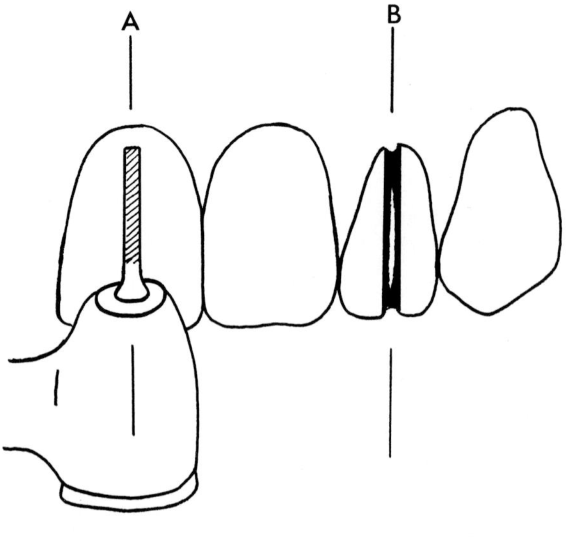

Figure 14–1 Removal of upper anterior bridge. The slit in the labial surface of the central incisor abutment should be made parallel (along line A) to the slit made in the lateral incisor abutment (along line B).

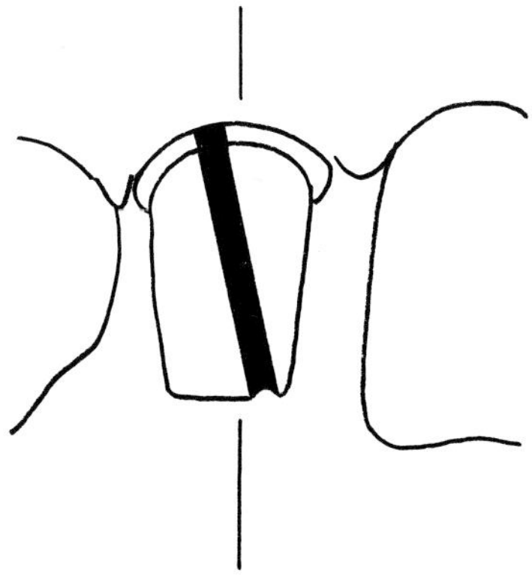

Figure 14–2 If the groove that remains after a crown has been removed by slitting is not parallel to the walls of the abutment preparation, it will interfere with the insertion and withdrawal of a new restoration. The malaligned groove illustrated should be filled with polycarboxylate cement.

as parallel as possible to the long axis of the prepared tooth to facilitate subsequent repreparation and impression making. Otherwise the groove that occurs in the abutment preparation as a result of cutting through the crown may interfere with proper insertion and withdrawal, unless it is obliterated by filling with cement (Fig. 14–2).

Any attempt to reprepare the surface of the abutment tooth to a deeper level so that the groove will be eliminated may lead to a pulp exposure. The dentist should be careful to keep this type of groove to a minimum depth as he proceeds to cut through the crown material. In most instances, the edges of the groove should be smoothed and the groove left as is and considered part of the abutment preparation. In fact, the groove adds to the retentive form of the preparation and the retention of the new crown in that it helps resist rotational forces.

A blunt instrument is placed into the slit and twisted to spread the crown apart slightly and loosen it. The same procedure is applied to the other abutment teeth of the restoration to be removed. In removing crowns and bridges the dentist should be careful not to use force great enough to fracture an abutment tooth. Some dentists have a heavier hand than others when pushing, pulling, or using a reverse mallet. Of course, applied force is not easy to measure. One way to insure against breakage is to completely divide a crown in half. This may be a wise procedure for a fragile abutment tooth, one that is periodontally involved, or one that is critical to the construction of a fixed restoration. Sometimes, depending on its thickness, the crown may be removed with minimal force when it is only half divided by a slit on the buccal and part of the occlusal surface. The force that may be applied for the removal of crowns and bridges and the amount of slitting necessary are directly related to biophysical factors such as length, taper, diameter, resistance to deformation, fit, and accessory grooves.

In the years before the advent of high-speed tooth reduction apparatus, the removal of cemented restorations was arduous, difficult, and unpleasant. Today metal crowns are easily cut, without vibration, with a carbide bur in an air turbine, as is porcelain with a diamond stone in the same instrument.

The Hole

A hole made in the occlusal surface of a crown exposes tooth structure that may be used as a pressure point for the mechanical elevation of the crown. Elevation is accomplished by threading a stainless steel screw into the hole until it contacts the underlying solid tooth structure. If the threads of the screw "bite" into the gold, and contact is made with the solid bearing area of the tooth, continued turning of the screw with a wrench will separate the crown from the tooth. Two or more abutments of a fixed bridge may be loosened in turn by this procedure. The Jelenko Inlay Remover* is a simple device that threads a screw into a hole in an inlay or a crown. The screw is turned and threaded into the hole in a crown by the forceful turning of a knurled knob at the end of a housing that extends the mechanism outside of the mouth (Fig. 14–3). The shortcomings of these methods are as follows:

1. Under the force of continuous rotation, the screw may perforate the pulp chamber.
2. An adequate thickness of gold is necessary for the threads of the screw to obtain a "bite." This is not always feasible.
3. The torsion induced by turning the screw with a wrench may damage the periodontal structures.

Another method involves a predrilled hole, a screw that fits easily into the hole, stainless steel claws mounted on a yoke, and a miniature reversible ratchet wrench to tighten the screw against the tooth structure. This method has similar shortcomings plus a much higher cost. The claws are designed to grip under the margins of a crown, but very often there is not enough marginal area available for a definitive grip. Also, the mechanism is bulky and may be difficult to apply in some areas of the mouth. The leverage provided by the length of the ratchet wrench may excessively burden the periodontal membrane.

Despite the shortcomings of these procedures, in selected cases they achieve a fair amount of success in the removal of cemented crowns and bridges. It should be remembered, however, that the effectiveness of these methods and others strongly depends on the aforementioned factors that influence removal.

In writing about the removal of cemented crowns and bridges, Karnoff[1] states: "Jack-screws have proved disappointing in most cases; we rarely find enough thickness of occlusal gold to engage the screw threads."

The Reverse Mallet Crown and Bridge Remover

The reverse mallet is an adjunct in the removal of crowns and bridges. It employs a sliding weight that moves along the length of a thick metal shaft. A variety of points are available for attachment to

---

*J. F. Jelenko & Company, Incorporated, New Rochelle, NY 10801.

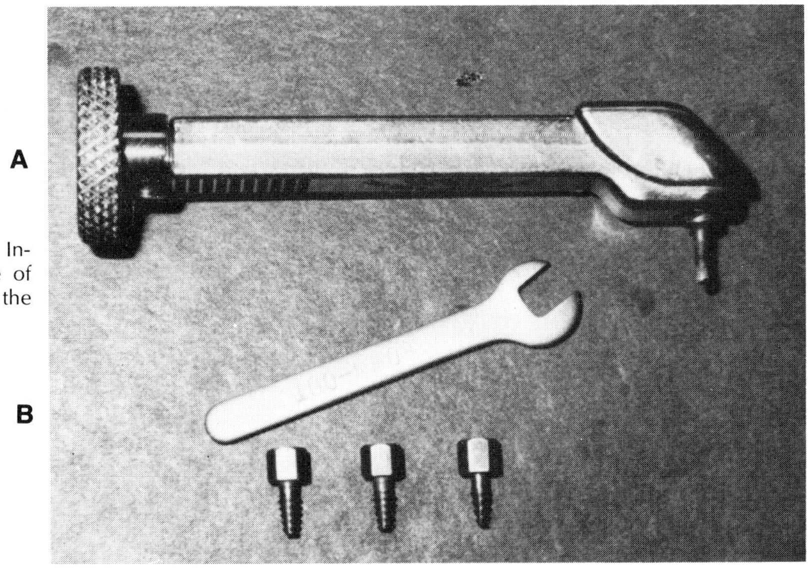

Figure 14–3 *A*, The Jelenko Inlay Remover. *B*, An example of screws and wrench used for the removal of inlays and crowns.

the working end of this instrument. One point is designed for placement under a margin of a crown, and another for interproximal placement. With a point of the removal instrument in one of these positions, the sliding weight is tapped forcibly against the opposite end of the instrument to loosen the restoration. It is difficult to gauge the correct amount of force to use with this type of instrument; too little force may not be enough for removal, too much may fracture an abutment tooth. If the removal force exerted by this instrument is applied to one end of a bridge (Fig. 14–4), it may cause rotation and breakage

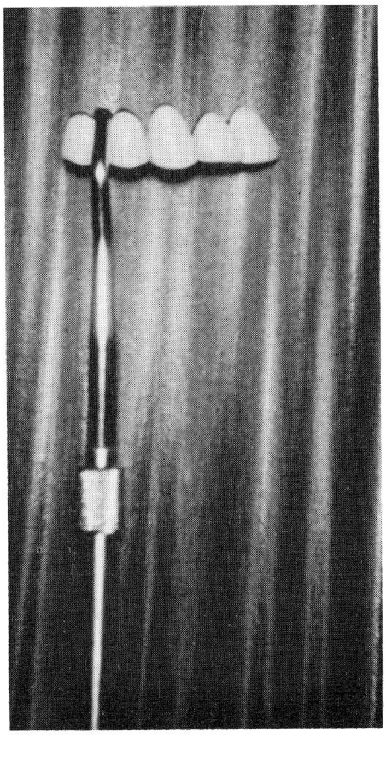

Figure 14–4 A reverse mallet should not be used to remove cemented crowns and bridges. It is especially hazardous if applied to one end of a fixed bridge, as breakage may occur at the other end.

of the abutment at the other end of the bridge when loosening is accomplished. Actually, it would make more sense mechanically and biologically to use *two* reverse mallets simultaneously, one at each end of the bridge (Fig. 14–5). However, this would be a cumbersome and impractical procedure. Therefore, it is best to limit the use of the reverse mallet to the removal of restorations that have been partially loosened by slitting or other means, so that the potential for breakage is minimized. *It should never be used to initiate removal.*

The reverse mallet can be a dangerous instrument if used without extra care and discipline. It may inflict damage not only to the abutment teeth involved but also to the teeth in the opposite jaw, and to the gingival and facial tissues as well.

Practical Considerations in the Removal of Cemented Restorations

1. After a crown has been removed, undesirable grooves and other discrepancies that remain may be filled with polycarboxylate cement. This cement will stay in place without resorting to retentive undercuts.

2. The use of a reverse mallet is not effective prior to the slitting of crowns; however, after the abutment crowns of a bridge have been slit, gentle tapping with a reverse mallet may accomplish removal.

3. Components of bridges and splints may be repaired and replaced without removing the entire prosthesis. For details of

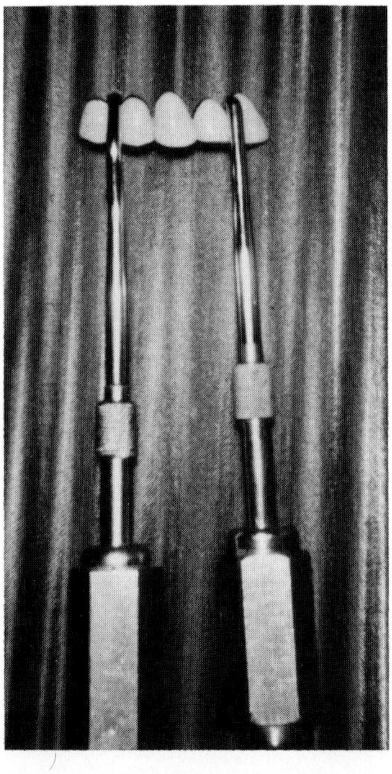

Figure 14–5 Although the use of two reverse mallets as shown here would be a more cogent approach to removal, it is best to avoid using these instruments to initiate removal of cemented restorations.

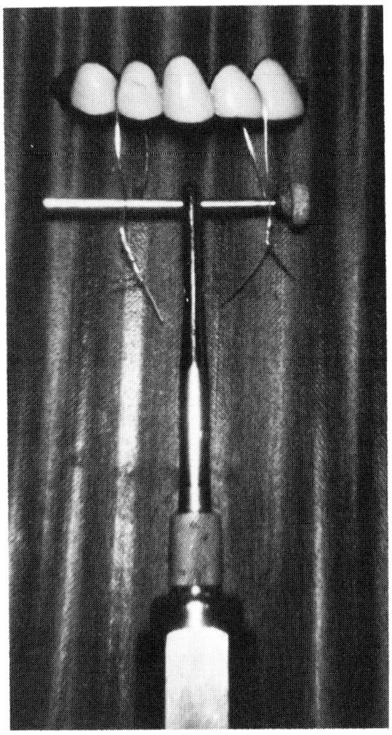

Figure 14–6 The use of the reverse mallet at a newly established central area is not recommended.

the mechanics involved the dentist is referred to other crown and bridge textbooks.[2, 3]

4. Drilling a hole through any cemented crown involves the risk of perforating the pulp chamber of the tooth. A high-speed bur that progresses through the thickness of a crown may continue to progress with accelerated speed when it reaches the softer underlying tooth structure, which supplies less resistance to its cutting efficacy.

5. Certain removal procedures are easier said than done. For example, the often suggested method of threading dental floss, wire, or paper clips under pontics to create a central area for the application of the reverse mallet seldom accomplishes removal (Fig. 14–6).

6. Fixed restorations that are not too badly damaged or distorted by slitting and removal forces may be repaired and utilized as temporary coverage during subsequent restorative therapy. Repair is accomplished by reseating the prosthesis in the mouth and applying self-curing acrylic resin to close the slit and to restore the contour of each abutment crown. After removal, shaping, and polishing, the repaired prosthesis may be replaced in the mouth, using a temporary cement that is selected according to the biophysical factors involved so that future removal will be facilitated. The old long-span or extensive fixed prosthesis that has been removed from the mouth and repaired with acrylic resin makes a more substantial temporary bridge as far as reten-

tion and function are concerned than does the usual self-cured acrylic resin temporary bridge.

7. When a hole is required in the occlusal surface of a crown for removal purposes, it is often suggested that the dentist find the thickest part of the occlusal surface to locate the hole. However, this area is difficult to find. X-rays are of no value in this determination. Therefore, the central area of the occlusal surface that has been thinned by the carving of occlusal anatomy should be avoided, and the hole established on the rising incline of a thick cusp.

8. As a safety precaution during removal procedures, a strand of dental floss (tape) should be threaded under and around a bridge or a splint prior to the application of removal force. The ends of the floss should be secured outside the mouth. This will prevent the restoration from suddenly springing out of the mouth or into the patient's throat. A gauze pad positioned lingually to the restoration may also be helpful in the removal.

SUMMARY

Perhaps in the future a non-traumatic method will be devised for the removal of cemented fixed restorations, utilizing a small amount of electronic energy, ultrasonic vibration, or some other phenomenon. Until then, cemented restorations must be partially destroyed if they are to be removed without damage to the underlying abutment teeth. The prime consideration in the removal of cemented restorations is to preserve the integrity of the underlying abutment teeth.

Today in dentistry the slitting of abutment crowns with high-speed, vibrationless apparatus is probably the least traumatic method for the removal of cemented fixed restorations. A few guidelines for success are as follows:

Slits should be parallel to the long axis of the abutment preparation and to each other.

A slit should be accomplished with a minimum of penetration and indentation of the underlying abutment tooth surface.

Slits made through the acrylic resin veneer of a crown may be easily repaired with self-curing resin after removal, and the restoration may then be used as a temporary restoration and cemented with a temporary cement.

REFERENCES

1. Karnoff, E. M.: Removing cemented crowns and bridges without destroying them. N. Y. J. Dent. *45*:158, 1975.
2. Tylman, S. D.: Theory and Practice of Crown and Fixed Partial Prosthodontics. 6th ed., St. Louis, The C. V. Mosby Company, 1970.
3. Weinberg, L. A.: Atlas of Crown and Bridge Prosthodontics. St. Louis, The C. V. Mosby Company, 1965.

fifteen

Factors For Prevention In Crown and Bridge Therapy

It is gratifying to be able to restore a disease-riddled mouth to health, but certainly it is better to prevent disease and promote health rather than to repair the damage produced by disease. Since this is the era of preventive dentistry, we should all join the "In Group."

Maynard K. Hine

An ounce of prevention is worth more than any amount of cure. This great truism has been acknowledged for centuries. Prevention negates therapy! Nevertheless, for many years in dentistry the majority of effort was directed toward developing and improving the technology for dental repair, and a lesser effort was aimed at preventing the *necessity* for dental repair. Today, the profession is deeply engrossed in reversing these considerations.

After fixed restorative therapy is accomplished, two enemies of oral health continue to undermine the endeavor. The culprits, of course, are dental caries and periodontal disease, dental caries being more prevalent in youth and periodontal disease in later years. Protection and insurance against the deleterious effects of these diseases upon fixed prostheses and the remaining dentition should derive from oral hygiene, nutrition, and other considerations.

Oral hygiene is the phase of preventive dentistry that has received the most attention. However, there are many other facets of prevention that should be considered in proper perspective, such as fluorides, dietary counseling, pit and fissure sealants, *and even certain preventive considerations in restorative dentistry.* For example, what good is the meticulous accomplishment and successful placement of excellent crowns and bridges if the surrounding hard and soft tissues are not maintained in a state of good health? The ultimate success or failure and durability of the fixed restoration depend on its foundation—the gingival tissues and the underlying bone. A faulty or improper diet is harmful to these tissues. No dentist wants his crowns and bridges to be framed with pathology. Proper nutrition, then, is a requirement for prevention in crown and bridge therapy. Concern for subsequent periodontal health after restorative dentistry and biologic evaluation of fixed bridges prior to final cementation are other preventive considerations. In fact, the dentist should endeavor to *incorporate as many preventive factors as possible into restorative treatment.* Preventive considerations in crown and bridge therapy are as follows:

1. *Oral hygiene.* The removal of plaque should be a continuous and never-ending endeavor to prevent caries and periodontal disease.

2. *Sanitation.* The interproximal spaces and the areas under pontics should be designed for easy cleansing. This may be considered a mechanical contribution to effective oral hygiene.

3. *Nutrition.* Control of food habits is required to maintain the health of the bone and tissues that frame the fixed prosthesis.

4. *Biologic evaluation of bridges prior to final cementation.* This tentative placement to assay tissue reactions, fit, and contact points is called temporary cementation. It allows adjustments and refinements that enhance the biologic compatibility of the prosthesis and the tissues.

5. *Antibacterial and anticariogenic factors.* Since all restorations have a potential for leakage, a cement with antibacterial properties may function as a secondary line of defense against bacterial invasion. Silicophosphate cements possess anticariogenic properties by virtue of the fluoride they contain.

6. *Microleakage.* An improvement of the marginal seal will help prevent recurrent caries.

7. *Periodontal conditions.* The contours and location of crown margins, and other soft tissue considerations play a part in the prevention of periodontal conditions.

8. *Oral habits.* Fingernail biting, lip biting, pipe smoking, tongue thrusting, bruxism, and abnormal swallowing should be curtailed, for they threaten the longevity of fixed restorative measures.

ORAL HYGIENE

Oral hygiene education is probably the most important preventive measure today. Except for water fluoridation and the inauguration of preventive measures in restorative therapy, the successful application of procedures for preventing caries and periodontal disease is greatly dependent on the cooperation of patients. Patients should be instructed in all aspects of oral hygiene and other beneficial preventive measures, but expectations of and demands on patients should be reasonable.

Patients should also be informed that completed crowns and bridges will not last indefinitely. As time passes, acrylic resin veneers may change color and abrade away; gingival recession may occur, and some of the cementum of the restored teeth may become exposed; caries may progress in these exposed areas, or interproximally, or on the roots and occasionally advance up and under a fixed retainer. After a *specified length of time,* maintenance, occlusal adjustments, prophylactic measures, and other care constitute a new and separate part of therapy. Recognition of the *time and expense* for this "new and separate part of therapy" may motivate the patient to greater cooperation in the home care required for oral hygiene. Instruction in the use of the toothbrush, dental floss, and the water-pic, and in nutrition should fall on eager ears. Restorations are placed with care by the dentist. The patient must now "carry the ball" and be instilled with a positive awareness that "his" care determines the extent of his oral health and the durability of the restorative therapy.

Good oral hygiene should be established if fixed prosthodontics is to be successful. It is the most efficacious measure in the prevention of periodontal disease. Good oral hygiene requires that plaque be removed at least once a day by brushing and using dental floss and possibly other adjunctive materials such as disclosing agents and oral irrigating devices. Interdental cleaning devices and stimulators such as soft wood sticks, plastic or rubber points, and interdental brushes may also be beneficial.[1] Fixed bridges require special oral hygiene care. Dentists should recommend the type and design of toothbrushes and their proper use. Most toothbrushes are bristled with nylon filament, although some are still made with hog bristles. It should be noted that nylon toothbrushes will abrade acrylic resin veneers quite rapidly, and their use, therefore, should be limited to porcelain, metal and natural teeth. Flossing presents more of a problem, since spaces between some teeth do not exist because of solder joints, and the floss must be threaded beneath the bridge. *All bridges and splints should be designed and fabricated to allow passage of dental floss between abutment teeth and between pontics and tissues.* Nevertheless, every effort should be made with any available materials to clean under, around, and between all fixed restorations and natural teeth.

Dental Floss

There is clinical evidence that toothbrushing *alone* does not adequately remove dental plaque from the proximal surfaces of the teeth.

Dental floss is a good adjunct to toothbrushing. When floss is worked into the crevice between tooth and gingiva, it not only removes oral debris but also *interrupts* plaque formation.

A new type of dental floss has been developed that contributes very effectively to the interproximal cleansing of both natural teeth and crowns and bridges. SUPER FLOSS* is a seventeen inch strand of floss, a segment (approximately 3½ inches) of which has been

---

*Educational Health Products, Incorporated, 221 Mill Road, P.O. Box 24, New Canaan, CT 06840.

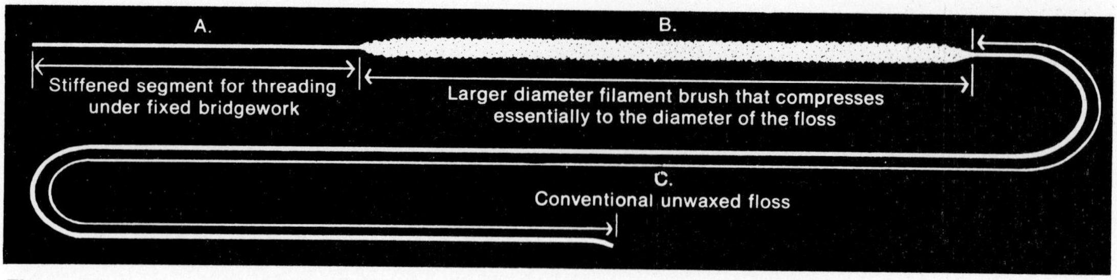

Figure 15–1 A new type of dental floss for interproximal cleaning of both natural teeth and crowns and bridges. It has a thickened segment that conforms to the mesial and distal walls of crowns and bridges or natural teeth.

exploded into a spongy filament brush of larger diameter than the floss (Fig. 15–1). This variable diameter dental floss is unwaxed, highly shred resistant, and very strong. The unitary construction allows the floss segment and the *compressible brush segment* to work together as a single cleansing unit. After the floss segment is slipped through a contact point the brush segment may be pulled into the interproximal space. Now it is used as an interproximal toothbrush. By pulling back and forth on the ends of the floss strand, the spongy brush segment will very effectively remove plaque and food debris from adjacent tooth surfaces. This floss conforms to the mesial and distal tooth (or crown or bridge) surfaces and provides a gentle compression against the interdental papilla. This action not only opens the sulcus and cleanses under the free gingival margin but also strengthens gingival tone by stimulating an increased blood flow to the area.

When applied to a fixed bridge or splint, each firm end of the floss strand is stiff enough to penetrate and thread through a small interproximal space from buccal to lingual.

Another new type of dental floss has been introduced.[2] This new agent is called "dental cleansing tape." It is made of a Dupont elastomer called Hytrel, and although strong and elastic, it is also thinner and softer than conventional floss made of nylon, silk, or cotton. It is designed to combine the functions of dental floss with the polishing and cleansing actions of a toothbrush and dentifrice. The floss may be coated or impregnated with a polishing agent and flavor similar to available toothpastes.

A study designed to determine the reaction of a group of dental practitioners to this new interdental cleansing material showed the overall response to be highly favorable.[3]

Other Oral Hygiene Aids

Oral Irrigating Devices

Water devices that give a pulsating or steady stream of water are helpful in maintaining oral health. They remove loose debris from areas that cannot be cleansed with a toothbrush, such as under fixed bridges and between crowns and splints.

Interdental Cleaning Devices

Tapered narrow points of wood, plastic or rubber may be used to remove food particles and to stimulate gingival tissues. Examples of products for this purpose are as follows:

1. STIM-U-DENTS
   Stim-u-dents, Incorporated
   Detroit, MI 48238.
2. P/S Polisher/Stimulator
   Oral B Company, Fairfield Road
   Wayne, NJ 07470.
3. Pick-A-Dent
   Denticator Company
   San Francisco, CA 94101.

Mouth Rinses and Chewing Gum

The chewing of gum and the use of mouthwashes have not been shown by adequately controlled clinical studies to contribute to oral health. Their use simply results in the clearance of some loose oral debris from the mouth. However, there is increasing interest directed toward the use of mouth rinses and chewing gum as vehicles for antiplaque agents.

Chewing gum, sugarless or not, should be avoided after crown and bridge therapy. Some brands adhere tenaciously to acrylic resin veneers. However, a greater threat to oral health comes from the hydraulic pressures exerted on various confined areas of tooth structure by the chewing-gum mass. These forces may drive plaque, debris, and caries into a deeper invasion of the hard and soft tissues.

ELIMINATION OF THE CARIOGENIC FLORA

Fixed partial dentures permit rapid accumulation of bacterial plaques in difficult-to-clean areas. When these restorations are installed in a cariogenic flora, the result can be disastrous. Therefore, an initial objective in all restorative procedures should be the elimination of cariogenic flora without delay. If this is done, even noncleansed restorations do not produce rampant caries, and even poor restorations have a longer life.

1. Remove all bacterial plaque from every enamel surface with a non-abrasive prophylaxis paste containing fluoride.
2. Suggest the substitution of non-cariogenic foods for caries conducive foods containing sucrose in order to modify the oral flora.
3. Make enamel surfaces resistant to acid action by impregnating these surfaces with topical fluorides.
4. Motivate a program of home care to keep the cariogenic plaques from returning. Instruct the patient in the use of a disclosing solution or tablet to prevent plaque accumulation.
5. Open into, and remove the infected layer of all dentinal carious lesions. Restore these areas with a zinc oxide and eugenol in-

termediate filling material such as Interstate's Semi-Final* or Caulk's IRM.** Sedative filling materials (zinc oxide and eugenol formulations) promote healing of dentin and pulp. Massler[4] states: "The cariogenic flora becomes depressed or even eliminated in 48 hours after the removal of all infected cariogenic plaques from all enamel and dentinal surfaces." The best time to get rid of the cariogenic flora is just before crown and bridge procedures are started. This will contribute to the longevity of the restorations in a caries free environment.

SANITATION

It is not enough to make crowns and bridges that fit, function, and look well, they must also be designed to be clean. Sanitation refers to the cleaning (oral hygiene) of crowns and bridges and to *certain inherent characteristics that allow for ease of cleaning.* If a fixed prosthesis cannot be cleaned it becomes unsanitary and will cause periodontal disease and discomfort.

Therefore, crowns and fixed partial dentures may contribute to or detract from the sanitation of the oral cavity. When placed in the mouth they provide surfaces of various degrees of smoothness, spaces (interproximal) of different sizes, and various crevices and contours. All these, coupled with the spaces formed between pontics and tissues, are potential sites for trapping food, debris, and plaque.

Fixed restorations should be cleaned with a toothbrush, and require dental flossing, not only between all contacts but also *under all pontics.*

The following are practical considerations to minimize sanitation problems:

Interproximal Space

If the interproximal spaces between pontics and abutments are too small it will be difficult to pass dental floss between them for cleaning purposes. Also, food and debris get trapped in small spaces and are not easily brushed away. Large interproximal spaces, however, fill up more readily but are easily and quickly cleaned out by movements of the tongue, lips, and cheeks, and by rinsing and suction. Also, the patient can easily thread dental floss through the larger spaces. One end of the floss should be rolled into a ball, which is then pulled through the space to clean it and burnish away plaque.

A question remains: How large should the interproximal spaces be made? If too small, sanitation is impaired. If too large, esthetics are compromised. The answer depends on the dentist's recognition of the factors involved. Anterior restorations should not have extra-large spaces or the cosmetic effect will suffer. However, the spaces

---

*Interstate Dental Company, New Hyde Park, NY.
**L. D. Caulk Company, Milford, DE.

should be large enough for dental floss to pass through. It is occasionally necessary for the patient to utilize a threading device to pass the dental floss through the available spaces. Janar NUPONS Bridge and Splint Cleansers* and Johnson and Johnson's ZON Dental Bridgc Clcancrs** are both effective ways to conquer space (small interproximal space) (Fig. 15–2). Also, SUPER FLOSS,† a new type of dental floss with a spongy brush segment, may be easily threaded between splinted crowns and under bridge pontics. Posterior fixed bridges may have larger interproximal spaces, but they should still be small enough to satisfy the patient's esthetic requirements.

The axial contours of crowns and bridges, regardless of material used, should restore the original anatomy of the teeth. Proximal walls should not impinge on the interdental tissues. If they do, the soft tissues are irritated by the pressure and periodontal breakdown is initiated. Moreover, the periodontal lesion becomes chronic and is perpetuated because the interproximal area cannot be cleaned. Microbial plaque is trapped, and the gingival tissues become inflamed not only in response to the poor contours of the restoration but also in response to the residual bacterial mass.

The architecture of the interproximal embrasures should be made to meet anatomic and physiologic requirements and, at the same time, allow for sanitary considerations.

Multiple unit or long-span porcelain over metal fixed prostheses occasionally violate the anatomic, physiologic, and sanitary needs of proper fixed restorative therapy. The rigidity of metal understructures requires the overall span of metal to be thick enough to resist flexion. This is usually accomplished by the fabrication of wider and deeper contact areas and, therefore, smaller interproximal spaces result. Here again the potential mechanical benefits must be balanced against biologic and preventive considerations.

---

*Janar Company, Grand Rapids, MI 49501.

**Johnson & Johnson, New Brunswick, NJ 08903.

†Educational Health Products, Incorporated, New Canaan, CT 06840.

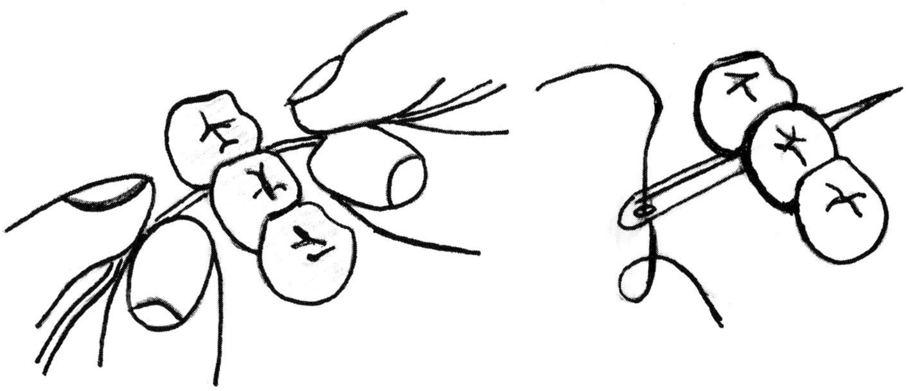

Figure 15–2 Floss alone or with a threading device should be routinely passed between teeth, crowns, and pontics to maintain effective oral hygiene.

The Extent of Interproximal Reduction

Dentists should keep in mind the need to make room for the "seven layer cake" that will ultimately occupy the space between adjacent teeth restored with porcelain-over-metal crowns. Actually, there are eight layers of restorative material between two full crown preparations. Occupying the interproximal space—from the distal of one crown preparation to the mesial of the next tooth, also a crown preparation—will be the following layers, cement, metal, opaque, porcelain/porcelain, opaque, metal, cement. Somewhere between these eight layers of restorative material there must be space for the interdental papilla to exist in a passive state. It should not be evicted. The successful accomplishment of this biologic requirement is heroic, and requires careful planning, preparation, and fabrication in the course of crown and bridge therapy.

Pontic-Tissue Relationship

Regardless of the design of a fixed bridge pontic, its tissue-facing surface should not be in pressure contact with the soft tissues of the edentulous area, nor should it be too far away from these tissues. Pontics should only face tissues with smooth, well-polished surfaces. They should barely contact or, if so, only passively. Again, anterior pontics have esthetic needs that differ from posterior pontics. A pontic that contacts tissues too heavily will not only contribute to gingival irritation but will also hinder the passage of dental floss for removal of bacterial plaque and food particles. Occasionally, tissue that is contacted too tightly by a pontic will proliferate up and around the gingival area of the pontic. This is generally accelerated by the lack of sanitation inherent to the situation, and may lead to the ultimate failure of the fixed prosthesis.

Occasionally, despite good fit, placement, contour, and polish, tissues under pontics of fixed bridges respond poorly and become irritated and inflamed. If oral hygiene is good, and bony support adequate, so that no local cause may be attributed to the soreness, suspicion may be cast toward ill-health, senility, or chronic debilitating disease to account for the unhealthy mucosa. However, some patients in apparently good health present soft tissues that appear normal but respond with soreness when close to pontics. These may be subclinical cases of nutritional deficiency or hormonal imbalance. The dietary deficiency should be corrected by prescribing vitamins and other supplements, and the patient should be referred to an endocrinologist if hormonal imbalance is suspected.

Other endogenous factors must be considered. Without a doubt there is a relationship between systemic conditions and gingival tolerance. Diabetes mellitus, pregnancy, puberty, and the gingival hyperplasia caused by drugs (such as diphenylhydantoin in the treatment of epilepsy) all may contribute to a poor pontic-tissue relationship regardless of considerations for sanitation.

In summary, the tissue-facing surface of a fixed-bridge pontic must be adjusted to allow easy passage of dental floss for sanitation and have a smooth, well-polished contour to avoid irritation if settling of the bridge occurs or if tissues proliferate. Sanitation is an important factor for prevention in crown and bridge therapy. It warrants proper considerations for the design of interproximal spaces and pontic-tissue relationships. But above all, it calls for cleanliness. Food, plaque, and debris should be removed from fixed restorations on a daily basis. Just as dishes are washed after every meal, so too should teeth be brushed and crowns and bridges cleaned. A wide variety of simple devices* is available for the extra chore of cleaning under a fixed bridge with dental floss. No fixed bridge should be cemented permanently without demonstrating to the patient the use of one of these devices to thread dental floss interproximally so that it may be passed under the pontic(s).

Removal of Excess Cement

The various luting agents for the final cementation of fixed restorations cause different problems in the removal of excess cement. The retention of a spicule of excess zinc phosphate cement may cause gingival irritation and may harbor debris and plaque; therefore, every speck of excess must be removed fastidiously. In doing so, the dentist must exert special care not to scratch the polished surfaces of the restoration. A scratched casting is less sanitary than a polished one.

Unlike zinc phosphate cement, alumina EBA cement does not require the meticulous removal of excess material. Large interproximal pieces of cement should be removed, and also other fragments located near or in contact with the gingival tissues. However, films or smears of this cement (usually on the lingual surface) may be allowed to remain. If the dentist attempts to remove this excess with instruments, the highly polished surfaces may become scratched. If left alone, they will self-destruct (remove themselves) in a day or so through food abrasion and thermal changes and possibly enzymic or microbiologic activity. However, any excess of cement containing eugenol must be removed from an acrylic resin surface as completely and as quickly as possible as a preventive measure against subsequent damage to the resin.

Plastic cements, acrylic or polycarboxylate, require special considerations in the removal of excess. If removal is not accomplished before these resins approach the rubbery stage of partial polymerization, cementing material may be inadvertently pulled out from under a margin. This will leave a void or a rough edge, which will act as a deterrent to sanitation and periodontal health. After complete hardening, excess resin cement may have to be ground away; this is difficult and may result in rough and unsanitary areas.

---

*NUPONS, Janar Company, Grand Rapids, MI 49501.
ZON, Johnson & Johnson, New Brunswick, NJ 08903.
SUPER FLOSS, Educational Health Products, Incorporated, New Canaan, CT.
BRIDGE AID, Floss Aid Corporation, Santa Clara, CA 95052.
EEZ-THRU, J.O. Butler Company, Chicago, IL 60611.
FLOS PIK, Janar Company, Grand Rapids, MI 49501.
FLOSS CADDY, Oral Health Products, Incorporated, Tulsa, OK 74135.

Silicone grease* is recommended as a practical aid (Fig. 15–3) in the removal of excess cement. *Prior to cementation* the fixed bridge or splint is covered with a film of silicone grease. A small amount is placed in each interproximal space and a thin film is smeared on the buccal and lingual surfaces. *Caution!* Keep the silicone grease away from the margins and exert care not to push any of this lubricant into the insides of the castings while handling. Do not use abolene oil or mineral oil as a lubricant. Any mobile material may flow where it is not wanted. Petroleum jelly, carding wax, and other agents have been used to facilitate the removal of excess cement, but silicone grease is more effective.

Design of Fixed Prosthesis

Sanitation refers not only to the cleaning of fixed restorations but also to characteristics that allow for ease of cleaning and others that *decrease the need for cleaning*. For example:

1. Good contact relationships between all teeth (natural or abutment casting) contribute to sanitation.
2. Well-designed embrasures and contours deter food impaction and facilitate sanitary measures.
3. Veneer design for molar abutment castings. Acrylic resin veneers on molar crowns should be limited to the minimum area of the buccal surface that is required for esthetics. They need not be extended farther distally than approximately four fifths of the buccal surface of first molars, three quarters of second molars, and two thirds of third molars (Fig. 15–4). These designs are based on the premise that polished gold is cleaner and attracts less plaque and food debris

*Opotow Dental Silicone, Teledyne Dental, Palo Alto, CA 94304.
RM Silicone Grease, Rocky Mountain Dental Products Company, Denver, CO.
ProCem Silicone, Professional Products Company, San Diego, CA 92112.

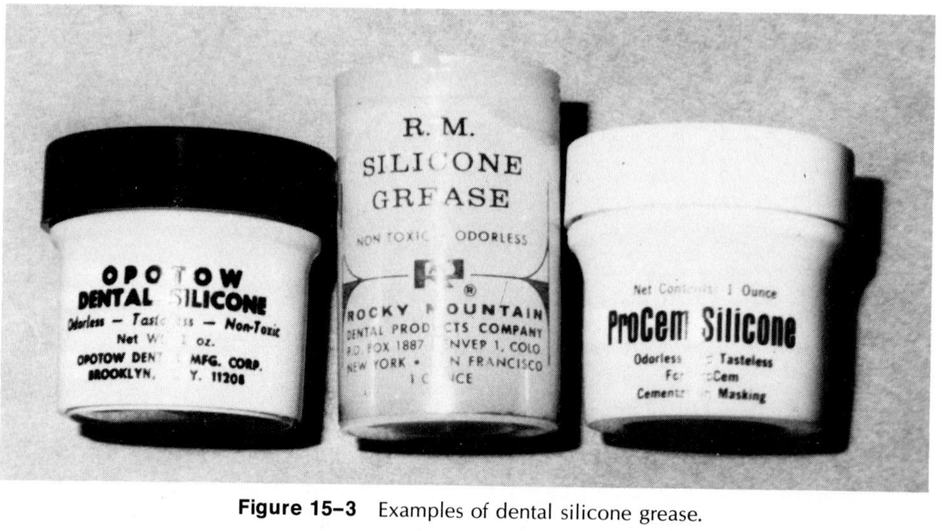

Figure 15–3 Examples of dental silicone grease.

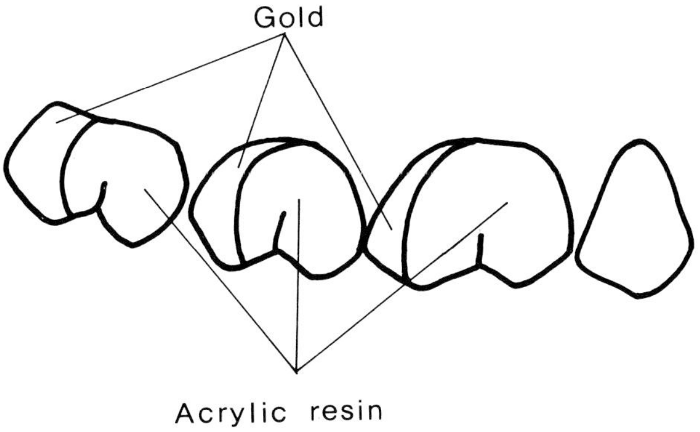

Figure 15–4 Acrylic resin veneers will provide the necessary esthetic values without covering the entire buccal surface of molar crowns. From the first to the third molar, there is a decrease in acrylic resin and an increase in cleaner gold.

than acrylic resin. Gold also maintains its polish and luster longer than acrylic resin. Also, the distal margin of contact between acrylic resin and its gold housing in the casting is less likely to attract food debris if its position is not confined to the distal interproximal embrasure.

An acrylic resin veneer that is wrapped around the distal buccal surface of second and third molars contributes nothing to esthetics. These areas cannot be seen when the patient smiles or talks. Gold is cleaner! Acrylic resin veneers on the buccal surfaces of molar crowns should be limited to the mesial fraction of the casting, for they serve no other purpose than to disguise a small area of gold. The polished distal area of a gold molar crown will be cleaner if a marginal line of contact with acrylic resin is not present.

NUTRITION

Nutrition is the process by which living organisms obtain and use nutrients from food for the maintenance of function and for the growth and repair of tissues. An understanding of the science of nutrition includes an understanding of the composition of foods and a knowledge of the proper food selection for an adequate diet. Nutrition includes not only the intake of an adequate and balanced diet but also the digestion and transportation to the tissues of essential food elements, and utilization of these elements by the body cells.

One very important aspect of preventive crown and bridge therapy that has been neglected is that of the effects of nutrition on the periodontium. Good nutritional analysis and guidance are indispensable for the effective prevention of dental disease.

The dentist who recognizes and teaches the importance of nutrition can help his patients derive the fullest benefits from crown and bridge therapy. Proper nutrition will help the fixed restoration to function in an environment of healthy bone and soft tissues. Even the pulpal health of the abutment teeth may be influenced by adequate nutrition. And, of course, of utmost significance is the role of proper nutrition in minimizing the formation of plaque on, near, and about the crowns and bridges. This is a vital consideration in preserving the existing dentition as well as in the longevity of the repair.

Regardless of its palatability, food is masticated poorly when teeth and occlusion are faulty. Difficulty in the proper mastication of food, obliging the patient to change to a soft diet, can have serious physical health effects. The tendency to favor "softer" foods may result in a substantial increase of carbohydrate foods in the diet. However, even dentitions that are successfully repaired with crowns and bridges function somewhat less effectively than natural teeth. Patients who have lost many teeth and who are using fixed partial dentures show a wide variation in functional efficiency. As a result, the stomach has more work to do, and discomfort and indigestion may occur. This leads to changes in digestive chemistry and modifications of pH, saliva, plaque formation, and enzymic activity, and these changes challenge the integrity and longevity of fixed partial prostheses.

Many patients are stubborn and resistant to change in their eating habits. Eating habits of a lifetime are not easily altered. In many instances they are difficult to modify because they have deep emotional origins. Nevertheless, when necessary, the dentist must motivate a patient to modify these habits. He must appeal to the patient's sense of reason. He must point out the underlying consequences if the patient does not change. And, of course, he must highlight the benefits of better food habits.

A most important goal for the dentist is to influence the patient *to reduce his intake of cariogenic sucrose,* especially between meals. Sucrose, especially in the form of sticky confections, candies, and cookies, aids in the rapid growth of cariogenic organisms. The patient's diet is best changed by substitution, not by chiding or ridicule. "Substitution" is the key word. Substitute for sucrose with non-cariogenic starches and sugars such as in apples, oranges, nuts and potato chips.

The patient should also be cautioned to minimize his intake of processed foods. Processing of natural foods increases sucrose content and greatly increases cariogenicity. For example, non-cariogenic peanuts, grapes, and whole wheat become caries conducive peanut butter, raisins, and white bread.

It would be ideal if all dental personnel involved in counseling were to set an example and be highly motivated by developing a continuous interest in their own nutrition.

Nutritional Guidance

1. Have the patient record his food intake of the previous 24 hours to get an idea of what he actually eats.
2. Evaluate the diet with regard to adequacy.
3. Present a prescription for an acceptable personalized diet. Make careful and judicious substitutions.

Sugar and Phosphoric Acid in Carbonated Beverages

Patients should be warned about the harmful effects of soft drinks. They may dissolve teeth! Carbonated beverages contain large amounts of refined sugar, as much as five teaspoons in one eight-ounce bottle.[5] They also contain large quantities of phosphoric and citric acids, which etch and erode tooth enamel. In fact, these same acids are used in various techniques to modify tooth enamel. For example, a dilute solution of phosphoric acid is used in the acid-etch technique, and it does its job of etching the enamel *in less than two minutes.* Even mild acids in citrus fruits may erode tooth enamel; lemon juice, for example, but the stronger acids in soft drinks are far more destructive.

Carbonated beverages such as Coca Cola, Pepsi Cola, and Dr. Pepper clearly designate *sugar and phosphoric acid* among the ingredients listed on the container. When crown and bridge therapy has been accomplished, these ingredients challenge the solubility of the cement line and the caries resistance of the remaining supragingival and subgingival tooth structure.

When crown and bridge therapy has been completed it is especially important to suggest that the following foods be avoided: highly refined and overcooked foods, processed foods, fast foods, pastries, carbonated beverages, chewing gum (even sugarless gum), candy (especially sticky types), and lemon juice.

Suggestions for good between-meal foods are as follows: celery, radishes, cucumbers, apples, oranges, peaches, cheese, plain milk, and potato chips (real potatoes, non-processed).

Nutrition influences the two principal oral health problems, dental caries and periodontal disease. In fact, nutrition can selectively influence the types of bacteria, their proliferation (dental plaque), and the degree of dental caries.[6] Fluoride, phosphates, combinations of the two, and some trace elements may provide a local anticariogenic effect. Sucrose has been designated the most cariogenic food factor. Sugar-loaded candy, foods, and beverages, and frequent between-meal intake of such foods, are conducive to dental caries. Nevertheless, dentists should be careful not to oversimplify the situation by assuming that a one-to-one relationship exists between sugar and dental caries. It is not sugar alone. It has been shown that the manner in which sucrose is used is more important than the total amount eaten.[7] Research evidence indicates that variables other than the sucrose content of foods can be of importance in causing caries.[8] There are indications that foods may show wide differences in cariogenicity, aside from their sugar content.

The dentist should combat the between-meal eating of snack foods. The patient should be told which foods are highly cariogenic, and foods of low cariogenicity should be suggested to replace them.

Nutrition is but one of the many preventive factors that influence the success or failure of restorations fixed in the human mouth. The dentist should recognize that a well-balanced diet of essential nutrients is vitally essential to the general health of his patient and to the success of the crowns and bridges he has utilized in the treatment of the patient.

Since nutrition counseling is an important part of many dentists' patient education programs, the American Dental Association Bureau of Dental Health Education has revised and expanded its pamphlet *Diet and Dental Health* to help dentists teach their patients about diet. A sample copy of this pamphlet and other publications dealing with nutrition may be obtained without cost from the Bureau of Dental Health Education.

BIOLOGIC EVALUATION OF BRIDGES

A few decades ago fixed bridges were mechanical devices that were cemented into place shortly after fabrication. Today, the final cementation of a fixed partial denture should be accomplished only after biological compatibility has been verified to some degree. Fixed bridges are foreign bodies. When placed in the mouth to replace missing tissues, they are a type of implant. Being an implant, each fixed bridge requires some evidence that it is biologically acceptable to its environment. If it is inserted and allowed to function for a trial period, the reaction of the host may be evaluated and changes may then be made to improve biologic acceptance.

The biologic evaluation of bridges allows for improving soft tissue relationships with pontics, overextension of retainers, accuracy of fit, occlusal relationships, contact points, and esthetics. This embraces many preventive considerations.

How is biologic evaluation accomplished? The answer is temporary cementation. The temporary cementation of fixed bridges for a trial period is the only way to obtain a biologic assessment. Despite the problems involved, this tentative placement to assay tissue reactions and other relationships provides better crown and bridge therapy.

ANTIBACTERIAL AND ANTICARIOGENIC FACTORS

The use of antimicrobials coupled with other measures of caries control seems to offer the most promise of eventually eliminating dental caries. There is, however, no antimicrobial agent available today that will selectively destroy cariogenic organisms. Nevertheless, research is progressing along these lines; and a clinical study[9] has demonstrated an antibiotic, Vancomycin, that suppresses *Streptococcus mutans*, an organism that has been implicated in human dental caries. Other research has suggested that acidulated phosphate gel may have a direct antibacterial effect on the same organism. The antibacterial agent with the greatest potential as a preventive modality under investigation today is chlorhexidine.[10] It has marked plaque-inhibiting ability.

Meanwhile, most of the methods for the control of caries are designed to increase the resistance of a tooth to the caries process by the utilization of fluoridation. Silicophosphate cement is an old example of this, for it possesses anticariogenic properties by virtue of the fluoride it contains. Jerman[11] states: "The lack of permanent seal and the prevalence of recurrent decay place increased emphasis on the cariostatic properties of all restorative materials."

Since all restorations have a potential for leakage, a cement with antibacterial properties may be designed to function as a secondary line of defense against bacterial invasion.

MICROLEAKAGE

An improved marginal seal, since it is directed towards eliminating recurrent caries and premature loosening of fixed restorations, is a preventive consideration in crown and bridge therapy.

The margins of restorative materials that are in contact with tooth structure do not seal the area. Therefore, leakage occurs and may allow the ingress of oral fluids, bacteria toxins, soluble ions, and debris. This is referred to as microleakage. It may lead to pulpal sensitivity, caries, staining of margins, and pulp pathology. To prevent microleakage a restorative material should combine chemically with the tooth surfaces and should also expand and contract to the same degree as the tooth during temperature changes. No dental restorative material has this ability. There is no filling material, cement, or other type of restorative material available in modern dentistry that will effectively seal the interface between a tooth and a restoration in the oral environment. Because of the lack of a chemical bond between restorative material and tooth structure, microleakage is a constant factor for failure. The degree of microleakage is a measure of the acceptability of a restorative material.

Crowns and bridges depend on a cementing material to preserve the integrity and health of prepared tooth structure by providing a seal against the ingress of deleterious agents. Here, success is partially dependent on the solubility of the cement in the fluids of the oral environment. Unfortunately, the most insoluble cement falls victim to the ravages of thermal change, deformation, and other phenomena.

In fixed restorative dentistry the solubility of the cement is just one of many factors that influence the marginal seal. Other factors to be considered are as follows:

1. Accuracy of the fit of the restoration
2. Temperature fluctuations
3. Thermal conductivity of restorative material
4. Cementation technique
5. Strength of the tooth-cement-restoration "mechanical" bond
6. Cavity varnish
7. Deformation
8. Film thickness
9. Capillary action

Many of these factors have been discussed at length in dental literature; however, too few observations have recognized the influence of capillary action. Capillary penetration exists between restorative materials and tooth structure.[12] The degree of penetration is influenced by the narrowness of the crevice, the surface tension of the liquid (oral fluid), and the extent to which it wets the solid surfaces. Decreasing the size of the crevice by improving the adaptation of the restorative material will increase capillary pressure and penetration. Paradoxically, this poses a significant threat to the marginal seal of *well-fitting restorations* as compared to ill-fitting restorations having poor adaptation.

Since marginal leakage is an inherent shortcoming of dental restorative materials, the clinician must appreciate the importance of protecting the pulp under all restorations. The best way to do this is with proper cavity lining materials. Varnishes of copal resin, and liners of calcium hydroxide and zinc oxide/eugenol cements decrease leakage when applied to the walls of dentin adjacent to the pulp. However, zinc phosphate cements were not found to decrease leakage into the dentin.[13] Since zinc phosphate cement is a porous, permeable liner and has an acidic effect on the pulp, its use is contraindicated for pulp protection.

Microleakage is a serious threat to preventive dentistry. The clinical skills of the dentist and his knowledge of the physical and chemical nature of restorative materials play important roles in minimizing this problem.

PERIODONTAL CONDITIONS

The inadequate reproduction of proper anatomical form in artificial crowns has always been related to periodontal disease. The relationship of proper tooth contours to the surrounding gingivae has been stressed as important to periodontal health.[14–16] Indeed, the gingival tissues are presumed to be protected by the deflective convexities of tooth structure.[17] Apparently the concept of deflective crown contour has always been accepted, based on fanciful thinking rather than research. Actually, both a proximally overcontoured restoration and one with buccal and lingual cervical bulges may contribute to periodontal disorders. Recent research reports[18, 19] support the concept that deflective anatomy in the gingival third of the facial and lingual surfaces of restored teeth bears *no relation to gingival health.* Yuodelis, Weaver and Sapkos[20] have observed excellent gingivae response with flattening the facial and lingual contours of restorations. Gingival tissues do not require protection from the cervical bulges of crowns.

Dimensions, contours, contact points, proximal surfaces, and marginal ridges have received an appropriate amount of discussion in dental literature. So too, have crown margins. However, much more has been stated about the location of the crown margin than about its contour or other modifications. Without a doubt, the contours and the placement of crown margins influence the periodontal health of the tissues adjacent to a fixed prosthesis.

Crown Margins

The marginal contact of a cast gold crown cemented to the prepared margins on a tooth is always less than perfect. Here are the reasons:

1. No casting is totally exact.
2. The film thickness of the cement introduces a discrepancy. Venting may reduce the error but will not totally obliterate it.
3. Hydraulic pressure "kickback" during cementation causes faulty positioning of the casting. Again, venting is only partially helpful.
4. If the cementation procedure is not absolutely perfect in technique and timing of application, marginal fit is impaired.

Where Does the Gingival Margin Go?

This is an age-old question. The placement of the "less than perfect" margin is slightly controversial as to its relationship with the gingival tissues. Should it be below the gingiva? And if so, how far below? Or should it be supragingival? Much has been said for each possibility. Some dentists, for insurance, "sweep it under the carpet." Going too far into the gingival sulcus is poor policy. It brings a larger amount of foreign material into more intimate contact with tissue that may not tolerate its presence. The slightest amount of tooth mobility during function causes movement of the restorative material against the tissues in the sulcus. This may lead to irritation and the chronic inflammatory reaction that is responsible for framing many restorative endeavors with unhealthy gingival tissues.

The placement of gingival margins should be influenced by the clinical requirements for esthetics, retention, contour, and inhibition of plaque retention. The proper position for a gingival margin when esthetics is of prime concern is *slightly into the healthy gingival crevice.* Usually, the esthetic requirements of anterior jacket crowns need special consideration in the placement of the subgingival margin. Abutments of a cantilever bridge also require special considerations regarding the placement of gingival margins because of the unusual forces involved. However, in no situation should gingival margins be placed at or near the alveolar crest.

The Nature of the Margin

Of equal importance to the position of the margin is the nature of the margin. Is it sharp or rough or is it rounded and smooth? Any part of a margin that is rough and unpolished will contribute to the biologic failure of the restoration. The best fitting casting with proper margin placement may cause gingival irritation if the margin is *too sharp*, or too knifelike. The inherent discrepancy after final cementation (fit, cement film, hydraulics, cementation technique) keeps the sharp edge from a smooth juxtaposition with the prepared tooth structure. In other words, the sharp edge stands away from a smooth, nondetectable coalescence with the tooth. *The gingival tissues draped over this knife edge or pressed against it by food or tongue suffer constant irritation.*

Carpenters can saw, sand, and plane two pieces of wood into a smooth union with an undetectable junction, but dentists cannot blend metal, porcelain, or plastic to subgingival tooth structure with a similar smoothness. It just cannot be done. The gingival margins of a crown in position on a tooth cannot be ground or burnished to be flush with tooth structure, especially interproximally. The junction between the restoration and the prepared tooth structure *will always form a crevice*[21] with one sharp edge—the edge of the crown—and the potential for the retention of bacteria and calculus. Subgingival bacterial retention associated with calculus appears to be more important to disease than does plaque. Here is a dual threat to gingival health.

Margin Modification for Gingival Health

Before cementation the best-fitting crown margin is usually a sharp one. After cementation, the ultimate cement film thickness and related hydraulic phenomena create a discrepancy, and the sharp margin is now oriented into a new position that may irritate the gingival tissues.

Early in dental education, great respect is taught for the fine, ultrathin, razor-like margins of castings. The finer the margin, the greater the protection that is warranted. Paradoxically, this is concern for a negative value—for the very feature that may undermine a cast restoration biologically. As mentioned before, sharp margins cause gingival irritation regardless of how well they fit. *Periodontal health is enhanced by the rounding, dulling, and polishing away of sharp margins.* This should be accomplished *even at the expense of losing marginal coverage.* Since, as stated before, margins are not perfect anyway, it would be better to lose a little marginal integrity in order to gain healthy tissue tolerance. And tissues are far more tolerant to the rounded, smooth edge than to the sharp one.

Although porcelain is considered to be well tolerated by the gingiva, it may also be very irritating if the smallest sharp edge or burr is overlooked by the dentist. Also, placing porcelain margins more than slightly into the gingival sulcus (which is almost always done to ensure a good cosmetic effect with anterior restorations) may cause periodontal disease. After clinical research involving porcelain crowns on upper anterior teeth, Mannerberg[22] reports: "Despite an apparently clinically acceptable result, it appears that the porcelain crown whose cervical border is placed down to half the depth of the gingival pocket implies a risk for permanent inflammatory irritation of the gingiva."

The margins of all crowns, including temporary acrylic coverage, should be edge-polished. The open end, margins and all, should be *boldly* placed against the polishing wheel of a lathe and *blunted ever*

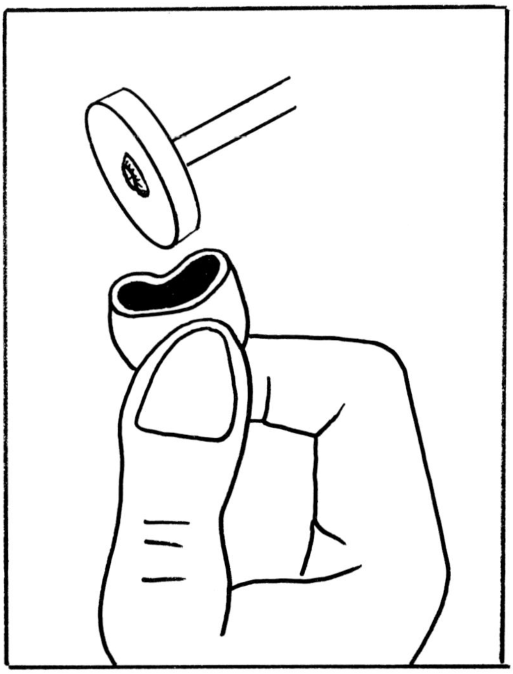

Figure 15–5 The margins of all crowns, including temporary acrylic resin crowns, should be polished to negate sharp edges. The edges of the margins are in more intimate contact with the periodontal tissues than any other part of a fixed prosthesis. Polished smoothness is more essential here than anywhere.

so slightly to negate sharp edges, and then polished to a high luster (Fig. 15–5).

This suggestion may raise a few eyebrows and elicit a bit of controversy, but the proof is the pink, firm, and healthy tissues that frame fixed restorations treated in this manner.

Modify Crown Margins for Better Tissue Tolerance

Acrylic Resin Crowns. Utilizing light pressure, apply a rubber wheel directly across and perpendicular to the margins (Fig. 15–5). In a similar manner, polish well with wet pumice at slow speed, and apply Lustershine* polishing agent at medium speed.

Gold Crowns. Using light pressure, apply a rubber wheel** directly across the sharp margins. In a similar manner, apply tripoli at slow speed to all margins and then high shine all margins with rouge. With the fingertips, touch around the margins of the crown lightly, allowing the sensitivity of the fingers to detect sharp or rough areas.

Porcelain Crowns. Remove sharp edges with a smooth-cutting stone. Use a medium-abrasive Dedeco† rubber wheel and then a fine-polishing Dedeco† rubber wheel. The margins of porcelain-over-metal crowns are also modified in this manner. Sensitive fingertips are a great aid to biologic compatibility.

---

*Accurate Set, Incorporated, Paterson, NJ 07501.
**Jelenko rubber wheels, J. F. Jelenko & Company, New Rochelle, NY 10801.
†Dental Development & Manufacturing Corporation, Brooklyn, NY 11238.

What Goes on in the Gingival Sulcus?

There is a dynamic relationship occurring within the confines of a gingival sulcus that is subject to many subtle *changes and movements. Before a restoration and cement are introduced* to the gingival sulcus of a prepared tooth, there exist therein certain moving parts and changing phenomena:

1. The mobility of the tooth (in function or otherwise)
2. The movements of the gingival tissues caused by pressure from food, tongue, lips or cheeks
3. The changing pH
4. Capillary action
5. Deposition of plaque and calculus

Restorations and cement invade this very narrow arena. These are tolerated and remain in healthy coexistence if they don't bring irritating margins with them, and if the cement and cementation technique allow for accurate seating. Because all this activity is concentrated into such a small, problematic space, the dentist is cautioned to encroach *only very slightly into the sulcus* with the margins of the cemented restoration and to be especially careful not to introduce margins that are sharp, rough, or unpolished. *The smooth, polished edge* is a prime requirement, and the saving grace of a crown margin.

In summary, the health of the gingival crevice containing restorative dental material depends on the following:

1. Fit and adaptation of the restoration
2. Type of restorative material (metal, porcelain or plastic) and degree of porosity
3. Depth of gingival encroachment (length of crown margin)
4. Width of gingival encroachment (thickness of crown margin)
5. Shape of gingival encroachment (sharp or blunt)
6. Smoothness of gingival encroachment

ORAL HABITS

Teeth and fixed restorations may be moved by the pressure of the muscles and soft tissues surrounding them. Oral habits cause a large amount of malocclusions.[23] In the early years of life, preventive or interceptive orthodontics deals with the prevention of incipient conditions that may produce malocclusion. In later life, oral habits may contribute to the failure of crown and bridge therapy if not intercepted and controlled. There are already enough great stresses in the oral cavity; those imposed by harmful habits must be controlled. Masticatory forces and other normal muscular actions create diverse pressures against fixed restorations.

Two noxious oral habits that are detrimental to crown and bridge therapy are bruxism and teeth clenching. Another, the "reverse swallowing" tongue habit may contribute to malocclusion and dental caries.[24] Gum chewing has been reported to be responsible for temporomandibular joint disturbances.[25] Smoking and alcohol may also be harmful to restorations—smoking for its contribution to plaque and stain, and alcohol for its solvent effect on certain restorative materials. Alcohol, nicotine, and tars may also act as irritants to the gingival tissues. Giddon[26] states that potentially harmful oral habits may develop from the intake of noxious vapors, liquids, and air currents that modify the moisture content or temperature of the mouth. He points out that "perhaps the most insidious of these is smoking, which, according to recently summarized studies,[27] is related unquestionably to acute necrotizing ulcerative gingivitis and probably to other oral diseases."

Many dentists have had esthetic, well-constructed restorations fail for unknown reasons. Occasionally upper anterior teeth that have full crowns are suddenly afflicted with periodontoclasia or a fanning out of the dentition. Even splinted upper anterior teeth or fixed bridges involving three to six teeth may be tilted forward en masse. These problems can be avoided if the muscle problems that cause them are understood. Malocclusion may result from a deviate swallow, and early recognition of this pattern of muscle activity is essential to successful crown and bridge therapy. If corrections are not accomplished prior to restorative treatment, the original problem may recur and sabotage the end-result.

Added to the aforementioned harmful oral habits are fingernail biting, lip biting, pipe clenching, tongue thrusting, and abnormal swallowing, which should also be controlled by proper guidance, including myofunctional therapy and possibly psychiatric assistance. The oral habit that poses the *greatest threat* to the longevity of crown and bridge therapy is *bruxism.*

The Battle of Bruxism

Bruxism is a civil war and its battlefield is the oral environment. Once again it is a battle between the North and the South, and it portends evil and destruction to both upper and lower armies and their associated surroundings and components of repair. To bring peace and equilibrium to this foray requires recognition of the definitive nature of the problem, and understanding of the potentials for its resolution with special emphasis on a new modality: dental biofeedback.

Exactly what is bruxism? And how does it threaten crown and bridge therapy? Bruxism is defined as a clenching of the teeth associated with forceful lateral or protrusive jaw movements which result in rubbing, gritting, or grinding together of the teeth, usually during sleep.[28] This nonfunctional gnashing, grinding, or clenching of the teeth is sometimes referred to as a habit, usually associated with emotional stress, tension, anxiety, fear, frustration, or fatigue. Bruxism may cause abnormal wear patterns on the teeth, and frequently results in occlusal traumatism.[28] What does it do to crowns and bridges? In some cases it annihilates them, in others it destroys them slowly and subtly, and both the dentist and patient are unaware of the reasons for restorative failure. *Bruxism is a powerful phenomenon and may fracture, wear, and loosen teeth, crowns, and bridges.* It may also accelerate periodontal disease and contribute to temporomandibular joint distress. It is a stress-induced muscle activity that may occur at night or even during the daytime. If bruxism, clenching, or dysfunctional use of the muscles of mastication is clearly recognized, it is usually attributed to malocclusion or psychological factors, and various traditional remedies are utilized. These are equilibration, tranquilizers, muscle relaxants, night guards, and psychological counseling. Too often these procedures result in only partial or temporary relief, much to the chagrin of the patient and dentist. The underlying state of tension is not resolved by the traditional remedies.

Dental Biofeedback

The patient with bruxism must learn to relax his or her muscles, especially those of the jaw. This is accomplished through electromyograph (EMG) feedback training.[29] Afterward the patient learns to maintain thorough relaxation of oral muscles even without the EMG feedback (Fig. 15–6).

Cannistraci[30] records it this way:

Recent discoveries about the nature of muscle activity have led to an ef-

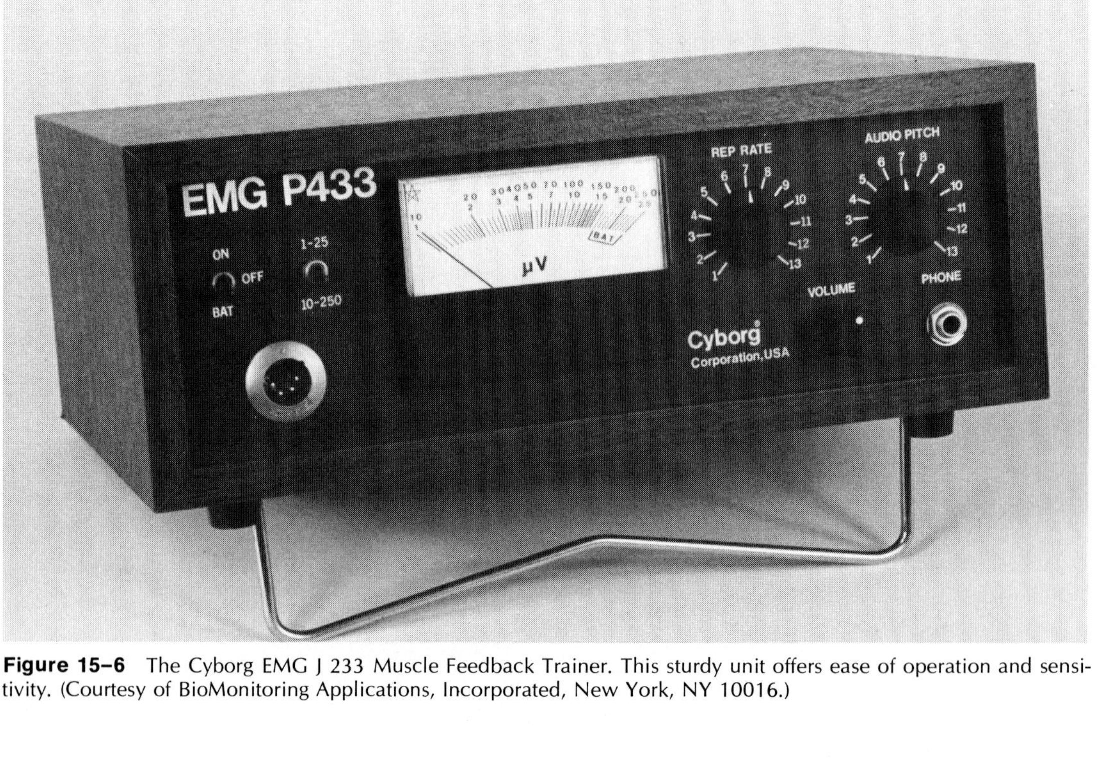

Figure 15–6 The Cyborg EMG J 233 Muscle Feedback Trainer. This sturdy unit offers ease of operation and sensitivity. (Courtesy of BioMonitoring Applications, Incorporated, New York, NY 10016.)

fective new approach for reducing tension. With this method, the patient learns to exercise voluntary control over usually subconscious jaw-muscle activity. Unlike most traditional procedures, self-regulation permits the individual to participate constructively in treatment and, with the new personal skill he develops, to prevent the problem from recurring. By applying the acknowledged link between mental and physical processes, this method places an important resource at the disposal of both dentist and patient.

Biofeedback training for voluntary relaxation of the masticatory system represents a significant advance in both treatment and prevention of many common dental disorders. Extensive clinical experience demonstrates that it promotes successful cure by bringing the patient's inherent learning capability to bear on these problems. As a preventive technique, it allows the patient to develop and retain healthy muscle habits. Therefore, this new application of biofeedback technology has a clear place in the practice of modern dentistry.

Halitosis

Patients with fixed bridges and splints, and others about to receive them, frequently express concern about mouth odors. They worry about oral areas that are difficult to keep clean. Since the space under a pontic or between the splinted components of a fixed restoration may gather fermentable debris, the patient occasionally resorts to candy mints, Life-savers or cough lozenges to insure a socially acceptable breath. Sometimes this becomes a habit. Breath, good or bad, is thus masked, but *teeth, crowned or otherwise, may be devastated by the sugar habitually deposited in the gingival crevices.* Indeed, as a direct result of the attempt to refresh the breath the remaining natural teeth and crowns and bridges are bathed at frequent intervals in a sugar solution that is destructive to cervical, interproximal, and subgingival tooth structure.

Some patients using floss, toothbrush and adjunctive aids maintain a mouth restored with crowns and bridges in a state of good oral hygiene. Nevertheless, they still have halitosis. Since there is no chemical test for the detection of odor, a person must depend on someone else to warn him of objectionable breath. It should be pointed out that although most instances of halitosis can be diagnosed and treated by the dentist, there are many instances in which the cause is systemic and requires treatment by a physician. Systemic conditions such as sinus disease, postnasal drip, tonsillar infections, pharyngitis, bronchitis, pulmonary diseases, diabetes, or gastrointestinal disturbances may induce or contribute to halitosis.[31] However, as mentioned before, most mouth odors originate from dental conditions. Periodontal disease, ulcerative lesions, fistulous exudates, and malignant tumors may be etiologic or contributory. Because bad breath is considered a symptom, not a disease, therapy should be directed toward removing the causative factors.

Patients concerned about bad breath should be informed as follows:

1. Good oral hygiene should be their prime concern.
2. Odor-producing foods, tobacco, and alcohol, which frequently contribute to fetor oris, should be avoided.

3. Certain foods that may not be easily digested by the individual, such as cucumbers, pickles, or cabbage should be restricted.

4. During sleep the reduced activity of the tongue and the reduction of the flow of saliva allow the bacterial flora to be more active, resulting in "morning mouth." Nearly every human has an unpleasant breath after sleep.

5. Mouth breathers generally suffer from halitosis. Dried saliva may have a bad odor.

6. Mouthwashes and flavorful toothpastes may temporarily mask the condition for limited periods of time.

7. *Caution:* Do not use candy, Life-savers or chewing gum to cope with the problem of bad breath.

8. Avoid breath-control agents containing sugar substitutes. These sugar alcohols seem to offer no advantage as substitutes for sucrose in snack foods.[32] They may still contribute to caries.

9. Agents such as Mann's Breath Deodorant* may be recommended to substitute for sugar-containing substances. Since this product can be obtained only through dental supply houses, the dentist may dispense small amounts to patients who present a breath problem.

PREVENTION IN RELATION TO GENERAL DENTAL PRACTICE INCLUDES

1. Dental plaque control
   a. toothbrushing
   b. dental flossing
2. Application of fluorides
3. Nutritional counseling
4. Saliva analysis
5. Education and motivation of patient

PREVENTION PERTINENT TO CROWN AND BRIDGE THERAPY INCLUDES THE ABOVE, PLUS

1. Good restorative procedures to decrease microleakage
2. Design of restorations to facilitate oral hygiene
3. Periodontal considerations of crown contours and margin form and placement
4. Antibacterial and anticariogenic factors
5. Control of harmful oral habits

---

*Mann Chemical Corporation, Louisville, KY 40202.

REFERENCES

1. Germo, P., and Flotra, L.: The effect of different methods of interdental cleansing. J. Periodont. Res. *5*:230, 1970.
2. Jaffe, P.: Dental cleansing tape. N.Y.J. Dent. *43*:245, 1973.
3. Lipton, J. A.: Dentists' reaction to a new preventive agent. N.Y.J. Dent. *45*:253, 1975.
4. Massler, M.: Changing concepts in prevention and treatment of dental caries. N.Y.J. Dent. *39*:82, 1969.
5. Sugar, enemy of good nutrition, Part 2. Consumer Bulletin, March, 1961, p. 41.
6. McBean, L. D., and Speckmann, E. W.: A review: The importance of nutrition in oral health. J. Am. Dent. Assoc. *89*:109, 1974.
7. Gustafsson, B. E., et al.: The Vipeholm Dental Caries Study: The effect of different levels of carbohydrate intake on caries activity in 436 individuals observed for five years. Acta Odont. Scand. *11*:232, 1954.
8. Bibby, B. G.: The cariogenicity of snack foods and confections. J. Am. Dent. Assoc. *90*:121, 1975.
9. DePaola, P. F., et al.: Temporary suppression of *Streptococcus mutans* in humans through topical application of Vancomycin. J. Dent. Res. *53*:108, 1975.
10. Edelstein, B. L.: The scientific basis of prevention. N.Y. State Dent. J. *41*:18, 1975.
11. Jerman, A. C.: Silver amalgam restorative material with stannous fluoride. J. Am. Dent. Assoc. *80*:787, 1970.
12. O'Brien, W. J.: Capillary action around dental structures. J. Dent. Res. *52*:544, 1973.
13. Going, R. E.: Microleakage around dental restorations: A summarizing review. J. Am. Dent. Assoc. *84*:1349, 1972.
14. Wheeler, R. C.: Complete crown form and the periodontium. J. Prosthet. Dent. *11*:722–734, 1961.
15. Goldman, H. M., and Cohen, D. W.: An Introduction to Periodontia. 4th ed., St. Louis, The C. V. Mosby Company, 1969, p. 47.
16. Weinberg, L. A.: Esthetics and the gingivae in full coverage. J. Prosthet. Dent. *10*:737–744, 1960.
17. Kornfeld, M.: Mouth Rehabilitation. Vol. 1, St. Louis, The C. V. Mosby Company, 1967, pp. 95–100.
18. Perel, M. L.: Axial crown contours. J. Prosthet. Dent. *25*:642, 1971.
19. Perel, M. L.: Periodontal considerations of crown contours. J. Prosthet. Dent. *26*:627, 1971.
20. Yuodelis, R. A., Weaver, J. D., and Sapkos, S.: Facial and lingual contours of artificial complete crown restorations and their effects on the periodontium. J. Prosthet. Dent. *29*:61, 1973.
21. Eissmann, H. F., Radke, R. A., and Noble, W. H.: Physiologic design criteria for fixed dental restorations. Dent. Clin. North Am. *15*:543–568, 1971.
22. Mannerberg, F.: Gingival changes following porcelain crown therapy. Odont. Revy *22*:155–162, 1971.
23. Gingold, N. L.: Oral habits and preventive orthodontics. N.Y.J. Dent. *44*:148, 1974.
24. Saladino, P. J.: Reverse swallowing. J. Prosthet. Dent. *17*:219, 1967.
25. Elman, E.: Gum-chewing and the temporomandibular joint. J. Am. Dent. Assoc. *71*:1416, 1965.
26. Giddon, D. B.: Psychophysiology of the oral cavity. J. Dent. Res. *45*:1627, 1966.
27. Goldhaber, P., and Giddon, D. B.: Present concepts concerning the etiology and treatment of acute necrotizing ulcerative gingivitis. Int. Dent. J. *14*:468, 1964.
28. Boucher, C. O.: Current Clinical Dental Terminology, St. Louis, The C. V. Mosby Company, 1963, p. 51.

29. Budzynski, T., and Stoyva, J.: An electromyographic feedback technique for teaching voluntary relaxation of the masseter muscle. J. Dent. Res. 52:116, 1973.
30. Cannistraci, A. J.: Procedures for voluntary stress release and behavior therapy in the treatment of clenching and bruxism. 1975, New York, Biomonitoring Applications, Inc. (Tape).
31. Accepted Dental Therapeutics, 35th ed., Chicago, American Dental Association, p. 295.
32. Navia, J. M., et al.: Caries promoting properties of sucrose substitutes in foods: Manitol, xylitol and sorbitol. IADR Abstract No. 611, 1974.

sixteen
Appendix

MATERIALS FOR CROWN AND BRIDGE THERAPY

Some of the dental products referred to in the text are listed below in alphabetical order. For each product the questions will be What is it? and What is its use? The answers, derived partially from information supplied by the manufacturer and partially from dental literature, will be further augmented by comments provided by the author. The comments are based on the author's opinion and experience in handling the material, and also on research evidence documented in dental literature.

Adaptic	Fynal	Opotow Crown & Bridge Paraben
Cavit	Hydroxyline	Polyjel
Cavitec	Hypo-Cal	Pulpdent
Copalite	Impregum	Ramitec
Durelon	Imput	Semi-Final
Dycal	Jel-Sol	Temrex Cement
Epoxylite CBA	Opotow Alumina EBA Cement	
Fluoro-Thin		

ADAPTIC

Johnson & Johnson Dental Products Company
New Brunswick, NJ 08903

What is it?

Adaptic is a composite resin restorative material composed of a resin system similar to the one pioneered by the laboratory of the National Bureau of Standards (Bowen's formula), and a natural crystal quartz filler. The resin system matrix (usually referred to as the BIS-GMA resin binder) is filled with a large amount of the inorganic filler, and the result is a restorative resin with more desirable properties than any unfilled resin.

What is its use?

Adaptic is basically a filling material, but may also be used for post and core techniques, and to rebuild an abutment preparation to proper contour. Dentists seem to prefer the paste form of the composite resin to the powder-liquid systems. Adaptic matches tooth structure very well, polymerizes rapidly, and provides a harder restoration that seems capable of resisting abrasion better than resins such as unfilled acrylic.

Comments

Adaptic, one of the first group of composite resins developed, has become one of the popular resin restorative materials in dentistry. All of the currently available composite resins, including Adaptic, are irritating to the pulp, as are acrylic resins and phosphoric acid cements. Protection is usually provided by a calcium hydroxide base. However, in a painful tooth, zinc oxide and eugenol cement may be used as a protective base under Adaptic and will not inhibit polymerization as it does when placed under an acrylic resin material. Some cavity varnishes may not be suitable for use under Adaptic because of possible chemical interaction. A recent investigation[1] suggests that "Copalite could be used in conjunction with Adaptic restorations, provided that it supplies sufficient protection to the pulp against the penetration of bacteria and possible chemical irritants."

Many dentists have been tempted to use a composite resin such as Adaptic instead of amalgam for an esthetic Class II restoration. Some manufacturers have intimated that their composite resin products are adequate in Class I and Class II restorations; indeed, they may be when esthetics is the main consideration, the preparation is conservative, and the compromise is fully acknowledged by both patient and dentist. Clinical studies comparing composite resin to amalgam in Class II preparations[2] indicate that secondary caries or fracture is no greater with a composite than with an amalgam, and marginal integrity may be better over the time intervals (up to three years) recorded. However, *the significant issue is wear.* The composite resins' lack of resistance to wear has been observed in both Class I and Class II restorations. As a result of wear, occlusal surfaces, especially marginal ridge areas, are modified in anatomical form. No commercial composite resin product seems to be any better than another as far as low resistance to abrasion is concerned.

REFERENCES

1. Grajower, R., et al.: Compatibility of a composite resin with pulp insulating materials. A scanning electron microscope study. J. Prosthet. Dent. *32*:70, 1974.
2. Phillips, R. W., et al.: Observations on a composite resin for Class II restorations: Three-year report. J. Prosthet. Dent. *30*:891, 1973.

CAVIT

Premier Dental Products Company
Norristown, PA 19401

What is it?

Cavit is a ready-mixed temporary filling material in a tube. It is manufactured in Germany by ESPE. It contains zinc oxide, calcium sulfate, zinc sulfate, glycol acetate, polyvinyl acetate, polyvinyl chloride-acetate, trienthanolamine, and red pigment, but no eugenol. The setting reaction is initiated in part by saliva; the reaction of water with calcium sulfate and zinc oxide–zinc sulfate produces the set.[1]

What is its use?

Cavit is used as a temporary filling, as a root canal sealer between treatments, and as a material to fill in undercuts on teeth in the mouth prior to impression making. Cavit is not a medication, but may be used to seal a medication in a cavity.

Comment

Cavit is a temporary filling material with a high linear expansion that apparently is caused by water sorption.[1] This expansion may account for its sealing effectiveness against interface penetration.[2] If placed in a dry cavity preparation, Cavit may cause pain.[1, 3] It is not a satisfactory cementing material for temporary crowns because of its film thickness and high hygroscopic expansion.[1] Cavit does not have antibacterial properties or the ability to sedate tooth structure or to obtund pain. It dehydrates dentin.[3]

Do not heed the manufacturer's suggestion to swab eugenol on a tooth and then cover it with Cavit. Eugenol alone is not beneficial to cut tooth structure—only the *combination of zinc oxide with eugenol* provides a material that will sedate tooth structure with minimal effect (see Chapter 8, p. 154).

REFERENCES

1. Widerman, F. H., Eames, W. B., and Serene, T. P.: The physical and biologic properties of Cavit. J. Am. Dent. Assoc. *82*:378, 1971.
2. Parris, L., et al.: Effect of temperature change on the sealing properties of temporary filling materials. Oral Surg. *17*:771, 1964.
3. Johnson, G., and Brännström, M.: Dehydration of dentin by some restorative materials. J. Prosthet. Dent. *26*:307, 1971.

CAVITEC

Kerr Manufacturing Company
Romulus, MI 48174

What is it?

There has been a lot of confusion related to what this product is or is not. It is often mistaken for Cavit (Premier Dental Products

Company) and vice versa because of the similarity in name; it has been erroneously listed as an EBA cement by the Council on Dental Materials and Devices (ADA)[1]; and there has been a significant change in its formulation in recent years.

Cavitec is a zinc oxide and eugenol cement that is supplied in two collapsible tubes. In 1968 the composition was stated to be as follows:[2]

Accelerator—	polymerized resin	61%
	eugenol	30%
	mineral oil	7.5%
	other miscellaneous ingredients.	
Base—	zinc oxide	75%
	mineral oil	10.5%
	sulfathiazole	12%
	other miscellaneous ingredients.	

In 1971 the results of a study[3] at the Eastman Dental Center, Rochester, NY, pointed out that "there are no advantages to be gained in pulp recovery by the use of sulfathiazole in a zinc oxide and eugenol cement base under dental restorations." Also, the question arose as to whether the sulfathiazole could sensitize a patient so that subsequent exposure to the drug would lead to an allergic reaction.

In 1973, the 35th edition of *Accepted Dental Therapeutics*, (ADA, 1973) lists Cavitec as an accepted preparation, but states a modified composition of the base with the deletion of sulfathiazole.

What is its use?

Cavitec is a zinc oxide and eugenol cavity liner recommended for use in deep cavities. It may be used as a base under silicate or amalgam fillings, and as a temporary filling.

Comments

Because of high surface tension and slight flow, Cavitec stays exactly where placed and does not flow to other areas on prepared tooth structure. This may be a desirable characteristic in some instances, for unlike many other zinc oxide and eugenol cements, Cavitec will not flow where it is not wanted. It is a relatively weak cement. Its compressive strength at 24 hours has been shown to be only 750 psi.[4] It may therefore be useful in the temporary cementation of finished fixed bridges.

REFERENCES

1. Council on Dental Materials and Devices, Additions to the list of classified dental materials and devices. J. Am. Dent. Assoc. *89*:656, 1974.
2. J. Am. Dent. Assoc.: *76*:1411, June 1968.
3. Reed, A. J., Sayegh, F. S., and Awwa, I. A.: The effect of sulfathiazole on pulp recovery after cavity preparation. Pharmacol. Therap. Dent. *1*:88, 1971.
4. Chong, W. F., Swartz, M. L., and Phillips, R. W.: Displacement of cement bases by amalgam condensation, J. Am. Dent. Assoc. *74*:97, 1967.

COPALITE

Cooley and Cooley, Ltd., Houston, TX
Harry J. Bosworth Company, Chicago, IL

What is it?

Copalite is a cavity varnish composed of gum copal, synthetic resins, and chlorbutanol dissolved in a volatile organic solvent.

What is its use?

Copalite is used to protect an abutment preparation from irritating acid materials, or to protect a newly formed cement margin from early dissolution. It is also effective in improving the marginal seal of restorative materials.

An applicator prepared with a small ball of cotton wrapped around its end is dipped into Copalite, and the varnish is applied to dry tooth structure.

Comments

Varnishes such as Copalite can help to reduce postoperative sensitivity, but they do not supply a film thick enough to provide thermal insulation.[1] Film thickness measurements have shown that Copalite may dry to a thickness of 2μm when applied to the surface of the tooth with a moistened brush.[2]

It is usually difficult to obtain an intact layer of this varnish, because there is a tendency for small holes to form as it dries. For this reason, two or three thin coats should be applied. The objective of the multiple layers of varnish is not to build up a thick layer, but to fill in the holes and provide a more complete coating for greater protection of the underlying tooth structure. The ability of a cavity varnish to block acid penetration depends on the continuity of the film formed; therefore, cavity varnishes will *reduce* but not totally prevent the penetration of the constituents of acid-containing cements into dentin.[3] Copalite does not have the same effect when applied in thick layers as in thin layers. A thin film may prevent microleakage, whereas a thick layer may decrease the integrity of the marginal seal because of its inability to flow out over the tooth surface and wet it. Varnishes become thicker when the solvents evaporate, and they evaporate quickly. Therefore, bottles should be tightly capped when not in use, and the time of opening should be minimized. Copalite should be thin. If it thickens, it should be thinned with the solvent provided. What seems thick to one dentist, however, may seem thin to another; therefore, since there is no precise way to measure this characteristic of varnishes, it is safer to stay on the thin side, for the danger lies in having the varnish too thick.[4] In crown and bridge therapy a thick film of cavity varnish applied to a prepared abutment tooth may limit complete seating of a crown by taking up some of the room required for the film thickness of the cementing agent. Also, in a short preparation with questionable retentive form even a thin film of cavity varnish may decrease retention by filling in some of the ultrasmall discrepancies that would otherwise be penetrated by the cement.

Going[5] points out that a layer of Copalite varnish applied over zinc oxide-eugenol or calcium hydroxide effectively fulfills all the requirements of a good cavity liner.

REFERENCES

1. Braden, M.: Heat conduction in teeth and the effect of lining materials. J. Dent. Res. *43*:315, 1964.
2. Eames, W. B., and Hollenback, G. M.: Cavity liner thicknesses and retentive characteristics. J. Am. Dent. Assoc. *72*:69, 1966.
3. Swartz, M. L., et al.: Role of cavity varnishes and bases in the penetration of cement constituents through tooth structure. J. Prosthet. Dent. *16*:963, 1966.
4. Johnston, J. F., Phillips, R. W., and Dykema, R. W.: Modern Practice in Crown and Bridge Prosthodontics. 3rd ed., Philadelphia, W. B. Saunders Co., 1971, p. 362.
5. Going, R. E.: Cavity liners and dentin treatment, J. Am. Dent. Assoc. *69*:415, 1964.

DURELON

Premier Dental Products Company
Norristown, PA 19401

What is it?

Durelon is a resin cement that utilizes an aqueous solution of polyacrylic acid (made from acrylic acid). It is a polycarboxylate cement. The powder is mainly a specially activated mixture of magnesium and zinc oxides, and is quite similar to that of zinc phosphate cement.

What is its use?

Durelon is recommended as a cementing medium for fixed restorations, as a base for pulp protection, and to repair the contour of prepared abutment teeth. It is also useful for orthodontic procedures.

Comment

Durelon was the first commercial polycarboxylate cement available to dentistry. Claims that Durelon will provide true adhesion to moist dentin are not substantiated by *in vivo* testing. Nevertheless, it is a valuable asset to fixed restorative therapy, for it is the only type of cement that will adhere to prepared tooth structure long enough to be of practical assistance. In biologic evaluations polycarboxylate cement has been shown to be mild and nonirritating to the dental pulp. In this respect it is similar to zinc oxide and eugenol cement. But we must emphasize that it does not obtund pain, and it does not provide antibacterial activity. Therefore, claims that this cement has the same biologic effect on the dental pulp as zinc oxide and eugenol are misleading.

Durelon liquid is available in a syringe-like calibrated glass tube and in a squeeze-bottle container. The liquid in the glass tube is much easier to dispense than that in the squeeze bottle. The tube may also offer a longer shelf life.

Durelon is not recommended for pulp capping, since it does not stimulate reparative dentinogenesis and calcific bridging at the exposure site, and it lacks an antibacterial effect.[1,2,3]

REFERENCES

1. McWalter, G. M., El-Kafrawy, A. H., and Mitchell, D. F.: Pulp capping in monkeys with a calcium-hydroxide compound, an antibiotic, and a polycarboxylate cement. Oral Surg. *36*:90, 1973.
2. El-Kafrawy, A. H., et al.: Pulp reaction to a polycarboxylate cement in monkeys. J. Dent. Res. *53*:15, 1974.
3. McWalter, G. M., El-Kafrawy, A. H., and Mitchell, D. F.: Long-term study of pulp capping in monkeys with three agents. J. Am. Dent. Assoc. *93*:105, 1976.

DYCAL

The L. D. Caulk Company
Milford, DE 19963

What is it?

Dycal is a calcium hydroxide composition with a self-setting mechanism. It consists of two components: a base paste and a catalyst paste, both of which are supplied in collapsible tubes for convenient dispensing and safe storing. The base contains 1,3 di(2-hydroxy benzoate butane), the ingredient which reacts with calcium hydroxide, and pigments.[1] The catalyst contains calcium hydroxide, zinc oxide, and zinc stearate, all suspended in an organic vehicle, Santicizer 8.[1]

What is its use?

Dycal is used to supply calcium hydroxide to deeply prepared tooth structure to maintain the vitality of pulpal tissues in cases of pulp exposure or near exposure. Dycal stimulates the formation of a dentinal bridge over the exposed pulp.[1,2] In near-exposure areas, it stimulates the formation of secondary dentin.

Comment

The claim that calcium hydroxide formulations exert a persistent stimulating effect on the dental pulp, resulting in its eventual obliteration was not supported by recent research with Dycal.[2]

Because of its water solubility, Dycal should not be allowed to remain on the margins of restorations, and should not be used as a temporary filling.

REFERENCES

1. Sawusch, R. H.: Dycal capping of exposed pulps in primary teeth. J. Dent. Child. *30*:141, 1963.
2. McWalter, G. M., El-Kafrawy, A. H., and Mitchell, D. F.: Long-term study of pulp capping in monkeys with three agents. J. Am. Dent. Assoc. *93*:105, 1976.

EPOXYLITE CBA 9080

Lee Pharmaceuticals
South El Monte, CA 91733

What is it?

Epoxylite CBA 9080 is a crown and bridge cement derived from the modification of a composite resin material. It is based on the adduct of diglycidyl ether of bisphenol A and methacrylic acid. This class of resin, which contains various mineral fillers, is the basis for modern composite restorative materials. This base resin is diluted to a viscosity considered to be workable for a crown and bridge application with a low viscosity dimethacrylate monomer.[1]

What is its use?

Epoxylite CBA 9080 is especially indicated for difficult retention problems involving endodontically treated teeth, for the cementation of posts and cores, and for the recementation of old fixed prostheses that must be salvaged for economic reasons. Composite resin cement is probably the strongest, most insoluble, and most durable cement available. It is also translucent.

Comment

Composite resin cements, despite advertising claims, are not adhesive. It has also been shown that the cavity cleanser, a concentrated citric acid solution recommended to enhance the adhesive ability of the composite resin cement, will increase the undesired pulpal response.[2]

It is important to keep in mind that this cement has been shown to be irritating to the dental pulp, and that pulpal protection is always an important consideration when it is applied to vital teeth.

The mixed composite resin cement should look glossy and be flowable, and yet not be too thin or the end product will be unsatisfactory. A mix that is too thin will also have a very substantial delay in setting. On the other hand, if too much powder is used, and the mix is thicker, there will be a reduction of working time and an increase in film thickness.

REFERENCES

1. Lee, H., and Swartz, M. L.: Evaluation of a composite resin crown and bridge luting agent. J. Dent. Res. *51*:756, 1972.
2. Eriksen, H. M.: Pulpal response of monkeys to a composite resin cement, J. Dent. Res. *53*:565, 1974.

FLUORO-THIN

S. S. White Dental Products Division
Philadelphia, PA 19102

What is it?

Fluoro-Thin is a silicophosphate cement. It is approximately 90 per cent silicate and 10 per cent modified zinc oxide, by powder weight. The specially formulated silicate powder is claimed to allow a cement film thickness of less than 25 microns.

What is its use?

Although the low film thickness of Fluoro-Thin may make it suitable for the final cementation of all crowns and bridges, it is indicated primarily for the cementation of porcelain jackets. It is translucent, stronger than zinc phosphate cement, and possesses anticariogenic properties by virtue of the fluoride it contains in the silicate component.

Comment

Only this silicophosphate cement and one other (Lucent, L. D. Caulk Co.) meet the cementing media film thickness requirement of the American Dental Association Specification No. 21, Type 1.

Silicophosphate cements generally take a long time to set and are as irritating to the pulp as other phosphoric-acid-containing materials. Cavity liners should be employed when these cements are utilized. Despite the higher strength of this cement, it does not seem to retain castings any better than zinc phosphate cement. Vital abutment teeth should be coated with a thin layer of a copal type cavity varnish prior to contact with this cement. In fact, very careful pulp protection is necessary because of the low initial pH of these cements.

FYNAL

The L. D. Caulk Company
Milford, DE 19963

What is it?

Fynal is a resin-fortified zinc oxide and eugenol cement. The reinforcing agent is probably polymethyl methacrylate.

What is its use?

In selected instances in which the biophysical factors are favorable, Fynal may be used as a sedative, non-irritating final cement for finished crowns and bridges.

Comment

Fynal is not as strong and insoluble as EBA cements such as Zebacem (L. D. Caulk Company) and Opotow Alumina EBA (Teledyne Dental) and may be better used as a strong temporary cement. It is very adequate for use with acrylic resin temporary coverage on short preparations or long-span bridges, or in other situations requiring strong retention for temporary coverage.

HYDROXYLINE

George Taub Products, Incorporated
Jersey City, NJ 07307

What is it?

Hydroxyline is a calcium hydroxide cavity liner that provides a heavy concentration of calcium hydroxide suspended in an easy-flowing volatile solvent. When applied to tooth structure, it dries rapidly and sets to a tough, adherent, visible film. It creates a chemical and physical barrier against harmful ingredients of restorative materials.

What is its use?

It is used to provide a lining of calcium hydroxide on prepared tooth structure to protect the underlying pulp, and also to treat an exposed pulp.

Comment

Hydroxyline must be shaken or stirred thoroughly before use. If the material is used repeatedly or if the cap is not tightened on the bottle, thickening and drying will occur. If this should happen, add several drops of thinner, tighten cap, and shake vigorously. Hydroxyline should be applied to dry dentin in a thin coat with a fine brush or a cotton pellet. This calcium hydroxide liner provides an adherent coating that is not easily disturbed by the application of a cement or filling material.

HYPO-CAL

Ellman Dental Manufacturing Company, Incorporated
Hewlett, NY 11557

What is it?

Hypo-Cal is a radiopaque calcium hydroxide cavity liner supplied in a syringe with a blunt needle applicator tip and a micrometer screw feed that dispenses the material. Hypo-Cal contains 45 per cent calcium hydroxide, USP, 5 per cent barium sulphate, 2 per cent hydroxyethyl cellulose, and 48 per cent water. The applicator tip is supplied with a "Protecto-Flo cap" to prevent drying and clogging, and to disinfect the needle after each use.

What is its use?

It is used as a pulp protecting cavity liner for indirect pulp capping, for pulpotomy, and for pulp protection before cementation.

Comment

Hypo-Cal supplies a quick lining of calcium hydroxide without mixing, sticky caps, waste, or clean up. Since it contains no chemical setting agents, it must be air dried to harden. If it is applied too thickly, hardening will be delayed. It must be applied in thin layers. One problem with this method of application is that occasionally the material continues to run out of the end of the needle after the micrometer screw is no longer turned. It is, therefore, suggested that after each small turn a reverse turn should be made.

There is some doubt about the ability of the Protecto-Flo cap to disinfect the needle between applications to different patients. The time lapse between patients receiving applications of Hypo-Cal may be very significant as far as the time required for disinfection in the Protecto-Flo cap is concerned. When this device must be used on one patient soon after use on another, or if the dentist just wants to insure sterility of the needle, the following procedure is suggested:

1. Dip needle and needle attachment into a glass jar containing 65 to 70 per cent ethanol (ethyl alcohol) for one second.

2. Remove and flame briefly in a Bunsen-burner flame to kill microorganisms; the needle is then basically sterile and may be used in the mouth. Isopropyl alcohol should not be used in this procedure because it produces too much energy when it burns and may heat up the device excessively. Methanol, a light alcohol, evaporates too fast to be effective. Ethanol is just right for this procedure.

IMPREGUM

Espe GMBH, Seefeld, Ober-Bayern, Germany, and
Premier Dental Products Company, Norristown, PA 19401

What is it?

Impregum is a rubber impression material of a new chemical composition. It is an imine-terminated polyether crosslinked by an aromatic sulfonate ester. It is supplied in two collapsible tubes. One contains the base, which is a low molecular weight polyether containing ethylene imine terminal groups. The other tube contains the accelerator (aromatic sulfonic acid ester). The procedure for mixing equal lengths on a paper pad is the same as for the other rubber impression materials.

What is its use?

Impregum is used for crown and bridge impressions. It has a pleasant taste and odor and is easy to mix and clean up. It sets fast and has good dimensional stability in air, but less in water. It compares favorably with other elastic impression materials in mixing time, working time, and consistency.

Comment

Little difference has been shown between the use of a custom tray or a stock tray when utilizing a polyether impression material.[1] The dentist should be aware that there is less working time when using Impregum than when using a polysulfide impression, and should adjust his technique accordingly. Prolonged exposure to water should be avoided, and impressions should be dried soon after they are made to avoid dimensional change. Compared to other rubber impression materials Impregum has a high modulus of elasticity, which may make a complex impression difficult to remove. It has been shown that a polyether impression material is more susceptible to tearing in clinical circumstances than polysulfide impression material.[2]

Physical contact with the accelerator should be avoided during mixing, for the aromatic sulfonic acid ester may cause a skin irritation.[3] Also, to avoid any possible irritation to the mouth tissues, the two components should be very thoroughly mixed.

Regardless of this material's high affinity for water, it is probably the most accurate of all available rubber materials.

REFERENCES

1. Hembree, J. H.: Accuracy of elastomer impression materials. IADR, Abstract No. 57, 1974.
2. Braden, M., et al.: A polyether impression rubber. J. Dent. Res. *51*:889, 1972.
3. Craig, R. G., O'Brien, W. J., and Powers, J. M.: Dental Materials. St. Louis, The C. V. Mosby Company, 1975, p. 151.

IMPUT (BODY SILICONE)

Buffalo Dental Manufacturing Company
Brooklyn, NY 11207

What is it?

Imput (body silicone) is a silicone putty impression material. It has a heavy doughlike consistency before and immediately after mixing. It is a dark-brown color with the odor and taste of cinnamon. It is supplied as a large jar of body silicone and a small squeeze-bottle container of catalyst.

What is its use?

Imput (body silicone) impression material is used in both fixed and removable prosthodontics.

Comment

Imput was one of the first silicone elastomeric materials to be designated as "silicone putty." This material has a putty-like consistency and is provided in two forms: Imput Body and Imput Wash. The Imput Body material is one of the thickest and heaviest of all available silicone impression materials. It sets harder than any other silicone material. It is therefore better suited for obtaining a master impression for multiple-unit fixed restorations than the conventional full-mouth plaster technique. The mouth-hardened Imput Body has enough elasticity to spring out of undercuts on the adjacent, unprepared tooth without distortion and yet is firm and hard enough to hold transfer copings or castings securely in position within the impression. Using Imput Body instead of plaster of paris eliminates the time consuming "jig-saw" problem of putting together the pieces and chips of broken plaster. Dies may be firmly positioned in transfer copings with pressure, without the flexibility and springback characteristics of the regular rubber impression materials.

JEL-SOL

J. F. Jelenko & Company, Incorporated
New Rochelle, NY 10801

What is it?

Jel-Sol is a clear liquid formulation that is completely water soluble, non-inflammable, and harmless to acrylic, gold, porcelain, and skin.

What is its use?

Jel-Sol provides the most effective removal of zinc oxide and eugenol temporary cement from acrylic crowns, bridges, and splints. It also cleans this material from glass slabs and instruments.

Comment

Jel-Sol should be used as follows: pour enough Jel-Sol into a porcelain dish (on tripod over bunsen burner); immerse the restoration to be cleaned; bring Jel-Sol to the boiling point and allow the hot solution to remain for ten minutes, remove restoration and rinse in tap water; brush out and blow dry.

Note: The boiling point of Jel-Sol is low enough to prevent distortion of acrylic resin restorations. However, sufficient Jel-Sol should be used to completely cover the entire restoration being cleaned. *Do not* use Jel-Sol to clean temporary cement from aluminum shells.

OPOTOW ALUMINA EBA CEMENT

Teledyne Dental
Elk Grove Village, IL 60007

What is it?

Opotow Alumina EBA Cement is a zinc oxide and eugenol cement containing *o*-ethoxybenzoic acid in the liquid, and alumina and hydrogenated rosin in the powder. It is compounded according to the formulation developed at the National Bureau of Standards (see Chapter 8, Table 8–2).

What is its use?

It is used for the final cementation of crowns and bridges with crown retainers. It is also used as a sedative base under amalgam, silicate, and composite resin fillings. EBA cements provide good compressive and tensile strength for retention, low viscosity and surface tension that allows for accurate seating of castings, antibacterial properties, and the ability to obtund pain. Occasionally an EBA cement may be used for the temporary cementation of acrylic resin crowns and bridges to abutment teeth that are very short or of poor retentive form.

Comments

Opotow Alumina EBA Cement was the first commercially available EBA cement, and the first final cement to be strong and insoluble and yet biologically compatible with prepared tooth structure. This cement provides two features that zinc phosphate and polycarboxylate cements do not: 1) extended working time, and 2) sedative and anodyne action.

OPOTOW CROWN AND BRIDGE PARABEN

Teledyne Dental
Elk Grove Village, IL 60007

What is it?

Opotow Crown and Bridge Paraben is a combination of methylparaben, U.S.P. (methyl 4-hydroxybenzoate), and propylparaben, U.S.P. (propyl 4-hydroxybenzoate). These neutral esters of parahydroxybenzoic acid are white, fine powders that exhibit bacteriostatic and fungistatic activity at low concentrations against a wide variety of bacteria. They are nontoxic and soluble in eugenol and both are classified in Group A by the Council on Dental Therapeutics of the American Dental Association.

What is its use?

It is used as an additive to enhance the antibacterial and physical properties of zinc oxide and eugenol temporary cements.

It will modify a zinc oxide and eugenol impression material by increasing its fluidity. It may be used as a component of a root canal filling formulation or to give an antibacterial value to a calcium hydroxide cement.

It may also be used to thin the consistency of zinc oxide and eugenol mixtures maintained unset, with a desiccating agent, for subsequent use as temporary fillings.

A small amount (approximately 1 per cent) added to the mix of zinc oxide/eugenol cement utilized in temporary cementation will 1) lower the film thickness of the mixture and increase its flow; 2) allow for easier and *more complete seating* of temporary acrylic crowns, owing to decreased viscosity; 3) eliminate bad odors associated with the removal of temporary restorations; 4) improve the antibacterial activity of the cement; 5) lower the surface tension of the cement and give it greater penetrability; 6) increase the ultimate compressive strength of the cement; and 7) increase working time.

Comment

Opotow Crown and Bridge Paraben in a mix of zinc oxide and eugenol cement causes a delay in setting time. This allows for more working time in the temporary cementation of acrylic resin crowns. Without the paraben additive, the moisture in the resin may accelerate the setting of the zinc oxide and eugenol cement the moment the cement contacts the resin on placement in the crown. The immediate thickening and advancing viscosity may inhibit complete seating of a temporary fixed restoration. As a result, the occlusion may become high and require grinding for adjustment, and the margins may no longer be where they belong.

Opotow Crown and Bridge Paraben is an asset to restorative therapy. *It is very effective when used with Temrex Cement.* It should be added to a thin mix of this cement, which is applied to the acrylic resin temporary coverage, and *seated quickly* on the prepared teeth.

Temporary acrylic bridges and multiple unit splints that are in the mouth for more than a few days are inclined to pick up offensive odors, especially if there is some seepage; however, when the paraben additive is used in the cement the prostheses are odor-free on removal.

Although Opotow Crown and Bridge Paraben will modify all zinc oxide and eugenol mixtures to some degree, the reaction may be less effective with formulations containing a large amount of resin, rosin, or plasticizer.

Adding a small amount of Opotow Crown and Bridge Paraben during spatulation produces the following beneficial physical changes:

A decrease in	*An increase in*
consistency	fluidity
viscosity	plasticity
surface tension	flow

POLYJEL

L. D. Caulk Company
Milford, DE 19963

What is it?

Polyjel is a rubber impression material based on a new chemical system. It is an imine-terminated polyether crosslinked by an aromatic sulfonate ester. Polyjel is referred to as a polyether impression material, and is supplied in two collapsible tubes. One contains the base, which is a low molecular weight polyether containing ethylene imine terminal groups. The other tube contains the accelerator (aromatic sulfonic acid ester). The procedure for mixing equal lengths on a paper pad is the same as for the other rubber impression materials.

What is its use?

Polyjel is used to make impressions for the fabrication of fixed and removable prostheses. It has a pleasant taste and odor and is easy to mix and clean up. It sets fast and has good dimensional stability in air, but less in water. It compares favorably with other elastic impression materials in mixing time, working time, and consistency.

Comment

When a polyether impression material is utilized, there is little difference between use of a custom tray or a stock tray.[1] It is important to note that there is less working time when using Polyjel than when using a polysulfide impression, and the technique should be adjusted accordingly. Prolonged exposure to water should be avoided, and impressions should be dried soon after they are made to avoid dimensional change. Compared to other rubber impression materials Polyjel has a high modulus of elasticity, which may make a complex impression difficult to remove. It has been shown that a polyether impression material is more susceptible to tearing in clinical circumstances than polysulfide impression material.[2]

Physical contact with the accelerator should be avoided during mixing, for the aromatic sulfonic acid ester may cause a skin irritation.[3] Also, to avoid any possible irritation to the mouth tissues, the two components should be very thoroughly mixed.

Regardless of this material's high affinity for water, it is probably the most accurate of all available rubber materials.

REFERENCES

1. Hembree, J. H : Accuracy of elastomer impression materials. IADR, Abstract No. 57, 1974.
2. Braden, M., et al.: A polyether impression rubber, J. Dent. Res. *51*:889, 1972.
3. Craig, R. G., O'Brien, W. J., and Powers, J. M.: Dental Materials. St. Louis, The C. V. Mosby Company, 1975, p. 151.

PULPDENT

Pulpdent Corporation of America
Brookline, MA 02146

What is it?

This material is supplied in two forms, a cavity liner and a pulp capping paste. The liner is a fast-drying, premixed suspension of calcium hydroxide in an aqueous solution of methylcellulose. The pulp capping paste is the same material adjusted to a paste-like consistency.

What is its use?

These materials are used to protect the pulp from chemical irritation; to stimulate the formation of secondary dentin; as a dressing after pulpotomy; and to stimulate the growth of new dentin over vital exposed pulp.

Comments

The liner and the paste are not radiopaque. However, the pulp capping paste may be obtained in a radiopaque form.

RAMITEC

Espe GMBH. Seefeld/OBB.
Premier Dental Products Company
Norristown, PA 19401

What is it?

Ramitec is a polyether rubber material similar to the polyether impression materials Impregum and Polyjel. It is designed to be used for obtaining interarch relationships.

What is its use?

It is used instead of wax or other materials to obtain an occlusal (bite) registration. Unlike wax, it will not warp or distort during or after removal from the mouth. Its thin-bodied consistency allows closure unaltered by the mouth's proprioceptive reaction to an interfering material.

Comments

Ramitec is an esthetic material with a non-objectionable odor and taste. It may be applied to the teeth with a spatula, by injection, or in a bite tray. However, adaptation by finger pressure creates a problem; the material sticks to the finger and strings out even if the finger has been moistened with water, saliva or silicone grease. This problem may be solved by applying Non-Tac* to the fingers prior to adaptation.

SEMI-FINAL

Interstate Dental Company, Incorporated
New Hyde Park, NY 11040

What is it?

Semi-Final is a resin-fortified zinc oxide and eugenol cement that is formulated to be hard, tough and durable. Its composition is as follows:

Liquid	Eugenol	
Powder	Zinc oxide	31%
	Polycarbonate resin	62%
	Zinc acetate	7%

What is its use?

It is designed to be used as a sedative intermediate filling material. Semi-Final is a rapid-setting, easily placed restoration that relieves pain and *lasts longer than the typical temporary filling.* It may also be used as a base under amalgam or composite resin fillings such as Adaptic.

Comment

Semi-Final does not provide a mixture suitable for temporary or final cementation. It is too thick and non-flowable. Its thickness, however, makes it easy to handle, and it will not flow or slump after application to upper teeth.

Semi-Final is probably the hardest setting zinc oxide and eugenol cement available. Twenty minutes after hardening, a sizable pellet taken from the mixing pad is almost unbreakable by hand. It acts as a durable, bactericidal restoration for hospital, school, or government clinics having caries control programs.

TEMREX CEMENT

Interstate Dental Company, Incorporated
New Hyde Park, NY 11040

---

*Accurate Set Incorporated, Paterson, NJ 07501

What is it?

Temrex Cement is a zinc oxide and eugenol cement. The powder is a specially prepared zinc oxide, U.S.P., with a small percentage of accelerator. The liquid is pure eugenol, U.S.P., with a trace of rose oil. No resins, rosins, or plasticizers are in the formulation.

What is its use?

It is utilized for temporary cementation of temporary acrylic crowns, splints and bridges; for sedation of deep, sensitive cavities and crown preparations; for cementation of temporary crown forms; and for temporary cementation of long-span permanent bridges with abutment preparations that may be very short or lack adequate retention form.

Comment

This zinc oxide and eugenol cement sets harder and is stronger than most other temporary cements. Its retentive ability is superior to other zinc oxide and eugenol temporary cements.[1] Temrex Cement has a very low film thickness,[2, 3] and allows the complete and accurate seating of well-fitting temporary crowns and bridges.

Zinc oxide and eugenol cements have the most favorable biologic properties of all cements and are the least irritating to the pulp. They minimize microleakage and provide thermal and galvanic insulation.

Temrex Cement, as do all zinc oxide and eugenol cements, inhibits microbial growth. This antibacterial value is increased with a paraben additive. The paraben also increases its strength, setting time, and fluidity.[2]

Both the powder and the liquid have an unlimited shelf life. The liquid is usable and just as effective if its color is modified to yellow or brown.

In the cementation of well-fitting temporary crowns, use a small amount of a thin mix to line the inside walls. It is not necessary to fill the crowns with cement. Be sure they are *dry*!

In the cementation of loose-fitting crown shell forms use a larger amount of a thicker mix to fill the *dry* crowns.

The mixed Temrex Cement should be applied to *dry* tooth structure for better retention and palliative action. Immediately after cementation or application to tooth structure, dryness need not be maintained. Water or saliva will not interfere with the set. In fact, a *warm* water rinse will hasten the set.

When cementing temporary acrylic resin restorations, *excess Temrex Cement should be removed from external surfaces of the resin as soon as possible after insertion* with cotton rolls or gauze squares. This will minimize or prevent any untoward action of the eugenol component of the cement on the acrylic resin.

Temrex Cement is not recommended for the final cementation of finished crowns and bridges.

REFERENCES

1. Oldham, D. F., Swartz, M. L., and Phillips, R. W.: Retentive properties of dental cements. J. Prosthet. Dent. *14*:760, 1964.
2. Horn, H. R.: Improved cementation. J. Am. Dent. Assoc. *63*:813, 1961.
3. Norman, R. D., Swartz, M. L., and Phillips, R. W.: Studies on film thickness, solubility and marginal leakage of dental cements. J. Dent. Res. *42*:950, 1963.

INDEX

Note: In this index, page numbers in *italic* type refer to illustrations; page numbers followed by (t) refer to tables.